HUMAN NEEDS AND THE NURSING PROCESS

HUMAN NEEDS AND THE NURSING PROCESS

edited by

Helen Yura, Ph.D., R.N., F.A.A.N
Assistant Director
Division of Baccalaureate and Higher Degree Programs
National League for Nursing
New York, New York

Mary B. Walsh, M.S.N., R.N.
Associate Professor
Medical and Surgical Nursing
The Catholic University of America
Washington, D.C.

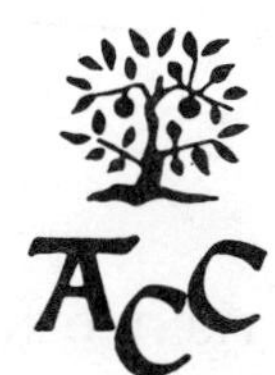

Appleton-Century-Crofts / New York

79 80 81 82 / 10 9 8 7 6 5 4 3 2

Prentice-Hall International, Inc., London
Prentice-Hall of Australia, Pty. Ltd., Sydney
Prentice-Hall of India Private Limited, New Delhi
Prentice-Hall of Japan, Inc., Tokyo
Prentice-Hall of Southeast Asia (Pte.) Ltd., Singapore
Whitehall Books Ltd., Wellington, New Zealand

Main entry under title:

Human needs and the nursing process.

Bibliography: p.
Includes index.
1. Nursing. 2. Nursing—Philosophy. 3. Human biology. I. Yura, Helen. II. Walsh, Mary B.
[DNLM: 1. Nursing care. WY100.3 H918]
RT42.H76 610.73 78-16148

0-8385-3941-6

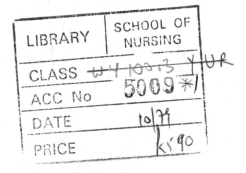

PRINTED IN THE UNITED STATES OF AMERICA

Contributors

Yura, Helen, Ph.D., F.A.A.N
Assistant Director
Division of Baccalaureate
and Higher Degree Programs
National League for Nursing
New York, New York

Walsh, Mary B., M.S.N.
Associate Professor
School of Nursing
Catholic University
Washington, D.C.

Carty, Rita M., D.N.Sc
Associate Professor
George Mason University
Fairfax, Virginia

Hoskins, Lois M., M.S.N.
Assistant Professor
School of Nursing
Catholic University
Washington, D.C.

Oland, Lynne, M.S.N.
Instructor
School of Nursing
Catholic University
Washington, D.C.

Sculco, Cynthia D., Ed.D.
Associate Professor
School of Nursing
Hunter College
New York, New York

Smith, Kitty S., M.S.N.
Associate Professor
George Mason University
Fairfax, Virginia

Spotila, Sister Loretta, M.S.N.
Clinical Nurse Specialist
St. Luke's Hospital
Cleveland, Ohio

Dedicated to Our
Nursing Colleagues

Contents

Preface

This book is based upon two significant points: (1) the nursing process is the core process for the practice of nursing; and (2) basic human needs—their maintenance, their fulfillment, their integrity—are the territory of nursing.

The purpose of this text is to present human needs as the territory for the utilization of the nursing process. It is hoped that the data bases developed from the assessment of these needs, the determination of wellness that might result from an analysis of these data, or the specific designation of nursing diagnoses stemming from partial or total failure to meet these needs will be beneficial to nursing educators and practitioners.

Strategies planned to reinforce the meeting of these needs or specific actions to offset need fulfillment deficits will be prescribed. The data base determined for a met need will serve as the expectation or goal for needs that have been unmet. The dimensions for implementation of strategies as well as expected outcomes will be presented. It is hoped that by this manner of presentation the expected data base for fulfilled needs will be developed, taking into consideration social, cultural, and economic factors.

To encourage the focus on basic human needs, with emphasis on maintaining the integrity between all needs, a group of selected nurses, knowledgable about specific human needs, developed papers according to the model outlined in the introduction. It was felt that this manner of presentation would assure a nursing focus, and help readers to grasp the relationship of basic human needs to the nursing process.

We hope that curricula and evaluative tools will eventually be developed with a human need focus, first to determine the expected or normal data base and then to develop a data base likely to appear when specific needs are unmet. This would simplify expectations concerning changes in client behavior and promote behavioral change in the direction of the expected or normal state (maximum wellness). Utilization of this model should provide the proper focus on health and normality, which is the goal of every individual. In addition, it assures a nursing focus for actions, evaluating the various medical sciences and medical therapies from the perspective of nursing.

The nursing process is heavily steeped in intellectual skills,as becomes evident in the presentations. The development of evaluative procedures based on human needs and the nursing process will not only ensure measurement and testing of nursing abilities, but will also allow for considerable flexibility. This flexibility can easily designate knowledge deficiencies and provide a basis for planning to offset them. It will also facilitate placement of individuals within curricula who have previous academic and/or nursing experience of various kinds. Knowledge of the nursing process remains central, since once the process is learned, it will continue to be the dominant mode of action. What changes in the nursing process is the data base—its scope, the number and specificity of nursing diagnoses, the action strategies to offset need deficits, the manner of implementation, and the level of sophistication for evaluation and the utilization of research results.

Hopefully this effort is only the first in a series of such human need presentations, bringing to the prospective nurse and the practicing nurse a wealth of information in order to assure that the highest level of health and nursing service is rendered to the public.

We are most grateful to the contributors of this text, who have much to offer to nursing colleagues and who willingly took on the task of presentation. In addition, the editors are grateful to the many nurses who have made the nursing process the core process of nursing both for today and for the future.

We also express our appreciation to Charles Bollinger and the staff of Appleton-Century-Crofts for the assistance and support given to us.

HY
MW

Introduction

The four phases of the nursing process (assessing, planning, implementing, evaluating) will be the framework around which each section will be developed. Two levels will be pursued: the first will be concerned with the healthy person, the aim being how to keep that person healthy in order to insure health maintenance, health preservation, and prevention of illness; the second level of development will involve human need violation.

First Level: Human Need Fulfillment (Wellness)

The *assessment* phase will establish the data base on which the later phases will be developed. Each author will define, according to the need being discussed, what is expected or required for that specific need to be met. Data will be derived from clinical situations to indicate what are the necessities for maintenance of this specific need fulfillment. Attention will be given to the differences in need fulfillment that occur in various age groups and at various stages of growth and development, in different sexes, in persons with different educational and cultural backgrounds, and in different socioeconomic situations. A variety of settings will be considered, and a variety of variables identified.

In the *planning* phase, the intended means of need fulfillment used by various persons will be identified. Questions for which answers will be sought include: What are the strategies necessary to bring about need fulfillment? How do persons anticipate what is necessary to meet perceived needs? Is the anticipation a planned activity?

The focus of the *implementing* phase will be to identify strategies carried out by the nurse and the client to accomplish need fulfillment. In order to carry out any deliberative plans the potentials of two persons or groups of persons are involved; one is the person experiencing the need, and the other is the person assisting in meeting that need. In some situations, a person may be quite independent of external forces in meeting a specific need; yet there may be occasions which necessitate less independence and varying degrees of dependence for need fulfillment.

In the cyclic process of nursing, there is an *evaluation* phase in which some checking must be done to determine whether the goals that were planned at the outset of the process have been achieved. Was the need met in this situation? If not, why not? If so, why? How can these actions be remedied, or repeated? A review of the strategies to determine their effectiveness is the only means by which the person and/or the agent can be sure that the outcomes resemble, or are the same as, the original data found on assessment. Constant surveillance is necessary in evaluating actions and determining the degree to which goals should be redefined or strategies replanned. If, on evaluation, the outcomes are not the same as identified in the initial assessment, or are not the desirable outcomes, then basic needs have been violated to some degree and a second set of data need to be collected.

Second Level: Human Need Violation

In *assessing* the ill person, when human needs are not being met, information is collected that provides evidence concerning the need and the extent to which it is being unmet. Having collected as many facts as possible about the person who is ill, a conclusion is drawn called the nursing diagnosis; that is, a statement of conclusions about which of the client's problems are amenable to nursing intervention.

The *planning* phase is one in which the nurse, or agent, devises and designs the strategies necessary to offset the defined deficits, or problems, of the client. When several deficits are discovered, priorities are established in order to focus on the most important first, proceeding to other, less important deficits later.

Implementation of the planned actions proceeds once the strategies are devised in terms of their importance to the client. The persons who are to carry out the actions are identified also. Often the client may carry out the action, but sometimes the client may be totally dependent on other agents to cope with his identified needs.

As action proceeds, the nurse and the client reflect upon and *evaluate* what has been done. They refer to the goals set at the outset of the process and determine whether there has been full or partial elimination of the deficit. Successful elimination of the deficit will place the client on the first level of the discussion, ie, the healthy plane, indicating that the goals have been met. If the goals have not been met to the degree desired, then the nurse and the client remain on the second level, revise goals and strategies, and continue to work together to accomplish a more desirable end.

HUMAN NEEDS AND THE NURSING PROCESS

Chapter One •

Prologue: Biologic Rhythms and Human Needs

Mary B. Walsh

In the temperate zones throughout the world nature provides man with a stunning display of cyclic activity each year. One cannot ignore the decrease of activity and growth in nature during autumn, when the leaves and shrubs change colors, when vegetables and plants in the gardens have completed their production season and are turning brown, changing to seed, and dying. The preparation for winter includes harbingers among the beasts that prepare for hibernation, pets whose fur coats become thicker and heavier, and birds that fly south to warmer climates. All signs suggest approaching change. Winter moves in, and then spring follows with a revival of life and a burst of new growth that is a welcome sight. The hot days of summer between refreshing spring and colorful fall complete the cycle.

But what about those parts of the earth where the cycles of temperature are not so apparent? Although they may not be clearly marked in some areas, cycles of life nevertheless exist in all parts of living matter. There are periods of increased growth, of rest and quiescence, of reproducing and dying. Some of the cycles are more obvious than others; some require close scrutiny, even microscopic observations, to observe the alterations in activity and the changing energy patterns.

The frequently quoted passage in Ecclesiastes cannot be disputed; there is the "time for birth and the time for death, the time for planting and the time for pulling up, . . . the time for sorrow and the time for joy . . . , the time for silence and the time for talk."[1]

Human nature, too, has a long history of cyclic activity. More than 2400 years ago, Hippocrates advised his associates to pay close attention to fluctuations in the symptoms of patients, to be aware of both good and bad days of his patients as well as those of health-caring persons.[2] The language, practices, and superstitions of man suggest a cyclic nature in human life, as evidenced by sayings such as "I have my ups and downs," "It's such a vicious cycle," "He has his good days and his bad days," "Don't mind her behavior—it's that time of the month."

Most people are aware of the changes in the moon occurring each month; the rarity of two full moons in any one month, as observed in June 1977, caused some comment among farmers; the theme of the "harvest moon" has been used by songwriters, lovers, and harvesters for many years. Some superstitions specify planting certain vegetables and not others during a full moon to insure a better crop.

An understanding of these rhythms has developed very slowly; early efforts to identify and explain cyclic activity was directed mainly toward plants and animals. As the age of technology created the demand for "shift-work" and the jet age sent man across time zones more rapidly than he had ever before crossed them, the study of rhythmic activity in humans has increased and research in biologic rhythms, especially circadian rhythms, is moving forward in an obvious way.

Although it is beyond the scope of this text to explain in detail all of the facets of biologic rhythms, a number of factors will be considered as selected human needs are discussed and as the client situations are presented and analyzed within the framework of the nursing process.

Maslow discusses the degree to which each human being is dependent on his own strengths and abilities to achieve gratification of his needs.[3] He is also dependent on other's strengths and abilities to help him achieve gratification; therefore, *intra*personal as well as *inter*personal dimensions are operative when analyzing oneself and when evaluating the degree of human need gratification. Although achievement of perfection is impossible, each person can improve himself to a level beyond his present one. The degree of improvement can range from very good to none at all, with a multitude of variables operating throughout this forward movement.

To relate the theory of body rhythms to a concrete model, one can visualize a number of circles located on a forward moving line. The line represents the direction of man's movement toward need fulfillment; it usually progresses in a positive way. Reality forces the analyst to realize that need fulfillment is not always achieved on a continual basis. There are times when regression rather than progression is the pattern. The circles on the path, representing the cyclic activity of life, may progress and regress periodically; neither is a continual or a perpetual state, but both are inherent in the life of every person and both exist constantly. For example, a housewife and mother who is conscientious about meeting her obligations to her family endures the monotony of daily chores, of rambunctious youngsters, and neighborhood conversation with admirable patience and tolerance. On most days, Ms. Wife–Mother copes quite well, but on some days the coping is sadly deficient. Just what is operating to account for the difference in ability to cope? There are several possibilities:

The weather can be a significant factor. How warm or cool is it? How humid? Is there rain on the way? Is it pouring rain now? Is the sun shining brightly?

Sleep can be a factor. How much sleep did Ms. Wife–Mother have? Was it a restful sleep? Was she worried? Was she overtired? Did one of the children waken her during the night?

Mood of family members can be a variable. Were the children irritable? Was Mr. W–M upset? Were there hyperactive and exaggerated behaviors among the family members?

Menstrual cycle can be a factor. Is this a "premenstrual" time? Does Ms. Wife–Mother identify increased stress just prior to the menstrual period? Is there physical discomfort due to increased retention of body fluids?

These are a few of the possible factors that can alter the direction or the size of the circles visualized on the forward moving line, and that can even change the shape from a circle to a flattened, prolonged form that will require time and adjustment to return to the true cyclic activity phases.

Human need gratification, therefore, is an important goal as man moves along the slow and difficult path to self-actualization.[4] Although perfection in this effort is continually aimed for and hoped for, few are able to reach it. The cycles of activity are continual and man's motivation for this perfection waxes and wanes, depending on a number of complex variables that operate within each individual. Although all parts of the cycle are not totally understood, it is by means of further analysis and identification followed by pursuit of areas for research that man's efforts and behavior will be better understood.

Historically, nurses have relied on anatomic and physiologic knowledge about man's body systems to provide the necessary base for providing client care. Rather than moving in an independent manner with fellow professionals, nurses have often assumed a role within the purview of the medical profession.

During the decade of the 1970s we are witnessing a change in nursing functions. There is now a refreshing view of the client as a self-sufficient, well person, who has certain human needs in common with his fellow-humans. The nurse plays a role in helping the client to maintain his state of wellness and to help him return to a state of wellness if and when a need occurs. In the process of nursing, both nurse and client experience the cyclic activity that is inherent in humanity. What effect does this cyclic activity have on the client? on the nurse? on the interaction between the two? on their interaction with others in the environment as well as with the environment itself, and vice versa?

The area concerned with biologic rhythms of the client and the persons assisting him is one facet of client care that was overlooked for many years. There is now an increasing awareness of the existence of body rhythms in all humans, clients, nurses, families, and coworkers.

This presentation will be concerned with biologic rhythms, what and where they are, how they are manifested, how the knowledge about biologic rhythms was used in one client situation, and the potential use of biologic rhythm data by the nursing and health care systems in the future as more information about it becomes available.

Rhythmicity

Rhythms exist in all living matter, including man. His body contains certain rhythms known as endogenous, or internal rhythms; the rhythmic activity in the environmental living matter is exogenous, or external in relation to man. Man's physiologic rhythms adapt to and are in harmony with the rhythms in his environment; however when removed from the environmental influences, man's rhythms do not disappear; they may become altered and lengthened in time, but they continue in a regular fashion.[5]

For a physiologic function to be considered rhythmic, there must be an identifiable pattern to the activity and the occurrence of this regularity by chance must be unlikely. The rhythms need not be repeated in exactly equal sequences, but there must be some regularity in the cycle for it to be considered truly rhythmic.[6]

The frequency of cyclic events varies from a few seconds to a number of years. As increasingly sophisticated means of measurement become available because of technologic advances, the data about body rhythms is becoming more plentiful. Meanwhile, the endogenous rhythms that can be measured include sensory acuity, blood pressure, heart rate, body temperature, electrolyte excretion, serum levels of corticosteroids, serum electrolytes, blood cell values (eosinophil and platelet levels), and urine constituents.[7] For research purposes, measurements can be made of the electrical activity of the human brain and the heart, as well as of hormonal secretion from the ovaries.[8] Other behaviors that can be studied include technical performance, sleep patterns, appetite, and gastrointestinal functions.[9]

The scientific study of these and other rhythms in man is known as *chronobiology*. Dr. Halberg, director of the Chronobiology Laboratories at the University of Minnesota Medical School, has pioneered this study. Chronobiologists evaluate body rhythms as well as the other time-related changes in man, including growth, maturation, and aging.[10] Dr. Halberg suggests that by means of such study, data can be obtained to secure a more effective use of therapeutic agents, and health personnel should be able to better define health and illness, with emphasis on the measures necessary to maintain health and prevent illness.[11] The purpose of using chronobiology is to achieve timely intervention; it may "become a powerful tool for . . . self-maintenance of personal health, enabling the individual to act in advance of catastrophic events. . . . We may thus substitute a chronobiologic ounce of prevention for many pounds of homeostatic cure."[12]

Aschoff suggests that there are four geophysical cycles in the universe: the tidal (circatidal), the day–night (circadian), the lunar (circalunar), and the seasonal (circannual).[13] These cycles provide time-oriented structures in the environment that are paradigms for biologic clocks that enable living matter to measure time and anticipate changes. Synchrony is essential between the geophysical cycle and any or all of man's circa-rhythms and this synchrony is achieved by certain environmental factors that become "time givers," or synchronizing agents that "entrain the endogenous self-sustaining oscillation within the organism."[14]

Each of the multiple parameters of the human body clock possesses its own rhythm and has an individual cycle of activity, different from, but in synchrony with, the cycle of the other parameters. The peaking and troughing of each normal rhythm forms a harmony of cycles just as a number of musical instruments create a symphonic harmony. These multiple parameters can be compared to the horses that children ride on a carousel. A specific path is followed by each horse; it goes up (peaks) and down (troughs) in a rhythmic way, but not all horses go up and down at once. The harmonious movement of a group of carousel horses would be disrupted if one horse established a rhythm of its own, out of harmony (synchrony) with the other horses. Chaos and arhythmicity would result. When one body rhythm goes out of harmony, chaos results in the entire system of body rhythms. This becomes manifested by symptoms of disease.

What Rhythmicity Is Not

The field of chronobiology is not to be confused with a popular theory being thrust on the public called the "theory of biorhythms." This pseudoscientific theory calculates and predicts physical, intellectual, and emotional rhythms, using a person's birthdate as the base. This formula for explaining human rhythms has no firm basis in science and the interchangeable language between the two, biorhythms and chronobiology, presents confusing ideas to the public. Prior to the mid-twentieth century, the term *biorhythm* was used to cover all theories about biologic rhythms. As the scientific study of these rhythms has grown more sophisticated, and as more intensive studies reveal the increasing complexity of the questions about biologic rhythms, the science of chronobiology has been identified. Chronobiologists place the theory of biorhythms in the same category as astrology. Dr. Franz Halberg states that he cannot argue about things he cannot measure and sees the biorhythm theories as being based more on emotion than on scientific fact.[15]

Those who support the biorhythm ideas offer formulae for cycles of different lengths; for example, a 23-day cycle, a 28-day cycle, a 33-day cycle; each of these is labeled according to physical, emotional, or intellectual cycles.

Dr. Wernli, a practicing physician, states he introduced the "Fliess Biorhythm Theory" at his clinic in Switzerland approximately two decades ago.[16] With no documentation from scientific or other references, Wernli devotes 72 pages to a discussion of how biorhythms are manifested in every person's life. An additional 32 pages contain photographs of well-known persons and a "rhythmogram" for a selected time period for each individual. Each "rhythmogram" has three cycles plotted pictorially, namely, a physical cycle, a sensitivity cycle, and an intelligence cycle. Each "rhythmogram" shows that the death of the person under discussion occurred on a "critical" day in his life—a day when at least two of the cycles were in a low, or trough phase, or at least moving downward into a trough. In some illustrations, all three cycles are in critical low phases.[17]

The formula of Wilhelm Fliess was published in the late nineteenth century. It is an unsophisticated formula that is not generally recognized by scientists. Had Freud not considered Fliess to be a great biologist, the formula may never have been known. Although neither sophisticated nor recognized, the underlying idea presented by Fliess may not be too far-fetched.

Department stores, airline terminals, train stations, and other places frequented by large numbers of people have available to the public a computerized machine on which, for 25 cents, a person can press a button to indicate his date of birth, and a record of his biorhythms will be printed and machine-fed to him.

Literature accompanying this display includes an order blank for the convenience of the consumer. Materials ranging in price from 1 dollar to 30 dollars can be obtained by sending a request and money to the indicated address. These materials include kits to chart and analyze biorhythms, texts to explain biorhythms, and a computer report of one's personal biorhythms.

Certainly the public is increasingly aware of the existence of rhythms, although the term biorhythms and chronobiology are not clearly differentiated in the mind of the layman.

Where the Control Center Is Located

If persons think deeply about man's cyclic activity, few would disagree that there is some kind of timing system operating in each human. This timing mechanism is taken for granted under normal conditions and man becomes aware of some type of rhythmic device that is related to his body functioning only when it becomes maladjusted. In an effort to more effectively readjust the human timing device, researchers have for some time been trying to find the location of the body clock. Historically, the search has resulted in much speculation about the relationships among the brain, the endocrine system, and behavior.[18]

The site of the body clock has not been definitely determined or agreed on by scientists; however, various studies have produced data that suggest possible clock locations; most studies, too, have resulted in as many questions as conclusions.

The pineal gland is one possible clock site. It is a small gland, shaped like a tiny pinecone, located deep between the two hemispheres of the brain.[19] Because of its sensitivity to light, it is thought that this gland may act as a type of "coupling device," and in this role may regulate the phases among some rhythms.

The adrenal gland cycle has appeared to have some "clocklike" features. Studies have shown that removal of the adrenals has abolished the rhythms of cell mitosis in new skin growth. Other studies of the adrenals have suggested alteration (specifically, amplitude) rather than an abolishment of the rhythm when the adrenals were removed.[20]

The hypothalamus has been a frequent target for study by those persons who are looking for the location of the body clock, probably because it is important in regulating so many body functions necessary for survival, such as respiration and body temperature. It is also crucial in the regulation of the appetite for food, desire for fluids, sexual drive, and other types of physical activity.[21]

Dr. Richter has done much work in studying the endocrine glands and their influence on body cycles. The pituitary, the adrenals, the thyroid, and other endocrine glands often show a clocklike activity that may be described as resembling the hands of the clock rather than the clock itself.[22]

These are a few of the many hypotheses about the location of the "body clock" in man, but no universally accepted conclusions have been reached. As the studies continue in pursuit of this elusive goal, the rhythmic activity of the human body becomes more and more apparent. Despite man's inability to identify its site, a timer is at work controlling the functions of each individual, whether sick or well.

Rhythmicity in Plants and Animals

For many years, plant and animal studies have been done to investigate the presence of internal rhythms and to determine the degree of influence exerted by external or environmental cues. Not surprisingly, plant and animal rhythms have been easier to study than have the rhythms of man. As a point of interest a few of the studies will be mentioned here. The literature contains many detailed studies, however, and a student who seriously wishes to pursue the study of human rhythms will discover many areas of plant and animal research from which to develop questions that can be related to the study of human rhythms.

One of Halberg's early studies, using mice, was carried out over a two-year period, during which the temperature changes of the mice were recorded. A 24-hour rhythm was detected. The mice were then blinded to eliminate light and dark cues and the rhythm of their temperature change speeded up to just over 23 hours, but the rhythm persisted despite removal of light and darkness cues from the external environment.[23]

The appearance of the groundhog in early February is a good example of one animal's cyclic activity. Dr. Albert, a researcher at the University of Maryland, has studied the clock that wakens the groundhog from its hibernation. It is quite unaware of the weather forecasting responsibilities placed upon him by man; instead, the male groundhog, the one whose clock wakens him first, is usually looking for a mate rather than for his shadow. Studies of the hibernation mechanism of animals such as the groundhog may prove valuable in future studies of man. Efforts are being made to discover how body thermostats are turned down, how other body functions are depressed, how this energy-saving mechanism is controlled, and how the body clock determines when it is time to waken the animal.[24]

The annual migration of birds and geese continues to puzzle scientists. Some speculations exist but little scientific knowledge has been identified to explain this annual demonstration. What kind of clock tells the birds to break up camp and fly south? Why do some species go south and others stay in the north? How do they navigate such a true and regular course? Why do some end their flight in Florida and others continue into the Caribbean? Whether or not the answers to questions such as these will help explain the mechanism of the human body clock remains to be seen.[25]

The umi-shida is a Japanese sea fern being studied by marine biologist Nicholas Holland. These sea ferns spawn one day a year in a rhythm that is so precise it intrigues the scientist who can do little more at present than speculate on the intricacies of the biologic clock of the umi-shida. Especially intriguing is the location of the clock; even if the sea fern is cut into many pieces, each piece that contains a gonad or an ovary spawns right on schedule, like "clockwork."[26]

The giant garden slug (*Limax maximus*) is being studied at the University of Maryland, Baltimore County, by Dr. Sokolove, a professor of biologic sciences. He has established that this animal exhibits an intrinsic rhythm, and despite removal of the "primitive eyes" of the slug, it responds rhythmically to a light–dark cycle, apparently through some unidentified extraocular photoreceptive system.[27]

These are but a few of the reports of studies of rhythmicity; much more knowledge is becoming available.

Rhythmicity in Man

The Origin of Rhythms

A number of theories have been advanced about the origin of human rhythms, including the following:

Rhythms are not present at birth but develop during the first year of life;

Rhythmicity depends on the level of neurologic maturity; the inference here seems to be that the clock is located somewhere in the central nervous system;

Each person is endowed with a set of biologic clocks as part of his inherited characteristics;

Rhythmicity is a set of learned responses that are dependent on environmental stimuli and the socialization processes for functioning.[28]

These are "hunches" suggested by those who have pursued the study of body rhythms and are continuing to search for more complete answers. Validation of these theories remains to be accomplished in the future.

The Biologic Rhythms of Infants and the Young

It has been established that different body structures and functions develop rhythmicity at different rates in the growing infant.[29] Hellbrügge, et al., studied the development of origin of physiologic rhythms in infants and recorded the following:

1. Only the periodicity of electric skin resistance, an indication of autonomic activity, is evident in the first weeks of life; this skin resistance is high in the morning hours and is low at night.
2. The rate of urine flow becomes evident in the second and third weeks of life; the flow becomes greater during the day than at night and is not correlated with fluid intake, apparently because the infant drinks nearly as much at night as he drinks during the day.
3. The body temperature rhythm does not become obvious until five to nine months of age. At the time it appears, it varies a degree or two over the 24-hour period as does the temperature of the adult.
4. Rhythmicity is evident at five to nine months of age in blood sugar levels, in urine constituents, and in urine flow.
5. Heart rate rhythm appears between 4 and 20 weeks of age.
6. Before 18 months of age, rhythmicity can be identified in potassium, sodium, and phosphate excretion; these ions are presumably active in nerve cell discharge.
7. Between 18 months and 2 years of age, creatinine and chloride excretion rhythms occur.[30]
8. Cortisol rhythm becomes evident at about three years of age.[31]

These studies, pursued at the University of Munich, presented some fascinating data. Some mothers will readily agree with one finding, namely that several rhythms are not synchronized with the 24-hour day–night period of the adult world. Researchers found that the newborn's pattern of sleep and waking, eye activity, body temperature, pulse, and excretion levels of potassium, sodium, and calcium were out of synchrony with the 24 hours. Most of these functions as well as behaviors were found to be ultradian rhythms; i.e., less, or shorter, than 24 hours. The 24-hour rhythm began to appear by the time the infant was 14 to 20 weeks old.

The fact that not all rhythms develop at the same rate suggests the absence of any one clock to govern the body rhythms.[32]

The Biologic Rhythms of the Aged

Some evidence suggests that as persons age, there is an increase in the internal desynchronization of rhythms. One rhythm that frequently is disturbed as one grows older is the sleep cycle. One possible explanation for this disturbance is the loss of contact with the synchronizing agents in the environment; also, it is possible that some of the rhythms may start to free run so that the rest–activity cycle of an individual goes out of phase with the day–night cycle.[33]

Authors differ in their opinions about alterations in body rhythms resulting from age. Such differences suggest that insufficient research is being done to arrive at valid conclusions about the effect of aging on body rhythms.

Bassler suggests that human growth hormone declines with age.[34] Perhaps this is a resonable conclusion to draw, but to establish the relationship between this decline and body rhythms, it seems necessary to ask: at what rate does the decline occur? at what chronological age does it begin to decline? when does it cease its decline? what are the hereditary factors that are operative?

Studies in Milan identified no circadian variation in the level of 17-hydroxycorticosteroids (17-OHCS) in the urine of older people. A very slight shift was noted in the time of the peak concentration; the peak occurred just slightly earlier than in a group of younger adults. This very insignificant peaking was attributed to a possible sleep disturbance. When abnormal urinary steroid rhythms appeared in older people, they were attributed to urinary tract infection that had not been previously identified.[35] Similar studies with a group of older people in New York City have revealed no abnormal or unusual rhythms in the 17-OHCS blood levels.[36]

One study conducted by a group of three persons at Utica College and the University of Iowa investigated the circadian rhythms of a group of young men and a group of older men, ranging in age from the 20s to the 60s. Four parameters were observed: body temperature, urine flow, heart rate, and potassium excretion. Each person was studied individually; light was controlled, food and water were measured, external disturbances were screened out, and muscle activity was limited by enforced rest periods. Of eleven young men, nine showed perfect internal synchrony. Of six elderly men, three showed no parallel between peaks and troughs of measured functions; i.e., they exhibited dissociation. Peak urine flow, for example, might occur at night when urine flow was low. Among depressed clients in the 40- to 60-year-old group, four out of five showed a great degree of desynchronization.

One question that arises is: which is the causative factor? Does the desynchronization (or irregular rhythm) cause the depression (or illness), or is the opposite true—does the depression cause the desynchronization?

As a person grows older, many events take place within the body of the person as well as in his environment that may have an effect on him and his functioning. Illnesses can occur, accompanied or caused by shock, fever, virus, etc.; social pressures and stresses change, habits may become less regular, and emotional stress may be present. Any one or several of these events may be the precursor of dissociated rhythms or desynchronization of rhythms.

The Rhythmicity of a Normal and Well Man

When Mr. B.O. Lodge was born 47 years ago, it is quite possible his mother was unaware of body rhythms; nevertheless, these rhythms were influential factors that were operating within his mother as well as in her environment; they played a crucial role in stimulating the onset of labor pains before the birth of Mr. Lodge. There may have been a full moon, or the time may have been the early morning hours; perhaps neither of these may have been true. It is not possible now to retrieve such data for analysis, but since Mr. Lodge's birth almost a half century ago, man has become increasingly aware that certain life circumstances and life events are worthy of more attention than was given to them in the past. Had Mr. Lodge's parents been aware of their body rhythms and had they kept more complete data about these rhythmic life events, Mr. Lodge would, no doubt, have been able to more thoroughly evaluate his own body rhythms in light of his heritage.

Not all questions about body rhythms can be answered within the framework of such knowledge; in fact, with more data available, it is possible that more questions will be raised than will be answered. However, it is useful to have as much data as possible in order to pursue the analysis and study of one's own body rhythms.

Situation

Mr. Lodge has been a relatively healthy person; he has had no serious illnesses during his life. His 40-hour work week as a supervisor in a clothing factory near his home provides for him a fairly regular work schedule and a consistency in the time he can spend with his wife and three teenage children. Family, relatives, friends, and co-workers of Mr. Lodge describe him as a pleasant, relatively stable person with an even temperament, a determined manner, who seldom gets upset or angry.

Mr. Lodge has recently been concerned about some changes in his behavior of which he has been aware. He senses that he has become less tolerant of the mistakes made at work by the employees, raises his voice at his teenagers for behavior he was previously able to tolerate with more patience, and his wife has suggested to him, half facetiously, that he is behaving like a "woman going through the change." At Mrs. Lodge's suggestion, they planned a visit to the neighborhood health clinic for an evaluation.

Biologic Rhythm Implications

Not so much is known about the male climacteric as is known about the menopause experienced by women. Nor is there as much information about the cyclic endocrine activity of males as is available about the monthly menstrual cycle of the female. As early as the seventeenth century, however, a physician identified a monthly fluctuation in weight of from one to two pounds in healthy men. In the twentieth century, much more data have become available about regular changes in the male, but much more remains to be learned.

As a result of a "hunch" about the cyclic endocrine activity of males, Danish endocrinologist Dr. Hamburger collected and analyzed his own urine for sixteen years. He was particularly interested in the fluctuation of adrenal hormones (17-ketosteroids), which can be detected in the urine.[37] When Dr. Halberg analyzed the results of Dr. Hamburger's study, he found that a monthly fluctuation was apparent in the levels of the 17-ketosteroids. Some Japanese scientists have also observed and reported this rhythmic fluctuation of adrenal hormones.[38]

Industrial psychologist Dr. Hershey studied the emotional rhythms of several industrial workers during a one-year period. He was concerned about the label attached to the behavior of these workers—suggesting that the working man was invariably a stable, immovable, unchanging person. Dr. Hershey's belief that there might be some variation in this labeled behavior led him to undertake the following study: for thirteen weeks, four times a day, he watched and interviewed each man of a selected group of men, and gave each a physical examination.[39] After the thirteen weeks, Dr. Hershey discontinued the watching and interviewing. For a period of time he asked the men to record and rate themselves on an emotional scale provided for them. A third phase of the study involved a series of observations and interviews with the families of the selected workers.[40]

The collected data were analyzed and plotted graphically by Dr. Hershey. A distinct pattern emerged from this analysis which showed:

1. One man, 60 years old, showed a nine-week cycle that included a gradual decline in his usual jovial, good natured behavior, during which time he was

critical of others, less apt to joke with his fellow workers and family, and was more withdrawn in his behavior than usual.

2. A 22-year-old man showed a 4.5-week cycle. While in the trough periods of this cycle he had a tendency to be apathetic and indifferent to his work and to his hobbies at home.
3. One man demonstrated a 4.5- to 6.5-week cycle; during the trough periods of this cycle, this man was irritable and magnified minor crises out of proportion.
4. One man showed a 5- to 6-week cycle; he experienced manic periods during which he was markedly outgoing and overconfident, whereas during the low periods he was drowsy, lethargic, slept a great deal, and wanted to sit quietly and be left alone. During the high periods he weighed less and slept less than during the low periods.[41]

Biologic Rhythm Alterations

Periodic or cyclic illnesses are recorded in medical literature although there is still insufficient emphasis on periodicity in medical education and practice. One famous example of a periodic illness is that of Mary Lamb, the sister of the English essayist Charles Lamb.[42] When Mary was 30 years old, it became evident that she suffered from periodic psychoses that occurred with regularity (38 times) over a 50-year period. Her brother was appointed her custodian and was able to observe the irritability that marked the onset of Mary's attacks; as soon as this was noted, Mary was hospitalized until she recovered; afterwards she was able to perform normally as a writer and as a hostess at social events. When symptoms of another attack appeared, the cycle of hospitalization and recovery was repeated and continued until her death at the age of 83.

Norwegian physicians Dr. Gjessing, Sr. and Dr. Gjessing, Jr. studied the biochemical mechanism of periodic catatonia.[43] Dr. Gjessing, Sr. observed a significant coincidence between his patients' radical change in behavior and a change in their physical appearance. Following a "hunch" about physiologic alterations, Dr. Gjessing initiated a number of physiologic measurements, including the measurement of nitrogen retention. He hypothesized that thyroid functioning abnormality was the basis for much of the observed catatonia. He "speculated that stress, brain damage, or perhaps metabolic shock due to some auto-immune reaction might damage a metabolic regulator and thus produce the clock-like symptoms of catatonia."[44]

The results of Dr. Gjessing's biochemical studies confirmed much of his belief about the role of nitrogen. The body usually regulates the balance of nitrogen, excreting via the liver approximately as much as it takes in. During attacks of catatonia, nitrogen was "over-excreted during the normal interval and retained during the phase of excitement."[45] Tests showed that levels of urinary ammonia were higher at the beginning of the catatonia attacks. Potassium and sodium chloride were excreted in greater quantities during the attacks. Thyroxin has prevented nitrogen retention and has successfully reduced symptoms in many patients; only when thyroid medication is not taken by these catatonia-prone persons do they have recurrent attacks.[46]

Daily recordings of temperature or of urine pigmentation over a ten-year period indicate regularity of changes in individuals studied and attacks of catatonia were predicted to within a day of their occurrence.

The English physician Dr. F. A. Jenner has studied one manic-depressive person for many years. The client is overactive and talkative for 24 hours, then moves into a sluggish period during which he urinates and excretes more but eats and drinks less than during the manic phase. A study of this man in a controlled setting showed him to have a 48 hour alteration of weight, urine volume, and red blood cell volume. The amount of fluid within and around cells shifted with his moods. On days during which he was depressed, the saliva sodium was low and saliva potassium was high; on manic days, the reverse was true. Dr. Jenner then isolated himself and the client in a room for 11 days, where meals were served to both of them and urine samples were collected from them. Lighting was regulated so the "day" was 22 hours long, although neither Dr. Jenner nor the client knew the length of the day. The moods of the client fluctuated between complete silence and hyperactivity and these moods adapted to a 22 hour day; that is, they alternated between lethargy and mania on a 44 hour cycle. However, water and electrolytes were excreted on a 24 hour cycle. The question remains unanswered: why did moods adapt to a 22 hour cycle and electrolyte excretion remain on a 24 hour cycle[47]

Nursing Assessment

Mr. Lodge and his wife were aware of an alteration in his usual behavior. The need to clearly identify the cause of this alteration led the couple to seek the services and help of the personnel at the health clinic.

A thorough physical examination and appropriate laboratory tests were done, and extensive examination of Mr. Lodge was completed. These tests showed no significant results, except (1) the behavior changes, relatively minor, but nonetheless present and noticeable in Mr. Lodge's behavior; (2) a high blood sugar level; (3) a low thyroid and high uric acid level. It was determined that Mr.

Lodge functioned at a "normal" level, that is, as he had been functioning for many years in his job, and in his pursuit of hobbies at home during the off-work hours. Mr. Lodge was duly concerned about these relatively minor alterations, and was eager and motivated to do what was necessary to remain as well as possible.

Nursing Diagnoses

After complete assessment by the nurse in the health clinic, the following nursing diagnoses were determined:

Mood alteration;
Less patient than usual;
More intolerant of others' pecadillos;
Hasty and irritable reactions, out of proportion to the event;
Tendency to be overweight;
Preference for foods high in carbohydrate;
Occasional burning on urination.

Nursing Orders

The nurse analyzed the data collected about Mr. Lodge during the assessment process and reviewed the nursing diagnoses that she had formed at the completion of the assessment; she decided that the two main areas needing attention were the nutrition of Mr. Lodge and his feelings about himself and his associates—his family, friends, and co-workers. The following nursing orders were prescribed:

Regularly observe Mr. Lodge's behavior when he comes to clinic; carefully record how agitated or how calm he is in response to more or less irritating situations. Encourage him to keep a daily log of his feelings, reactions to others, and response to negative work situations. With Mr. Lodge's knowledge, ask Mrs. Lodge to keep a daily log with twice a day (early morning and late afternoon) recordings of his manner, his tolerance level, and apparent stress in various situations.

Set up consultation with diet therapist; the aim of the nutrition plan is to control weight gain, reduce number of calories eaten each day to reduce high sugar absorption and limit foods high in cholesterol. Provide attractive foods that will satisfy appetite for high caloric foods, yet avoid deleterious effects and potential diabetes.

In combination with diet for prevention of diabetes development, incorporate foods that will reduce uric acid elevation to control possibility of gout development. Prescribe and discuss with Mr. Lodge the need for fluids, indicating the amount of fluids and type of liquids that would be most beneficial for him.

Refer Mr. Lodge to the physician for further evaluation of potential gout and kidney stone risk.

Strategy

The nurse met with Mr. and Mrs. Lodge to discuss the data collected over a three-month period and during Mr. Lodge's clinic visits. The focus of the discussion was to identify Mr. Lodge's strengths, namely, his affable nature and his ability to cope with various situations with reasonable patience and objectivity. Recognition of the occasional periods of irritability was not difficult for Mr. Lodge; he is a very reasonable man, not at all defensive, and he is interested in maintaining the good health he has enjoyed for many years.

The data indicated a beginning pattern in mood changes based on rhythmic changes due to age that was quite surprising to them. A presentation to the couple of some of the possible explanations of Mr. Lodge's behavior was well received. The nurse suggested that he:

Continue to keep a daily diary, or log, of moods and behavior;

Be consciously aware of subtle or sharp mood changes;

Deliberately reflect on the basis for the observed behavior and incorporate these rationales when describing behavior;

Return to clinic in three months to further discuss new data and determine future goals.

Rhythmicity of a Potentially Ill Man

Situation

The concern expressed by the nurse about the borderline results of the blood sugar, thyroid, and uric acid tests motivated Mr. B.O. Lodge to make an immediate appointment with the physician. The nursing assessment and diagnosis relative to his mood alterations were not discouraging; at least, he was not ill, and these mood swings were "within normal limits"; in other words, the variation in behavior could be expected at this age.

One of the results of an early visit with his physician was a medication prescription for Mr. Lodge that would control or prevent attacks of gout and a prescription for thyroid medication to supplement the normal secretion of thyroxin. When Mr. Lodge came to clinic to see the nurse again, a schedule of nourishment and activities was established that would enable him to cope with these relatively minor but potentially significant alterations in body functioning.

Biologic Rhythm Implications

Hormonal secretion rhythms are periodically out of phase and periodically in phase with other circadian rhythms. Although limited data are available in this area, there is some preliminary indication that depression coincides with the times when hormonal rhythms are out of phase.[48]

Is there a genetic factor that may suggest a relationship between Mr. Lodge's cultural background and his altered mood and blood levels? Dr. Simpson at the University of Glasgow studied two groups of people, Indians living in South America and British medical students living in Glasgow. He found high corticosteroid excretion between 9:00 A.M. and noon in the South American Indians and between noon and 3:00 P.M. in the Scottish medical students when the clock hour of midnight was used as a time reference. However, when the usual rest span of the group was used as a reference point, changes in the corticosteroid excretion occurred at a similar time within the rest–activity cycle of the two groups. It can be concluded that the corticosteroid excretion occurs in preparation for the activity of the day regardless of the culture or geographic location of an individual.[49]

Apparently there are no valid data to indicate that body rhythms vary among different people because of cultural differences. The person and his environment appear to be the crucial factors in differentiating rhythms.

Is there a relationship between Mr. Lodge's physical activities and his nutrition? If so, how can it be defined? A report of a study done in the 1920s suggests that activity during sleep can be related in some way to hunger. A group of medical students was studied; by means of devised measurements within a balloon in the stomach of each student, stomach contractions were observed to coincide with movements during sleep. The spontaneous bursts of activity recorded during the normal cycles of sleep coincided with recorded stomach contractions in such a way that there seems to be some relationship between this activity and hunger.[50] Other scientists have observed that sleep cycles of subjects and their desire for eating and smoking have coincided. With intensified activity of dreaming and moving about during sleep there is simultaneously an increased desire for eating and smoking. These findings raise several questions, one of which is: do these rhythms of activity and quiescence within the daily rhythm pattern of every individual bear some relationship to the "drive rhythms" of the central nervous system? When answers are determined for this question, perhaps there will be better explanations of problems related to obesity, to the unusual food preferences of pregnant women, and to the monthly variation in weight, more exaggerated in some persons than in others.

Biologic Rhythm Alterations

Among the data sought by the nurse in the client assessment is a determination of the pace maintained by the Lodge family and of how much stress they feel they experience. Dr. Holmes at the University of Washington has demonstrated a relationship between a person's health and the rate of change in his life.[51] By means of a validated scale, life changes were measured and rated to determine the amount of impact each had on a person's health. Findings indicated that persons who experience the most changes in life style will have about twice as much illness as persons whose lives have hardly changed. It is hypothesized that persons who are exerting themselves to adjust to change are exhausting some of their resistance potential and are therefore apt to become ill. "Adaptation has a physiological, biochemical meaning and every time we cope with something new the endocrine system must supply extra energy. . . . It is the pace of life, the rate of change that has predicted illness."[52]

The physician's prescription of medication for Mr. Lodge to prevent gout attacks was a valuable and essential means of preventing an uncomfortable and disabling metabolic imbalance. Nursing intervention requires an understanding of certain biologic rhythm variables operative in medication consumption. It has been suggested that "with care, drugs can be tailored to the beat of the body."[53]

Some experimentation was done with hypnotics taken at bedtime that did not sedate persons who were psychologically ill; the staff gave a fraction of a hypnotic dose in the midafternoon, a fraction in the evening, and a final fraction at bedtime. Persons who had been previously anxious were now eased into sleep with less sedation than was administered in one dose at bedtime.[54]

Not many drugs have been studied for their circadian rhythm properties. However, it is quite possible for drugs to influence the circadian rhythm of the body; it is also possible for the body to respond to medication with different intensity at different hours of the 24 hour period. For example, a fast-acting barbiturate can block the morning rise in hormone levels.[55] If Mr. Lodge is taking a medication for gout control, how can this knowledge of hormone blocking agents be used to plan his medication schedule? Based on his body rhythms, what time of day will be most effective for taking the medication? What other medications is he regularly taking (such as thyroid extract), or may he take (such as aspirin), and what can be the expected action among the different medications? If he takes all medications in the morning, will they be more effective than if taken in the evening? If the total dose is divided between morning and evening, can a different reaction be expected at each time?

As knowledge about biochemistry expands and as scientists become more alert to the significance of body rhythms, an increasing number of questions should arise in the minds of those who administer drugs. Whether the rhythm of the body is at a phase that is more or less receptive to the pharmacologic effect of a specific drug, or whether an administered medication alters or affects any one of the body rhythms are two questions that need careful scrutiny.

In addition to asking whether there is a particular time of day when a specific drug might be more or less effective, it is important to wonder whether a certain illness, disease, or pathology might change or even abolish the usual body rhythms.[56] On the other hand, is it possible that an altered rhythm might be the cause of illness or disease?

Nursing Assessment

The nurse supplemented her previous assessment by pursuing the following areas of inquiry, which she felt were most pertinent to the biologic rhythm area:

1. Mobility
   - A. In what physical activities do you regularly engage? With what frequency—daily? weekly?
   - B. How fatigued do you become during and after different types of physical exercise?
   - C. Is there any difference in the rate at which you fatigue? For example, does your exercise endurance last longer in the morning or in the afternoon, or in the evening?
   - D. Is there any dyspnea, or dizziness, or any discomfort during or following physical activity?
2. Food
   - A. How many meals do you eat each day?
   - B. What time of day do you eat?
   - C. When do you eat your heaviest meal?
   - D. Do you snack between meals? Regularly? Occasionally?
   - E. What type of food do you prefer at meals?
   - F. What foods do you dislike?

3. Fluids
   A. How frequently do you drink fluids during the day?
   B. What type fluids do you drink between meals?
   C. What fluids do you drink with your meals?
   D. Do you drink fluids at bedtime? Anytime after the evening meal? During the night?
4. Urine elimination
   A. What is your usual pattern of frequency of urination?
   B. Does the frequency vary with the amount of fluid intake? Type of fluid intake?
   C. Does pain or discomfort accompany urination?
   D. Is there ever more discomfort at night or during the day?
5. Bowel elimination
   A. What is your usual pattern of bowel evacuation?
   B. Do you regularly defecate in the morning or in the evening?
   C. Are the stools regularly semiformed? Hard? Watery? Soft?
   D. Is there any change in usual color of the stool?
   E. What factors appear to alter bowel habits? Sleep alteration? Change in physical activity? Overeating? Less fluids than usual? Fatigue? Altered meal times?
6. Sleep
   A. How many hours do you usually sleep each night?
   B. Do you waken during the night? Seldom? Often? Usually?
   C. Having wakened at night, do you have difficulty falling asleep again?
   D. What activities do you usually perform before going to bed?
   E. Do you nap during the day? In the evening?
   F. Can you identify any specific event or activity that you think interferes with your sleep?
7. Energy
   A. Do you consistently feel energetic or fatigued?
   B. Is your most productive work period in the morning, or in the afternoon, or in the evening?
   C. Are you able to think more clearly and creatively in the morning, or in the evening?
8. Perception of Self
   A. Are you less able to tolerate interruptions of your own plans at certain times of the day?
   B. Do you sense a feeling of family closeness consistently, or are there times when there are strained feelings?

C. Do you experience feelings of restlessness at any time during the day? The week? The month?
D. Are you able to communicate clearly on a consistent basis?
E. What factors seem to alter or improve your ability to communicate?

Nursing Diagnoses

The data collected by the nurse were examined and analyzed. Mr. and Mrs. Lodge submitted to the nurse their logs for the three-month period and the nurse included these data in her analysis. Having reviewed the recorded data, the following nursing diagnoses were identified for Mr. Lodge. He:

Experiences an energy lag in the late afternoon and early evening;
Has become habituated to eating candy bars and soft drinks between meals and at bedtime;
Has urinary frequency, once or twice each night with periodic increases in that frequency;
Experiences occasional constipation, apparently associated with stress.

Nursing Orders

Because the data are inconclusive and because there appears to be early indication of a pattern developing in Mr. Lodge's nutrition and elimination habits, the nurse recommended the following:

Continue the daily log by Mr. and Mrs. Lodge;
Eliminate between-meal snacks;
Reduce the amount of fluids taken after evening meals;
Establish routine time for retiring at night;
Avoid after-dinner nap.

Nursing Strategies

Mr. Lodge was not suprised when the nurse made these suggestions to him. He was surprised, however, to find the developing patterns that could be observed in the data he and his wife had collected in their daily logs. As the nurse identified for him the peaks and troughs of his energy periods, Mr. Lodge was able to relate these to his intake of food. The urinary frequency at night had a direct correlation to the amount and type of fluids he drank in the evening. Consistency in the time of retiring at night was positively related to those nights when he slept well.

Although a number of avenues remain to be explored, Mr. Lodge was encouraged that progress was being made in the analysis of his health status. The one major area to be examined was that related to his medication; just what effect will the gout and thyroid medications have on his usual activities, such as eating, eliminating, and sleeping? How will he respond to stressful situations at work and at home? Will the medication change his mood fluctuations?

Having agreed to pursue the continued recording of data, the nurse set an appointment for Mr. Lodge to return to clinic at the end of three months for further assessment of the data that he and his wife would continue to collect.

The Potential of Rhythmicity in Nursing

It is relatively easy to recite a definition of biologic rhythms. It is much more difficult, however, to answer the questions about the many complex facets of body rhythms. "Despite widespread research . . . the basis of circadian rhythms remains something about which we know very little."[57] Solutions to the problems posed in the investigations of biologic rhythms will not be realized until some future date. To incorporate the knowledge that is available about biologic rhythms into nursing practice today, the following goals seem appropriate:

Become aware of the existence of biologic rhythms in one's self, in one's associates, and in clients;
Use such awareness to pursue studies and gather data to help explain certain phenomena in client care;
Become acquainted with studies already completed, and with the literature available about the state of biologic rhythm knowledge at present;
Initiate a format, a schedule, or a plan that will insure the nurse's consideration of available rhythmicity data in client care.

Over a period of time, as many as 63 different types of human rhythms have been identified. The measurement of some rhythms requires elaborate instrumentation and sophisticated equipment for study. Other rhythms can be observed and measured with little more than the attention of the individual and a pencil and paper recording schedule.

A calendar diary of ourselves would no doubt show that we have a regular rhythmic cycle in weight, vitality, optimism, pessimism, work production, appetite for food, need for sleep, personality vibrancy or dullness, ambition and apathy, moodiness or complacency, lethargy and vigor. These are normal oscillations; when these fluctuations are exaggerated, there is interference in functioning and illness occurs.[58]

The following rhythmicity parameters can be measured by nurses and/or by clients and the practice of nursing will be enhanced and improved as recognition and measurement of these parameters are incorporated into the pursuit of the nursing process:

Time Perception

The client will probably experience a different time perception than the nurse. If they experience time perceptions that are almost identical, one can expect less friction and more compatibility during the pursuit of health for the client.

Persons with higher metabolic rates perceive clock time as passing more slowly than other persons. Children, whose metabolic rates are higher than adults, perceive time as passing slowly. As persons age, metabolic rates become slower and time seems to move more rapidly. Body temperature also affects one's perception of time. The higher the temperature, the slower clock time passes.[59] As one grows into maturity and adulthood, many bodily changes occur. One change is a decline in the rate of oxygen consumption and a resulting decline in the rate of metabolism.[60]

Temperature

Taking one's temperature is a relatively easy activity. Hospital routines usually define the specific frequency for taking each person's temperature. However, the taking and recording of temperatures has been such a perfunctory routine that little analysis of the records has been done. A wealth of data are available in the temperature recordings of hospitalized persons as well as in the personal records of any individual who has taken his temperature at regular intervals over a period of time. The rhythm method of birth control is based on temperature fluctuation and persons who have regulated family size by this means have excellent data for study. The following questions can be asked:

What is my temperature rhythm? What is my peak period of activity as indicated by the degree of my temperature? How can I anticipate the change in rhythm over a period of time? To what extent does the temperature rhythm fluctuate or change over a specific time period?

What is the normal temperature rhythm of the client? Is there a change in normal rhythm in the face of this illness? How does temperature rhythm alter with specific illness? Can the client's mood change be partially explained by the temperature fluctuations? Can temperature rhythm affect the client's appetite for food? In the presence of elevated blood sugar and uric acid levels, does temperature fluctuation vary? If so, in which direction? Does temperature fluctuation alter the sugar and uric acid levels or does the alteration of blood levels alter the temperature fluctuation?

Body temperature fluctuates by as much as two degrees within a day. The low usually occurs in the early morning; the high temperature of the body usually occurs in the late afternoon or early evening. Persons who experience a marked sensitivity to this rhythmic fluctuation of temperature are best known as "early birds" (larks) who work best during the day or "owls" who work best during the night.[61]

Blood Pressure

Taking one's own blood pressure is a relatively common practice today. The increasing number of Health Fairs in metropolitan communities and the availability of Free Clinics and other health care facilities provide many opportunities for blood pressures to be taken by qualified personnel. Even department stores and shopping malls have installed machines where customers can sit down, put a coin in a slot, put their arm in a cuff, and have their blood pressure revealed to them on a screen.

A single blood pressure reading is important. More important, however, is the periodic reading at a regular time and under the same environmental conditions. For example, a regular blood pressure reading each morning immediately on arising will provide a person with a pattern in readings over a period of time. This pattern, with its fluctuations, will be important to the person who is concerned with his rhythmicity. In addition to the early morning reading, a person can take a blood pressure reading just before going to bed at night to give an added dimension to his health status. For a person who must change his hours of sleeping because of work schedules, it would be important to compare the blood pressure rhythmicity while working days with the rhythmicity recorded while working nights.

Pulse Rate

Controlled external or environmental conditions are important in determining the rhythm of pulse rate. The introduction of mental stress, physical activity, eating, or other type of activity can alter the rhythmicity of pulse rate. To control such factors, the same plan can be followed as for the blood pressure readings. Pulse can be counted before arising and before retiring. Other time periods can be included to provide additional data about pulse rate, such as before and after meals, before and after selected physical activity, and before and after selected mental activity. The essential element in establishing rhythmicity is regularity in measuring the parameters and awareness of and control, when possible, of the surrounding variables.

Performance

The peak hours of efficiency in performing mental activity usually occur in the afternoon hours, with often a temporary dip in efficiency just after lunch. This dip occurs even if the noon meal is skipped, so it is not valid to blame the quality of the noon meal for the drop in efficiency.

Employee assignment schedules can be analyzed to determine the periods of more efficiency and better performance. The results of such analyses can be increased client and employee satisfaction, with less grumbling and fewer mishaps.

Analysis of one's own energy cycle can be done. Data can be collected that specifies peaks and troughs of energy periods together with identifiable operating variables. A daily log of moods, of feelings of ambition, or periods of sluggishness can provide a pattern to help one determine his work schedule. Scheduling oneself for creative types of activity when one is more refreshed and alert will probably result in productive activity. Recognition of the periods of the day when technical activities are more efficiently performed is productive and satisfying for employers and for employees.

Douglas suggests that knowledge of biologic rhythms has practical significance in studying, as well as promoting, efficiency and effectiveness in nursing care.[62] A curve of hormonal secretions can be plotted for each individual and by means of blood testing, the hormonal output is identified as being at its lowest in the early morning hours; it is at its peak at midday. By evening, around 6:00 P.M., resistance to stress is at the lowest level. These data suggest that creativity and efficiency are most likely to be apparent around the midday hours; data do show that more errors occur in nursing during the late afternoon and evening hours.

Douglas' admonition is to the leader—she should assess her own energy curve and seek a position that will allow her to make maximum use of her peak energy periods. Those who are responsible for placing and assigning personnel may do well to consider the studies about body rhythms in order to assist in the consideration of placing nurses on rotating shifts.

Although the biologic rhythm factor is important in assignments and in assessing one's own peaks and troughs of energy output, there are other factors to be considered: how rapidly can one adjust to alterations in time periods of assignments and responsibilities? Do some persons adapt more rapidly than others? To what extent do environmental factors play a role in body rhythm effectiveness, or in adaptation to change? Obviously, the simple plotting of body rhythm curves and knowledge of energy peaks and troughs is not the sole basis on which activities can be planned.

Nutrition and Elimination

Although environmental factors and external scheduling have powerful influences on a person's nutrition and elimination patterns, there are also innate patterns of hunger, thirst, and elimination. Periodic cycles of increased appetite for food are experienced by persons of any age and of both sexes. Little is known about the frequency of the increased and decreased appetites or about how often the cycle of peaks and troughs is repeated in a specific period of time. Increased knowledge about each person's pattern of appetite has implications for helping clients regulate food and fluid intake according to altered health or potential alterations. Social functions can be planned more effectively to make the occasions of eating and drinking more pleasant activities if these can be planned according to the rhythm of the host or hostess, at least.

Bowel and bladder elimination are dependent on intake of food and fluids, on stress or lack of it, on medications or absence of them, on sleep satisfaction or deprivation. Together with such identifiable influences, these functions possess a pattern unique to each individual. Recording the frequency, amount, and type of elimination activity provides valuable data that clients can use in regulating their own activities and that nurses can use in guiding the clients in a regulation of their functions.

Sleep

Just as the knowledge of rhythmicity is becoming incorporated into nursing, so is the increased knowledge about sleep becoming recognized as essential to the intellectual component of nursing. The nurse is aware of the importance of her own sleep cycles, and clients too are dependent on sleep for health. Patterns of sleep can be identified within the 24-hour period and over a time period of weeks or months. Identification of the variables that affect the quality of sleep are easier than the control of the variables; however, both are target areas for study. A first step in such a study, however, is discovery of one's own sleep pattern by means of regular recording of the length of the sleep periods and the quality of sleep. Analysis of such collected data reveals significant information that can contribute to better control of sleep patterns and understanding of the sleep cycles.

As various parameters of rhythmicity are studied, the variable of age becomes an important consideration:

What relation is there between rhythm desynchronization and the social schedule of the elderly? The usual work patterns are changed at retirement. Does this altered living pattern create alterations in body rhythms? Are the stresses of living greater or less than during the more physically active years? Are all older persons sensitive to the same degree to changes in schedules? Is it possible that some of the routines and rituals of the elderly are efforts to establish and/or maintain a healthier sense of well being that arises from a better established and more synchronized body rhythm?

Are body rhythms synchronized by a person's daily schedules? Just how important is social scheduling to any one person, and how can the answers to this question be applied to the older person generally?

In studying body rhythms of the infant and child, an early identification of the "timing" of the infant can possibly yield data that will give useful clues to what that person might expect as normal lifetime rhythms and synchrony. It has been noted that sleep patterns vary in the early years of life; some infants sleep 10 to 12 hours in a day; others sleep 18 to 20 hours. Some sleep soundly for long periods; others sleep with periods of wakefulness as a pattern. Profiles of these "different drumbeat" idiosyncrasies may "presage subtle differences of temperament and aptitude that are not yet articulated or defined in the language of time."[63]

It has been observed that the pulse, temperature, and certain urine excretion rhythms are implicitly coupled in their development; the rhythm of these parameters seems to develop at the same rate. Does this suggest that the heart and kidney body systems proceed at the same rate in their development? How does the rate of brain development relate to that of the other body organs?

Recording of Parameters

At present, most of the data recording about rhythmicity is done by pencil and paper graphs and records, either by machine or by man. It is not unreasonable to expect, however, that the means of measuring and recording health parameters will be relatively easy in the near future and each person will become responsible for better knowing himself and recording his own parameters. A business report in the Washington Post in June 1977, cites the availability of a $500 computerized wristwatch that reads the pulse of the person wearing it.[64] In the offing is a watch that will take temperatures, read the condition of the skin surface, and tell the wearer what his blood sugar level is. The predicted price of such a "computer" in the future is $20. This will be a welcome piece of equipment for diabetics, for example.

"Computers are shrinking in size and cost at a speed unmatched in their 25-year history."[65] It is predicted that the time will come when thousands of circuits can be made available on a board no larger than the thumb of an adult. With such circuitry available to record the data needed to keep track of health parameters, health care disciplines will be remiss unless they press for such technology to be used to maintain the health of humans.

As man learns and appreciates the significance of the body rhythms, he will be able to monitor each by means of computers and each person will become knowledgeable about the ranges that are normal for him. As parameters become less or greater than normal, the client's recording of these data to accompany his admission to a health care facility will provide a data base line immediately. How constructive this will be to arrive at a more reliable assessment and proceed with the nursing process with a more dependable foundation of data!

Summary

Rhythmicity is a cycle of events, a circular process, that is an invisible but essential part of all nature: plant, animal, and human. The length of the rhythms can vary from a few seconds to many years, but the rhythm of most interest to man is that which covers the 24-hour day, or circadian rhythm.

Various cues are significant to the initiation and the continuation of specific rhythms, whether biochemical in nature or limited to the presence or the absence of light. Various dimensions affect the rhythms, some of which relate to age and some to the sex of the person. The interrelationship between and among the various rhythms provides a field for continuing and continued research and study.

With the advent of technology and the jet age, man has been forced to recognize the existence of those rhythms that had always been present but were easily ignored. Whether the rhythmicity of the nurse or of the client is the focus of attention, both are important in increasing the health of the client and enhancing the relationship between nurse and client.

Inquiry during nursing assessment that will insure collection of data about the client's rhythmicity will be a major step forward in helping the client provide for his needs. The nursing process framework is the legitimate organizing structure that will enable the collection and the utilization of nursing knowledge and ability to effectively assist clients to meet their needs.

Knowing one's strengths and abilities, whether nurse or client, and knowing the usual baseline of biologic rhythm data will provide a more complete foundation on which the nurse can pursue client assessment and, in collaboration with the client, the planning and actions necessary to help in meeting his various needs.

References

1. Good News Bible. New York, American Bible Society, 1976, p 726
2. Luce GG: Biological rhythms in psychiatry and medicine. Chevy Chase, Maryland, National Institute of Mental Health, 1970, p 8
3. Maslow AH: Motivation and Personality. New York, Harper & Row, 1970, p 242
4. Ibid, p 242
5. Aschoff J: Circadian systems in man and their implications. Hospital Practice 11:51–57, May 1976
6. Halberg F: Implications of biologic rhythms for clinical practice. Hospital Practice 12:139–149, January 1977
7. Tom CK, Lanuza DM: Symposium on biological rhythms: introduction. Nurs Clin N Am 11:569–573, December 1976
8. Halberg, op cit, p 139
9. Bassler SF: The origins and development of biological rhythms. Nurs Clin N Am 11:575–582, December 1976
10. Halberg, op cit, p 139
11. Ibid, p 149
12. Ibid, p 149
13. Aschoff, op cit, p 51
14. Ibid, p 51
15. Russell C: You have a lot more than 'biorhythm' in your body. Washington DC, Washington Star, January 19, 1977, p A-1
16. Wernli HJ: Biorhythm. New York, Crown, 1976, p 22
17. Ibid, pp 96–128
18. Luce, op cit, p 100
19. Still H: Of Time, Tides, and Inner Clocks. Harrisburg, Pennsylvania, Stackpole, 1972, p 61
20. Luce, op cit, p 100
21. Richter CP: The role of biological clocks in mental and physical health. Mental Health Program Reports–3, Chevy Chase, Maryland, U.S. Department of Health, Education, and Welfare, National Institute of Mental Health, January 1969, p 404

22. Ibid, p 399
23. Russell, op cit, p A-1
24. Russell C: We may have a lot to learn from the groundhog. The Washington Star, Washington DC, February 2, 1977, p A-1
25. McCarthy C: Southward mystery. Washington DC, The Washington Post, October 10, 1976, p C-8
26. Saar J: The sex life of the umi-shida. Washington DC, The Washington Post, October 6, 1976, p B-1
27. Brill P: Biological rhythm: it works like a clock. Chronicle. Baltimore, Maryland, University of Maryland Graduate School 10:4–6, September 1976
28. Bassler, op cit, p 576
29. Bassler, op cit, p 577
30. Luce, op cit, p 38
31. Tom CK, Lanuza DM, op cit, p 571
32. Luce, op cit, p 38
33. Aschoff, op cit, p 56
34. Bassler, op cit, p 571
35. Luce, op cit, p 42
36. Ibid, p 42
37. Luce GG: Body Time. New York, Bantam, 1971, p 241
38. Ibid, p 241
39. Ibid, p 241
40. Ibid, p 242
41. Ibid, p 242
42. Ibid, p 246
43. Ibid, p 247
44. Ibid, p 248
45. Ibid, p 249
46. Ibid, p 250
47. Ibid, pp 251–252
48. Aschoff, op cit, p 55
49. Halberg, op cit. p 141
50. Luce, op cit, p 393
51. Luce, op cit, p 226
52. Ibid, p 227
53. Ibid, p 184
54. Ibid, p 188
55. Ibid, p 189
56. Aschoff, op cit, p 55
57. Brill, op cit, p 5
58. Luce, op cit, p 253
59. Ibid, pp 15–16
60. Ibid, pp 15–16
61. Russell, op cit, p A-1
62. Douglas LM: Review of Leadership in Nursing. 2nd Edition, St. Louis, Mosby, 1977, pp 38–39
63. Luce, op cit, p 43

64. O'Toole T: The smart machine revolution. Washington DC, The Washington Post, June 5, 1977, p 1
65. Ibid, p 1

Supplementary References

Alderson MJ: Effect of increased body temperature on the perception of time. Nurs Res 23:42–49, January–February, 1974

Beland-Marchak N: Circadian rhythms. Canadian Nurse 64:40–44, December, 1968

Bell S: Early morning temperatures. Am J Nurs 69:764–766, April 1969

Bünning E: The Physiological Clock. New York, Springer-Verlag, 1967

Colquhoun WP: Biological Rhythms and Human Performance. New York, Academic, 1971

Conroy RTWL: Jet travel and circadian rhythms. Nurs Times 68:370–372, March 30, 1972

Conroy RTWL, Mills JN: Human Circadian Rhythms. London, Churchill, 1970

Curtis GC: Psychosomatics and chronobiology: possible implications of neuroendocrine rhythms. Psychosom Med 34:235–256, 1972

Edelstein RR: The time factor in relation to illness as a fertile nursing research area: review of the literature. Nurs Res 21:72–76, January–February, 1972

Farrell BL, Allen MF: Physiologic/psychologic changes reported by USAF female flight nurses during flying duties. Nurs Res 22:31–36, January–February, 1973

Felton G: Effect of time cycle change on blood pressure and temperature in young women. Nurs Res 19:48–58, January–February 1970

Felton G, Patterson MC: Shift rotation is against nature. AM J Nurs 71:760–763, April 1971

Felton G: Rhythmic correlates of shift work. Communicating Nurs Res 6:73–89, December 1973

Felton G: Body rhythm effects on rotating work shifts. J Nurs Adm 5:16–19, March–April 1975

Gaston S, Menaker M: Pineal function: the biologic clock in the sparrow. Science 160:1125–1127, February 1968

Gorlick HS: Circadian rhythms affect nurse, patient, and therapy! RN 30:68–76, July 1967

Hall LH: Circadian rhythms: implications for geriatric rehabilitation. Nurs Clin N Am 11:631–638, December 1976

Hastings JW: The biology of circadian rhythms from man to micro-organism. New Engl J Med 282:435–441, February 1970

Hellbrügge T, et al: Circadian periodicity of physiological functions in different stages of infancy and childhood, Ann N Y Acad Sciences 107:361–373, September 1974

Hockenberger JM, Rubin MB: Cyclic occurrence of premature ventricular contractions in acute myocardial infarction patients: a pilot study. Nurs Res 23:489–491, November–December, 1974

Huber M: Identification of Circadian Rhythms in Five Known Cardiac Patients During Hospitalization. Masters Thesis, Washington DC, The Catholic University of America, School of Nursing, May 1969

Lanuza DM: Circadian rhythms of mental efficiency and performance. Nurs Clin N Am 11:583–594, December 1976

Maslow AH: A Memorial Volume. International Study Project, Inc. Menlo Park, California. Compiled with the assistance of Bertha G. Maslow. Monterey, California, Brooks/Cole, 1972

Mills JN: Human circadian rhythms. Physiol Rev 46:128–171, January 1966

Mitchell RE: Circadian rhythms. Postgrad Med 44:239–243, November 1968

Mullen E: The Effects of the Alteration of Periodic Factors of the Environment Synchronized Circadian Rhythms of one Human Being. Masters Thesis, Washington DC, The Catholic University of America, School of Nursing, 1968

Natalini JJ: The human body as a biological clock. Am J Nurs 77:1130–1132, July 1977

O'Dell ML: Human biorhythmology: Implications for nursing practice. Nurs Forum 14(1):43–47, 1975

Palmer JD: An Introduction to Biological Rhythms. New York, Academic, 1976

Richter CP: Biological Clocks in Medicine and Psychiatry. Springfield, Illinois, Charles C Thomas, 1965

Smolensky MH, Reinberg A: The chronotherapy of corticosteroids: practical application of chronobiologic findings to nursing. Nurs Clin N Am 11:609–619, December 1976

Stephens GJ: The time factor. Should it control the patient's care? Am J Nurs 65:77–82, May 1965

Stephens GJ, Halberg F: Human time estimation—a study with special reference to 24-hour synchronized circadian rhythms. Nurs Research 14:310–317, Fall 1965

Stephens GJ: Periodicity in mood, affect, and instinctual behavior. Nurs Clin N Am 11:595–607, December 1976

Strughold H: Your Body Clock. New York, Scribner's, 1971

Taub JM, Berger RJ: Acute shifts in the sleep–wakefulness cycle: effects on performance and mood. Psychosom Med 36:164–173, 1974

Tom CK: Nursing assessment of biological rhythms. Nurs Clin N Am 11:621–630, December 1976

Tooran LA: Physiological effects of shift rotation on ICU nurses. Nurs Research 21:398–404, September–October, 1972

Winget CM, et al: Circadian rhythm asynchronism in man during hypokinesis. J Appl Physiol 33:640–643, November 1972

Wurtman RJ: The effects of light on the human body. Sci Am 233:68–77, 1975

and metabolism of nutrients and the elimation of waste products. When considered in terms of the individual, the consumer, much more is involved: the production and availability of food, its selection and acquisition, and its preparation for eventual consumption. These depend on a wide range of factors including knowledge and education, finances, religious practices, values, age, sex and customs. The process of nutrition, as illustrated in Figure 2.1, involves the individual as a whole—physiologically, psychologically, socially, spiritually, and culturally.

According to Maslow's[3] theory of motivation, the need for food is one of the physiologic needs that is prepotent to all other needs. True hunger is based on a somatic need for food and as such can be isolated and studied. However, the act of eating itself may serve needs other than true hunger. Dr. Bruno Bettelheim

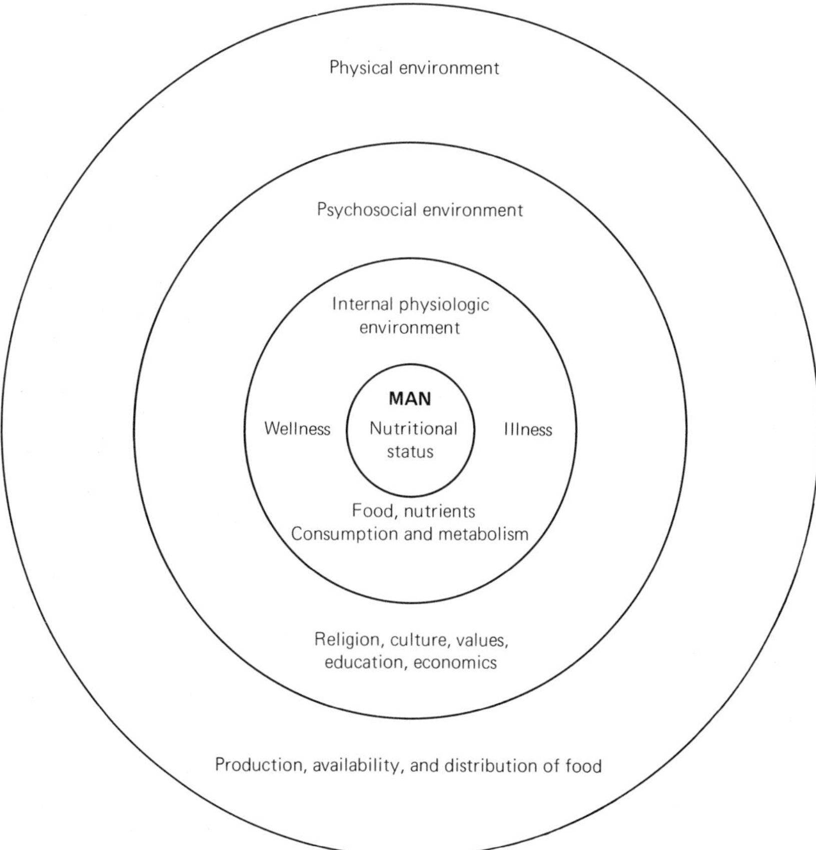

Figure 2.1: *Man and nutrition, environmental relationships.*

Chapter Two •

The Need for Nutrition

Lois Hoskins

> Man is first of all a nutritive process. He consists of a ceaseless motion of chemical substances. One can compare him to the flame of a candle, or to the fountains playing in the gardens of Versailles. Those beings, made of burning gases or of water, are both permanent and transitory. Their existence depends on a stream of gas or of liquid. Like ourselves, they change according to the quality and the quantity of substances which animate them. As a large river coming from the external world and returning to it, matter perpetually flows through all the cells of the body. During its passing, it yields to tissues the energy they need, and also the chemicals which build the temorary and fragile structures of our organs and humors. The corporeal substratum of all human activities originates from the inanimate world and, sooner or later, goes back to it. Our organism is made from the same elements as lifeless things. Therefore, we should not be surprised, as some modern physiologists still are, to find at work within our own self the usual laws of physics and of chemistry as they exist in the cosmic world. Since we are parts of the material universe, the absence of those laws is unthinkable.[1]

Nutrition as a Human Need

Nutrition as defined by Webster is "the process by which an organism takes in and assimilates food; anything that nourishes . . .the study of diet and health."[2] As a physiologic process, nutrition includes the ingestion, digestion, absorption, states, "Eating and being fed are connected with our deepest feelings. They are the basic interactions between human beings on which rest all later evaluation of oneself, of the world and of our relationship to it."[4] The motivation for eating, therefore, is not necessarily the need for nutrition. Other basic needs may be met through eating.

Nutritional concepts have been developed based on a knowledge of normal human needs for life and growth. Application of these concepts falls in the domain of nursing. The nurse, through utilization of the nursing process, supports and maintains healthy behaviors. Abnormal behaviors, intentional or unintentional, such as severe dieting or malabsorption, may lead to an unhealthy nutritional state. Such behavior violates satisfactory fulfillment of the basic nutritional needs of the individual. Nursing intervention may be necessary to assist the client to better understand his needs and to restore him to a normal or an optimal nutrition state.

Assessment of Nutritional Status

The subject of nutritional assessment has been receiving more attention both nationally and internationally in recent years than in the past, largely out of concern for the relationship of the world's population to the production and distribution of the world's food supply. The Joint Food and Agriculture Organization/World Health Organization (FAO/WHO) Expert Committee on Nutrition has held meetings and published papers addressing the issues. One of these, *The Assessment of the Nutritional Status of the Community* by Jelliffe[5] is an excellent resource for assessments. Another paper, edited by Christakis, *Nutritional Assessment In Health Programs*, [6] was prepared based on a conference sponsored by the American Public Health Association. A third publication recommended by this author is Fomon's *Nutritional Disorders of Children: Prevention, Screening, and Follow-up.*[7]

What areas need to be assessed to determine the nutritional status of a client? What are the criteria for a healthy nutritional status? Man's nutritional state will reflect the types of nutrients he takes in, the body's utilization of those nutrients, the body's output in terms of growth, energy, and waste. Therefore, the assessment will include a dietary study and physical and laboratory examination of the client. What factors influence the nutritional status of the client? Whitehead states, "Nutrition is the end product of the emotions and the intelligence as well as the food eaten."[8] To analyze the coping mechanisms and motivating factors with respect to a client's nutrition the assessment must include, in addition to the physical data, information about the client's psycho–social–cultural and spiritual needs and functions. Therefore, to effectively employ the nursing process with respect to the basic need of nutrition the nurse must do a total assessment of the client's behavior in all systems.

Dietary Assessment

It is important to obtain a detailed dietary history of the client. Probably the simplest method is 24-hour recall, that is, asking the client to relate everything he had to eat during the preceding 24 hours, or a typical day. He should specify not only what he ate but also the amounts eaten. The person may underestimate the importance of the size of portions of food he is eating. It may be of value to have some typical food measures available (tablespoons, cups) for comparison during this interview. In addition, a questionnaire may be used to establish a dietary pattern over time. Sample questionnaires are shown later with the client study. These should be modified to suit the age group or persons being interviewed.

Data otained from the dietary questionnaires can be used to determine the type and amount of nutrient intake. This can then be correlated with the recommended amounts from the basic food groups and also from the Recommended Dietary Allowances (RDA).[9] For a comprehensive guide to the composition of approximately 2400 food items, *Nutritive Value of American Foods,*[10] Agriculture Handbook No. 456 is recommended.

Physical Assessment

Physical assessment of the nutritional state will incude a review of all of the systems, because signs and symptoms indicative of changes in nutrition can be manifested in all of them. The WHO Committee has prepared a list of clinical signs that may be observed. Some of the signs are classified with a known value in nutritional analysis; others may or may not be of value but because they are suggestive of nutritional problems they indicate a need for further diagnostic study. Table 2.1 is an adaptation of these data.

Anthropometric methods of clinical evaluation are the most frequently used and significant measurements of nutritional assessment. Height or length and weight values should be taken on all age groups. The 1968 White House Conference on Food, Nutrition and Health recommended the following evaluations[11]:

	Neonates and Infants	*Preschoolers*	*School Age Through Adolescence*	*Adults and Aging*
Weight	X	X	X	X
Height*	X	X	X	X
Triceps Skinfold	X	X	X	X
Subscapular Skinfold				X
Head Circumference	X	X		
Chest Circumference	X	X		
Arm Circumference		X	X	X

*Recumbent length (crown–heel) is measured in the neonate and infant.

Skinfold thickness is a measure of the subcutaneous adipose layer and is used as an index of body composition of fat. Relating only weight for height does not distinguish between weight due to muscle mass and that due to fat. Athletes can be overweight without having excess fat. For use in measuring the triceps or subscapular skinfold the Lange or Harpenden calipers are recommended. A fold of skin and subcutaneous tissue is grasped and pulled away from the muscle at the back of the arm halfway between the acromium and olecranon processes. The calipers are applied to the fold immediately below the finger and read. Clinicians may become experienced in making the "pinch" test and inferring a judgment of body fat from it.

The measurements should preferably be recorded using the metric system and they must be accurate. McLaren[12] states that for accuracy the length should be within 0.5 cm; weight, 250 g; and skinfold thickness, 0.2 mm of the actual values. These measurements should be compared to tables to determine the client's relationship to others of his sex, age, and development. The author cautions the nurse to judge the tables she uses. Some tables are based on *average* weights, not *ideal*. It is suggested that the individual's weight at age 25 be considered an ideal weight for his adulthood. (Tables 2.2, 2.3, and 2.4) give heights and weights in children and adults. A table on skinfold measurements (Table 2.5) is presented as well.

A dental examination is also part of the nutritional assessment. The client should be questioned about his dental health habits and his mouth and teeth should be inspected. Some clients will require the consultation of a dentist.

Finally, biochemical data are needed to complete the physiologic assessment. Minimum data include the hemoglobin and hematocrit determinations. Tests for serum cholesterol, trigycerides, and blood glucose are desirable as well as urinary examination for protein and sugar content. Other laboratory examinations

Table 2.1 *Physical Signs Indicative or Suggestive of Malnutrition*

Body Area	Normal Appearance	Signs Associated with Malnutrition
Hair	Shiny; firm; not easily plucked	Lack of natural shine; hair dull and dry; thin and sparse; hair fine, silky and straight; color changes (flag sign); can be easily plucked
Face	Skin color uniform; smooth, pink, healthy appearance; not swollen	Skin color loss (depigmentation); skin dark over cheeks and under eyes (malar and supra-orbital pigmentation); lumpiness or flakiness of skin or nose and mouth; swollen face; enlarged parotid glands; scaling of skin around nostrils (nasolabial seborrhea)
Eyes	Bright, clear, shiny; no sores at corners of eyelids; membrances a healthy pink and are moist. No prominent blood vessels or mound of tissue or sclera	Eye membranes are pale (pale conjuctivae); redness of membranes (conjunctival injection); Bitot's spots; redness and fissuring of eyelid corners (angular palpebritis); dryness of eye membranes (conjunctival xerosis); cornea has dull appearance (corneal xerosis); cornea is soft (keratomalacia); scar on cornea; ring of fine blood vessels around corner (circumcorneal injection)
Lips	Smooth, not chapped or swollen	Redness and swelling of mouth or lips (cheilosis); especially at corners of mouth (angular fissures and scars)
Tongue	Deep red in appearance; not swollen or smooth	Swelling; scarlet and raw tongue; magenta (purplish color) of tongue; smooth tongue; swollen sores; hyperemic and hypertrophic papillae; and atrophic papillae
Teeth	No cavities; no pain; bright	May be missing or erupting abnormally; gray or black spots (fluorosis); cavities (caries)
Gums	Healthy; red; do not bleed; not swollen	"Spongy" and bleed easily; recession of gums
Glands	Face not swollen	Thyroid enlargement (front of neck); parotid enlargement (cheeks become swollen)

Skin	No signs of rashes, swellings, dark or light spots	Dryness of skin (xerosis); sandpaper feel of skin (follicular hyperkeratosis); flakiness of skin; skin swollen and dark; red swollen pigmentation of exposed areas (pellagrous dermatosis); excessive lightness or darkness of skin (dyspigmentation); black and blue marks due to skin bleeding (petechiae); lack of fat under skin
Nails	Firm, pink	Nails are spoon-shaped (kollonychia); brittle, ridged nails
Muscular and skeletal systems	Good muscle tone; some fat under skin; can walk or run without pain	Muscles have "wasted" appearance; baby's skull bones are thin and soft (craniotabes); round swelling of front and side of head (frontal and parietal bossing); swelling of ends of bones (epiphyseal enlargement); small bumps on both sides of chest wall (on ribs)—beading of ribs; baby's soft spot on head does not harden at proper time (persistently open anterior fontanelle); knock-knees or bow-legs; bleeding into muscle (musculoskeletal hemorrhages); person cannot get up or walk properly
Internal System		
Cardiovascular	Normal heart rate and rhythm; no murmurs or abnormal rhythms; normal blood pressure for age	Rapid heart rate (above 100 tachycardia); enlarged heart; abnormal rhythm; elevated blood pressure
Gastrointestinal	No palpable organs or masses (in children, however, liver edge may be palpable)	Liver enlargement; enlargement of spleen (usually indicates other associated diseases)
Nervous	Psychologic stability; normal reflexes	Mental irritability and confusion; burning and tingling of hands and feet (paresthesia); loss of position and vibratory sense; weakness and tenderness of muscles (may result in inability to walk); decrease and loss of ankle and knee reflexes

From Christakis (ed): Nutritional Assessment in Health Programs. American Public Health Association. Washington, DC, 1973, p 19. Reprinted from American Journal of Public Health 63 (Suppl), November, 1963, with permission.

Table 2.2 *Growth Standards for Girls from Birth to Age 18*

Age	Height (in) Percentiles			Weight (lb) Percentiles			Height (cm) Percentiles			Weight (kg) Percentiles		
	5th	*50th*	*95th*	*5th*	*50th*	*95th*	*5th*	*50th*	*95th*	*5th*	*50th*	*95th*
Birth	18.3	19.5	20.7	5.3	7.3	8.8	47	50	53	2.4	3.3	4.0
1 mo	19.5	21.0	22.5	6.6	8.3	9.8	50	53	57	3.0	3.8	4.4
3 mo	22.2	23.6	25.0	10.2	12.4	14.4	56	60	64	4.6	5.6	6.5
6 mo	24.6	26.1	27.6	13.4	16.7	19.8	63	66	70	6.1	7.6	9.0
9 mo	26.3	27.9	29.5	15.3	19.8	24.1	67	71	77	6.9	9.0	10.9
1 yr	27.6	29.4	31.2	17.4	21.7	26.0	70	75	79	7.9	9.9	11.8
2 yr	31.6	33.8	36.0	22.3	27.1	31.9	80	86	91	10.1	12.3	14.5
3 yr	35.3	37.5	39.7	26.3	32.3	38.3	90	95	101	11.9	14.7	17.4
4 yr	38.1	40.7	43.3	28.8	36.1	43.4	97	103	110	13.1	16.4	19.7
5 yr	40.6	43.4	46.2	32.2	40.9	49.6	103	110	117	14.6	18.6	22.5
6 yr	42.8	45.9	49.0	35.5	45.7	55.9	109	117	124	16.1	20.7	25.4
7 yr	44.5	47.8	51.1	38.3	51.0	63.7	113	121	130	17.4	23.2	28.9
8 yr	46.4	50.0	53.6	42.0	57.2	72.4	118	127	136	19.1	26.0	32.9
9 yr	48.2	52.2	56.2	45.1	63.6	82.1	122	133	143	20.5	28.9	37.3
10 yr	49.9	54.5	59.1	48.2	71.0	95.0	128	138	150	21.9	32.2	43.1
11 yr	51.9	57.0	62.1	55.4	82.0	108.6	132	145	158	25.1	37.2	49.3
12 yr	54.1	59.5	64.9	63.9	94.4	124.9	137	151	165	29.0	42.9	56.7
13 yr	57.1	62.2	66.8	72.8	105.5	138.2	145	158	170	33.1	47.9	62.7
14 yr	58.5	63.1	67.7	83.0	113.0	144.0	149	160	172	37.7	51.3	65.4
15 yr	59.5	63.8	68.1	89.5	120.0	150.5	151	162	173	40.6	54.5	68.3
16 yr	59.8	64.1	68.4	95.1	123.0	150.1	152	163	174	43.2	55.9	68.1
17 yr	60.1	64.2	68.3	97.9	125.8	153.7	153	163	174	44.4	57.1	69.8
18 yr	60.1	64.4	68.7	96.0	126.2	156.4	153	164	174	43.6	57.3	71.0

From Robinson and Lawler: Normal and Therapeutic Nutrition, 15th ed. New York, Macmillan, 1977.

Table 2.3 *Growth Standards for Boys from Birth to Age 18*

	Height (in)			**Weight (lb)**			**Height (cm)**			**Weight (kg)**		
	Percentiles			*Percentiles*			*Percentiles*			*Percentiles*		
Age	*5th*	*50th*	*95*	*5th*	*50th*	*95th*	*5th*	*50th*	*95th*	*5th*	*50th*	*95th*
Birth	18.4	19.8	21.1	5.9	7.5	9.1	47	50	54	2.7	3.4	4.1
1 mo	19.9	21.4	22.9	7.3	9.4	11.1	51	54	58	3.3	4.3	5.0
3 mo	22.6	24.0	25.4	9.8	13.4	16.0	57	61	65	4.4	6.1	7.3
6 mo	25.1	26.7	28.3	14.7	18.0	21.3	63	68	72	6.7	8.2	9.7
9 mo	27.2	28.7	30.2	16.8	21.4	25.1	69	73	77	7.6	9.7	11.4
1 yr	28.4	30.2	32.0	18.7	23.3	27.8	72	77	81	8.5	10.6	12.4
2 yr	32.1	34.6	37.1	23.3	28.3	33.3	82	88	94	10.6	12.8	15.1
3 yr	35.3	37.8	40.3	27.1	32.5	37.9	90	95	102	12.3	14.8	17.1
4 yr	38.3	40.8	43.3	30.0	36.1	42.2	97	104	110	13.6	16.4	19.2
5 yr	40.3	43.4	46.4	33.0	40.3	47.6	102	110	118	15.0	18.3	21.6
6 yr	42.8	45.9	49.0	36.0	44.7	53.4	109	117	124	16.3	20.3	24.2
7 yr	44.8	48.1	51.4	40.3	50.9	61.5	114	122	131	18.3	23.1	27.8
8 yr	46.9	50.5	54.1	44.4	57.4	70.4	119	129	137	20.2	26.1	32.0
9 yr	48.8	52.8	56.8	48.0	64.4	80.4	124	134	144	21.8	29.2	36.5
10 yr	50.6	54.9	59.2	51.4	71.4	91.4	129	139	150	23.3	32.4	41.5
11 yr	51.9	56.4	60.9	53.3	78.9	102.5	132	143	155	24.2	35.8	46.5
12 yr	53.5	58.6	63.7	60.0	86.0	113.5	136	149	162	27.2	39.0	51.5
13 yr	55.2	61.3	67.4	65.3	98.6	131.9	140	156	171	29.6	44.8	59.9
14 yr	57.5	64.1	70.7	75.5	111.8	148.1	146	163	180	34.3	50.8	67.2
15 yr	61.0	66.9	72.8	88.0	124.3	160.6	155	170	185	40.0	56.4	72.9
16 yr	63.8	68.9	74.0	97.8	133.8	169.8	162	175	188	44.4	60.7	77.1
17 yr	65.2	69.8	74.4	106.5	139.8	174.0	166	177	189	48.3	63.5	79.0
18 yr	65.9	70.2	74.5	110.3	144.8	179.3	167	178	189	50.0	65.7	81.4

From Robinson and Lawler: Normal and Therapeutic Nutrition, 15th ed. New York, Macmillan, 1977.

Table 2.4 *Desirable Weights for Persons Age 25 and Over* According to Frame (in Indoor Clothing)*

	Height		Small Frame (lb)	Medium Frame (lb)	Large Frame (lb)
	Feet	*Inches*			
Men †	5	2	112–120	118–129	126–141
	5	3	115-123	121-133	129-144
	5	4	118-126	124-136	132-148
	5	5	121-129	127-139	135-152
	5	6	124-133	130-143	138-156
	5	7	128-137	134-147	142-161
	5	8	132-141	138-152	147-166
	5	9	136-145	142-156	151-170
	5	10	140-150	146-160	155-174
	5	11	144-154	150-165	159-179
	6	0	148-158	154-170	164-184
	6	1	152-162	158-175	168-189
	6	2	156-167	162-180	173-194
	6	3	160-171	167-185	178-199
	6	4	164-175	172-190	182-204
Women‡	4	10	92- 98	96-107	104-119
	4	11	94-101	98-110	106-122
	5	0	96-104	101-113	109-125
	5	1	99-107	104-116	112-128
	5	2	102-110	107-119	115-131
	5	3	105-113	110-122	118-134
	5	4	108-116	113-126	121-138
	5	5	111-119	116-130	125-142
	5	6	114-123	120-135	129-146
	5	7	118-127	124-139	133-150
	5	8	122-131	128-143	137-154
	5	9	126-135	132-147	141-158
	5	10	130-140	136-151	145-163
	5	11	134-144	140-155	149-168
	6	0	138-148	144-159	153-173

*Metropolitan Life Insurance Company, New York.
†Height for men, with shoes on, with 1-inch heels; height for women with shoes on, with 2-inch heels.
‡For women between 18 and 25, subtract 1 pound for each year under 25.

can be requested when there are suspected deficiencies or if they are indicated by other diseases.

Christakis[13] suggests minimal, mid-level, and in-depth nutritional assessments depending on the objectives of the assessment and the problems encountered. He suggests different levels of personnel to do the evaluation based on

Table 2.5 *Obesity Standards for Caucasian Americans. (Minimum triceps skinfold thickness in millimeters indicating obesity)**

Age	Skinfold Measurements	
	Males	*Females*
5	12	14
6	12	15
7	13	16
8	14	17
9	15	18
10	16	20
11	17	21
12	18	22
13	18	23
14	17	23
15	16	24
16	15	25
17	14	26
18	15	27
19	15	27
20	16	28
21	17	28
22	18	28
23	18	28
24	19	28
25	20	29
26	20	29
27	21	29
28	22	29
29	23	29
30-50	23	30

Adapted from Seltzer and Mayer: A simple criterion of obesity. *Postgrad Med. 38:*A 101–107, 1965.

*Figures represent the logarithmic means of the frequency distributions plus one standard deviation.

their proficiency and background. The following tables are taken from this information (Tables 2.6, 2.7, 2.8, 2.9, and 2.10).

• *Client Situation*

Tom P. came to the doctor's office complaining of recurring sore throats. The doctor requested the nurse practitioner in the office to do a nutritional assessment of Tom. The following questionnaire was filled out by Tom (See pp. 54–59).

Table 2.6 *Levels of Nutritional Assessment for Infants and Children, Birth to 24 Months*

Level of Approach*	History		Clinical Evaluation	Laboratory Evaluation
	Dietary	*Medical and Socioeconomic*		
Minimal	1. Source of iron 2. Vitamin supplement 3. Milk intake (type and amount)	1. Birth weight 2. Length of gestation 3. Serious or chronic illness 4. Use of medicines	1. Body weight and length 2. Gross defects	1. Hematocrit 2. Hemoglobin
Midlevel	1. Semi-quantitative a. Iron-cereal, meat, egg yolks, supplement b. Energy nutrients c. Micronutrients—calcium, niacin, riboflavin, vitamin C d. Protein 2. Food intolerances 3. Baby foods—processed commercially; home cooked	1. Family history: Diabetes Tuberculosis 2. Maternal Height Prenatal care 3. Infant Immunizations Tuberculin test	1. Head circumference 2. Skin color, pallor, turgor 3. Subcutaneous tissue paucity, excess	1. RBC morphology 2. Serum iron 3. Total iron binding capacity 4. Sickle cell testing

In-depth Level	1. Quantitative 24-hour recall 2. Dietary history	1. Prenatal details 2. Complications of delivery 3. Regular health supervision	1. Cranial bossing 2. Epyphyseal enlargement 3. Costochondral beading 4. Ecchymoses	Same as above, plus vitamin and appropriate enzyme assays; protein and amino acids; hydroxyproline, etc., should be available
For Ages 2 to 5 Years				
	Determine amount of intake	Probe about pica; Medications	Add height at all levels; Add arm circumference at all levels; Add triceps skinfolds at in-depth level	Add serum lead at midlevel; Add serum micronutrients (vitamins A, C, folate, etc.) at in-depth level
For Ages 6 to 12 Years				
	Probe about snack foods; Determine whether salt intake is excessive	Ask about medications taken; drug abuse	Add blood pressure at midlevel; Add description of changes in tongue, skin, eyes for in-depth level	All of above plus BUN

From Christaksis G. (ed): Nutritional Assessment in Health Programs, p 46. American Public Health Association, Washington, DC. Reprinted from Am J Public Health 63 (Suppl), November, 1963, with permission.

*It is understood that what is included at a minimal level would also be included or represented at successively more sophisticated levels of approach. However, it may be entirely appropriate to use a minimal level of approach to clinical evaluations and a maximal approach to laboratory evaluations.

Table 2.7 *Levels of Nutritional Assessment for Adolescents*

Levels of Approach	History: *Dietary*	History: *Medical and Socioeconomic*	Clinical Evaluation	Laboratory Evaluation
Minimal Level	1. Frequency of use of food groups 2. Habits—patterns 3. Snacks 4. Socioeconomic status	1. Previous diseases and allergies 2. Abbreviated system review 3. Family history	1. Height 2. Weight	1. Urine, protein and sugar 2. Hemoglobin
Midlevel	1. Above 2. Qualitative estimate 3. 24-hour recall	1. Above in more detail	1. Above 2. Arm circumference 3. Skinfold thickness 4. External appearance	1. Above 2. Blood taken by vein for albumin (serum), serum iron and TIBC; vitamins A and beta carotene; RBC indices; Blood urea nitrogen (BUN); cholesterol; zinc
In-Depth Level	1. Above 2. Quantitative estimate by recall (3–7 days)	1. Above	1. Above 2. Per ICNND Manual 3. X-ray of wrist and bone density	1. Above 2. Blood tests: folate and vitamin C; alkaline phosphatase; RBC transketolase; RBC glutathione; lipids 3. Urine: creatinine; nitrogen; zinc; thiamine; riboflavin; loading tests (xanthurenic acid/FIGLU) 4. Hair root: DNA; protein; zinc; other metals

From Christaksis G (ed): Nutritional Assessment in Health Programs, p. 55. American Public Health Association, Washington, DC. Reprinted from Am J Public Health 63 (Suppl), November, 1963, with permission.

Table 2.8 *Levels of Maternal Nutritional Assessment*

Levels of Approach	History: *Dietary*	History: *Medical and Socioeconomic*	Clinical Evaluation	Laboratory Evaluation
Minimal	Present basic diet; meal patterns; fad or abnormal diets; supplements	Obstetrical: Age: parity; interval between pregnancies; previous obstetrical history Medical: Intercurrent diseases and illnesses; drug use; smoking history Family and Social: Size of family; "wanted" pregnancy; socioeconomic status	Prepregnancy weight; weight gain pattern during pregnancy; signs and symptoms of gross nutritional deficiencies	Hemoglobin; hematocrit
Midlevel	The above, plus sem[illegible]uantitative determinatio[illegible] of food intake	The above, plus occupational patterns; utilization of maternity care and family planning services	The above, plus screening for for intercurrent disease	The above, plus blood smear; RBC indices; serum iron; sickle preparation
In-depth level	The above, plus household survey data; dietary history; quantitative 24-hour recall		The above, plus special anthropometric measurements of skinfold, arm circumference, etc.	The above, plus folate and other vitamin levels

From Christaksis G (ed): Nutritional Assessment in Health Programs, p. 62. American Public Health Association, Washington, DC. Reprinted from Am J Public Health 63 (Suppl), November, 1963, with permission.

Table 2.9 *Levels of Nutritional Assessment for Adults*

Levels of Approach	History		Clinical Evaluation	Laboratory Evaluation
	Dietary	*Medical and Socioeconomic*		
Minimal	Present food habits; Meal Patterns; "Empty calories"; Dietary supplements	Name, age, sex Address Socioeconomic level Number in family Brief medical history (including family)	Height and weight; Blood pressure	Hemoglobin A simplified Dipstix® evaluation which would identify presence of protein and glucose in blood, urinary pH
Midlevel	Semiquantitative determination of food intake	Sequential history: Present health, past history, review of systems, family history, social history (e.g., Cornell Medical Index); Smoking history	Anthropometric measurements (skinfold thickness, etc.); brief examination by M.D. or physician's assistant; Chest x-ray as indicated	Evaluations for serum cholesterol, vitamin A, vitamin C, and folic acid; urine excretion for thiamine
In-depth level	Household survey data; Quantitative 24-hour recall; Dietary history; Diet patterns as they might influence lipogenic characteristics	All of the above; personal interview by physician; Family history of cardiovascular disease	Comprehensive health status evaluation by an appropriate health team, by or under supervision of a physician	Serum triglyceride level, plus those nutrients in midlevel; Urine or serum evaluation of pyridoxine status (vitamin B_6 nutriture); Evaluation of protein nutriture by height, weight, and chronological age indices; Serum essentials and non-essential amino acid ratios; Evaluation of vitamin B_{12} nutriture by serum analysis; Serum iron and serum iron binding capacity; Adipose tissue aspiration and fatty acid analysis by gas-liquid chromatography

From Christaksis G (ed): Nutritional Assessment for Health Programs, p. 65. American Public Health Association, Washington, DC. Reprinted from Am J Public Health 63 (Suppl), November, 1963, with permission.

Table 2.10 *Levels of Nutritional Assessment for the Elderly*

Levels of Approach	History: Dietary	History: Medical and Socioeconomic	Clinical Evaluation	Laboratory Evaluation
Minimal	1. Meals eaten per day, week; regularity 2. Frequency of ingestion of protective foods (four food groups) 3. Supplemental vitamins, protein concentrates, mineral mixes 4. General knowledge of nutrition, sources of information	1. Chronic illness and/or disability; occupational hazard exposure; use of tobacco, alcohol, drugs. 2. Symptoms such as bleeding, fainting, loss of memory, dyspnea, headache, pain, changed bowel and/or bladder habits, altered sight and/or hearing, condition of teeth, and/or dentures 3. Therapy (prescribed or self-administered) such as drugs, alcohol, vitamins, food fads, prescription items, eyeglasses, hearing aids 4. Names, addresses, and phone numbers of persons providing medical or health care; close family or friends 5. Lives alone, with spouse, or companion 6. Sources of income	1. Height and weight; cachexia; obesity 2. Blood pressure, pulse rate and rhythm 3. Pallor, skin color and texture 4. Condition of teeth and/or dentures and oral hygiene 5. Affect during interview and examination 6. Vision and hearing appraised subjectively and objectively by examiner 7. Any gross evidence of neglect	1. Hemoglobin 2. Blood and/or urine sugar 3. Urinalysis (color, odor, bile and sediment by gross inspection); pH, glucose, albumin blood, and ketones by stick test 4. Feces (color, texture, gross blood; occult blood by guaiac test)

(Continued)

From Christaksis G (ed): Nutritional Assessment in Health Programs, pp. 74–75. American Public Health Association, Washington, DC. Reprinted from Am J Public Health 63 (Suppl), November, 1963, with permission.

Table 2.10 *Levels of Nutritional Assessment for the Elderly (Continued)*

Levels of Approach	History: *Dietary*	History: *Medical and Socioeconomic*	Clinical Evaluation	Laboratory Evaluation
Midlevel*	In addition to the above; 1. Food preferences and rejections 2. Overt food fads 3. Meal preparation facilities and knowledge 4. Food budget 5. Usual daily diet: Protective foods: meats, dairy products, fruits and vegetables, cereals; Nutrients: protein, fat, carbohydrates, iron, water and fat-soluble vitamins, minerals, trace elements, and water; Empty calorie food: (alcohol, candy, sucrose)	In addition to the above: 1. Family history of spouse, parents and siblings, other relatives, persons living in same household 2. Pain: location, frequency, character, duration 3. Mental hygiene: attitudes, fears, prejudices, symptoms of psychoses, possible psychosomatic symptoms and signs 4. Income: amount and adequacy for nutrition, housing, health, utilities, clothing, transportation, etc.	In addition include: 1. Head and neck examinations (otoscopic, opthalmoscopic, dental and oral cavity, nose and throat) 2. Chest (inspection, palpation, auscultation and percussion, bi-manual examination of breast tissue) 3. Abdomen (inspection, auscultation percussion, and palpation) 4. Rectal and pelvic 5. Inspection and palpation of extremities (evaluation for temperature, edema, pulse, discoloration, ulcers) 6. Gross neurologic evaluation; motor and sensory	In addition include: 1. Serum lipids (including B-lipoproteins) 2. Serum iron and iron binding capacity 3. Urinalysis 4. Electrocardiogram 5. Peripheral blood smear for differential white blood cell count and red cell morphology 6. Chest film 7. Post-voiding residual urine by catheterization (if indicated)
In-depth*	In addition include: 1. 24-hour dietary recall, preferably for each of several widely separated days; analysis of nutrient intake; evaluation of adequacy e.g., relate to activity, body weight, labora-	In addition include: 1. System review 2. Social history 3. Economic history including specifics on sources and amounts of income 4. Mental evaluation (attitudes toward aging)	If indicated, include: 1. Complete sensory and motor neurologic examination 2. Sigmoidoscopy 3. Opthalmologic examination (opthalmoscopic examination with pupils dilated, refraction, dark adaptation, color perception, visual field examination)	If indicated, include: 1. Serum total protein and albumin; serum creatinine and/or blood urea nitrogen (BUN) 2. Roentgenographic evaluation of bones and joints suspected of being fractured, harboring infection

tory data, affect, etc. 2. History of past and present food preparation and practices 3. History of dining practices and facilities, including companionship	4. Audiometry	and affected by rheumatic and/or metabolic bone disease and/or metastatic or primary neoplastic disease 3. Glucose tolerance tests 4. Blood and/or urine vitamin assays for water-soluble and fat-soluble vitamins 5. Trace element assays of blood, urine, and/or tissue 6. Kidney–ureter–bladder (KUB) film for stones in urinary tract or gall bladder 7. Bacteriologic cultures of any chronic infections 8. Barium enema, upper gastro-intestinal series, gall bladder series and intravenous pyelography 9. Fluoroscopy of chest 10. Angiography for coronary arteries, aorta, peripheral vessels 11. Bone marrow for unexplained anemia 12. Renal clearance studies 13. Histologic evaluation of biopsies of tissue suspected of being neoplastic

*The aged, quite unlike children and youth, are the end result of lifetimes of physiologic aging, diseases, and disabilities and cannot be evaluated as if they belonged to younger cohorts. In the above table, it is assumed that Midlevel evaluation procedures may be carried out in ambulatory care settings and that in-depth level procedures may be conducted as hospital or research procedures. The placement of these in actual practice will depend on availability of facilities and personnel.

DIETARY QUESTIONNAIRE FOR ADULTS AND ADOLESCENTS*

Name *Tom P.* Sex *M* Date of Birth *3-4-59*
Address *Washington, D.C.* Marital Status *Single* Today's Date *6-2-77*

1. Grade of school completed? *11* 2. Still in school? *Yes*
3. Occupation *None* 4. Are you employed? *Yes* Full time? *No*
   Part time? *Yes*
5. Income level *$40.00/month* Sources of income *Rock band group and allowance from parents*
6. Are you pregnant? *N.A.* Stage? ______ Lactating? ______
7. If pregnant, have you changed the way you eat or drink? ______
   How? ______
   On whose advise? ______
8. Where do you usually get your food supplies? *Mother shops at local grocery stores, A & P, Giant*
   If home produced, what? ______
   Do you home preserve? What? How much? ______

   If purchased:
   Kind of store? *Large chain* Cash or credit? *Cash*
   Distance to store? *½ mile* Transportation? *Car*
   How often shop for food? *Mother shops 1-2 times week*
   Why? ______
   Are food stamps available? *No* Do you purchase? *No*
   How much do you pay? $ ______ Value get? $ ______
   Are donated or surplus foods available? ______ Do you use? ______
9. Do you feel you have adequate storage facilities for food in your home?
   Yes
10. Do you feel you have adequate cooking facilities? *Yes*
    Kind? *Electric stove* Working oven? *Yes*
11. Do you feel you have adequate refrigeration? *Yes*
    Kind? *Frigidaire*
12. Do you eat at regular times each day? *No*
13. How many days a week do you eat:
    A morning meal? *every day*
    A lunch or midday meal? *5-6*
    An evening meal? *every day*
    During the evening or night? *every evening*

*Adapted from Screening Children for Nutritional Status: Suggestions for Child Health programs. Washington, DC, GPO, 1971.[14] Similar tools appear in Christakis[6] and Fomon.[7]

14. How many days a week do you have snacks, and what do you have then?
    In midmorning *none*
    In midafternoon *every day after school, usually Pop-tarts*
    In the evening *2 times/week, snack cakes*
    During the night *none*
15. Where do you usually eat your meals?
    Morning *home* Midday *school or home* Evening *home*
16. With whom do you usually eat?
    Morning *alone or with brothers or sister* Midday *school friends*
    Evening *family*
17. How many times a week do you usually eat away from home? *just lunch at school, others very infrequent*
18. Would you say your appetite is Good?____ Fair? X Poor?____
19. What foods do you particularly dislike? *vegetables, some fruits*
20. Are you on a special diet? *No* If yes, what kind? ____
    Who prescribed? ____
21. Are there foods you don't eat for other reasons? *No*
22. Do you eat anything not usually considered food (e.g., clay, dirt, starch, other)? *No* If yes, what? ____
    When? ____ How much? ____
23. Do you add salt to your food at the table? *No*
24. Do you have difficulty chewing? *No*
25. *Food Use Record:*

	Food	*Doesn't Eat*	*Does Eat*	*Times per Week*	*Specify*
1.	Bacon		X		2–3 X month
2.	Tongue	X			
3.	Sausage		X		2 X month
4.	Luncheon meat		X	2 X	
5.	Wieners		X		2–3 X month
6.	Liver		X		less than 1 X month
7.	Chicken		X	1 X	
8.	Salt pork	X			
9.	Pork or ham		X	1 X	
10.	Bones (neck or other)	X			
11.	Meat in mixtures (stew, tacos, casseroles, etc.)		X	1–2 X	
12.	Beef or veal		X	5–6 X	
13.	Fish		X		2–3 X month
14.	Cheese and cheese dishes		X	2 X	

	Food	*Doesn't Eat*	*Does Eat*	*Times per Week*	*Specify*
15.	Eggs		X		2–3 X month
16.	Dried beans or pea dishes	X			
17.	Peanut butter or nuts		X	1 X	
18.	Fruit juice		X		2–3 X month
19.	Fruit		X		2 X month
20.	Cereal–dry		X	6 X	
21.	Cereal (cooked or instant)		X	1–2 X	
22.	Pancakes or waffles		X		1–2 X month
23.	Potato		X	2–3 X	
24.	Other cooked vegetables				Only corn 2 X week
25.	Raw vegetables		X	4–5 X	Tossed salad
26.	Macaroni, spaghetti, rice, noodles		X	2 X	
27.	Ice cream, milk pudding, custard or cream soup		X	1 X	
28.	Sweet rolls or doughnuts		X		3–4 X month
29.	Crackers or pretzels		X	1 X	
30.	Cookies		X		2–3 X month
31.	Pie or cake		X	4–5 X	
32.	Potato chips, corn chips		X	2–3 X	
33.	Candy		X		2–3 X month
34.	Soft drinks, kool aid, popsicles		X	7 X	
35.	Artifically sweetened beverage	X			
36.	Coffee or tea	X			
37.	Beer		X	1–2 X	
38.	Wine	X			
39.	Whiskey, vodka, rum, scotch, gin	X			

26. How many servings per day do you eat of the following foods?

	Number of Servings
Bread (including sandwich, toast, rolls, muffins) (1 slice or 1 piece = 1 serving)	*2*
Milk (including use with cereal or other foods) (8 ounces = 1 serving)	*4*
Sugar, jam, jelly, syrup (1 teaspoon = 1 serving)	*1*
Butter or margarine (1 teaspoon = 1 serving)	*1*

27. What specific kinds of the following foods do you eat the most often?

Fruit juices	______
Fruit	______
Vegetables	______
Cheese	______
Cooked or instant cereal	______
Dry cereal	X
Milk	X
Cream or cream substitute	______
Butter or margarine	______
Salad dressings	X

TWENTY-FOUR-HOUR RECALL (used by interviewer)*

Name ______________________________

Date and Time of Interview ______________________________

Length of Interview ______________________________

Date of Recall ______________________________

Day of the Week of Recall ______________________________

"I would like you to tell me everything you (your child) ate and drank from the time you (he) got up in the morning until you (he) went to bed at night and what you (he) ate during the night. Be sure to mention everything you (he) ate or drank at home, at work, school, and away from home. Include snacks and drinks of all kinds and everything else you (he) put in your (his) mouth and swallowed. I also need to know where you (he) ate the food."

What time did you (he) get up yesterday? ______________________________

Was it the usual time? ______________________________

What was the first time you (he) ate or had anything to drink yesterday morning?
(List on the form that follows)

Where did you (he) eat? (List on form)

What did you (he) eat and how much?

How was it prepared? (Raw, cooked, fried, broiled, boiled, etc.)

Time	*Where Eaten*	*Food*	*Type and/or Preparation*	*Amount Eaten*

*Adapted from Fomon, S.J.: Nutritional Disorders of Children: Prevention, Screening, and Follow-up. USDHEW, HSA No. 76-5612, 1976.[7]

(*Occasionally the interviewer should prompt the client:* Did you use salad dressing on your salad: what kind, and how much? Did you get up during the night for a drink of water? How many times did you drink water—at home, at work, *etc.*)

Was your intake unusual in any way, and if so how? ______________
What time did you go to bed last night? ______________
Do you (he) take vitamins or mineral supplements? ______________
If so, what kind? ______________
How often and how many? ______________

(*Again, help client by prompting*—multivitamins, Vitamin C, iron, *etc.*)

If this is an infant or young child, ask about feeding habits:

Is he bottle fed or breast fed? ______________
Can he feed himself? __________ Fingers? __________ Spoon? __________
Can he drink from a cup or glass by himself? ______________
Is he teething or apparently having sore gums? ______________

TOM'S PHYSICAL EXAMINATION REVEALED THE FOLLOWING:

Name *Tom P.* Age *18* Birth Date *3-4-59*
Sex *M* Ethnic Origin *White–Caucasian*

ANTHROPOMETRY:

Height *173 cm* Weight *61 kg* Triceps Skinfold *5 mm*
Head Circumference ______ Chest Circumference ______ Arm Circumference *28 cm*
Percentile level (relationship to age – height – weight charts)
age/height percentile = 25th age/weight percentile = 15th
age/skinfold percentile = 15th

Pulse *72* Blood Pressure *110/76*

Mark the following clinical signs positive (+) or negative (–).

GENERAL IMPRESSION: alert (+), responsive (+), apathetic (–), listless (–), irritable (–), hyper-responsive (–), pallor (–), cachexic (–).

HAIR: shiny (+), lustrous (+), dry (–), brittle (–), thin (–), dyspigmented (–), easily pluckable (–)

EYES: bright (+), clear (+), fatigue circles (–), pale conjunctiva (–), increased vascularity (–), Bitot's spots (–) (grayish, or yellowish gray dull dry lesions of conjunctiva), thickened conjunctiva (–), signs of inflammation of eyelids (–), conjunctiva (–), xerophthalmia (–)

LIPS: moist, good color, dry, angular lesions and scars, cheilosis (swollen, tense, puffy, buccal mucosa extends out onto lips)

GUMS: good pink color, swollen, bleeding, reddened, softened, receding

TONGUE: good pink color, absence or atrophy of some papillae, smoothness, scarlet or purplish color, fissured, swollen papillae

TEETH: straight, clean, no overcrowding, edentulous, absent teeth, carious, calculus, fluorosis (opaque – paper white specks of areas in enamel to brown stain and pitting)

GLANDS: no swellings of face, palpable enlargement of parotids, thyroid visibly enlarged

SKIN: good color, smooth, elastic, slightly moist, dry, thin, scaly, crackled, roughened patches, greasy, nasolabial seborrhea, inelastic dermatitis, petechiae, edema

FINGERS AND NAILS: pink color, smooth, clubbed, spooned, ridged, brittle

ABDOMEN: flat, swollen, hepatomegaly, splenomegaly

LOWER EXTREMITIES: firm muscles, good tone, calf tenderness, edema, flabby, tingling

SKELETAL: no malformations, bowlegs, knock-knees, chest deformity, beaded ribs, enlarged joints, winged scapulae, front or parietal cranial protrusion, persistently open fontanelles

INTERNAL SYSTEMS:

Cardiovascular: normal rate and rhythm, normal B/P, no murmurs, tacycardia, bradycardia, abnormal rhythm, elevated blood pressure, enlarged heart

Gastrointestinal: no nausea and vomiting, regular elimination, stools - brown - formed - semisoft, no anorexia, indigestion, constipation, flatulence, diarrhea

NERVOUS: normal reflexes, mentally alert, no sensory loss, apparent psychologic stability, motor weakness, confusion, loss of muscular control, paresthesias, mental irritability, inappropriate affect, loss of position sense, loss of vibration sense, loss of ankle and knee jerks

LABORATORY EXAMINATION:

Urine:	Color	*amber*	pH	*5*
	Acetone	*negative*		
	Sugar	*negative*		
Blood:	Hct	*45*		
	Hgb	*15gm%*		

OTHER: *Reddened, inflamed appearance of throat, no elevation of temperature, no earaches, some pain on swallowing, most prominent on arising in A.M. and improves during the day.*

Summary of Nutritional Assessment

Tom P. is an 18-year-old male who comes to the doctor complaining of persistent sore throat. On nutritional assessment he is found to be in the 15th percentile for weight and body composition of fat and the 25th percentile for height. He appears visibly thinner than the average boy his age. His eating habits are poor: he eats few fruits and vegetables, uses vitamin pills for supplements, and is not regular in his food habits.

Nursing Diagnosis

Tendency to underweight due to poor eating habits.

This completes the physical assessment of Tom P.'s nutritional state. If abnormal signs or symptoms had been found further tests would have been indicated. To find out the cause of Tom's poor eating habits the nurse would have to assess other areas. From this she could then plan intervention.

Violation or Alteration of Need for Nutrition

Any violation of the normal state of nutrition results in an abnormal state, or malnutrition. The definition of malnutrition used here is from Scrimshaw, et al, World Health Organization: "Malnutrition is the pathological state resulting from a relative or absolute deficiency or excess of one or more essential nutrients, this state being clinically manifested or detected only by biochemical, anthropometric, or physiological tests."[15] Four forms of malnutrition are recognized: undernutrition, specific deficiency, overnutrition, and imbalance. In states of undernutrition there is an inadequate consumption of food or calories and in overnutrition there is a caloric excess. In specific deficiency states there is an inadequate intake of an individual nutrient. If there is an imbalance a disproportion exists among essential nutrients with or without an absolute deficiency of any one nutrient. Malnutrition due to over or underconsumption is usually referred to as primary malnutrition and that due to other causes such as diarrhea, malabsorption, tuberculosis, etc. is called secondary malnutrition. Extreme undernutrition occurs in states such as marasmus and starvation.

Another important concept is that of body weight, which represents the total weight of fat, muscle, organs, bone, and fluids. Each of these must be considered when determining a person's ideal weight. An individual whose work involves strenuous physical activity may have increased muscularity and weight whereas someone with an ideal weight may have excess body fat. Obesity is not synonymous with overweight. Obesity refers to the accumulation of body fat in an excess considered detrimental for body health. It is usually considered to be 20 percent or more above ideal body weight. Overweight is a term applied to persons who are 10 to 20 percent above ideal weight. Underweight status is considered to be 10 percent below ideal weight and seriously underweight is 20 percent below.[16] The problem is to define ideal body weight. Presently an accurate measurement of the skinfold thickness is considered to be the best single measure of body fat. However, many more sophisticated techniques are available for the measurement.

Many factors may influence or relate to the development of overnutrition or to undernutrition, but the direct physical cause is an imbalance in caloric intake and caloric expenditure. Food is needed for growth, maintenance, and repair of the body; any intake greater than this is an excess and becomes fat.

$$\text{Energy input} > \text{energy output} = \text{Fat}$$

In the progressive countries overconsumption of calories is the most common form of malnutrition, whereas in the underdeveloped countries it is caloric undernutrition. Also, in the more developed countries overconsumption of refined carbohydrates with less dietary fiber and protein has added to the nutritional imbalance.[17]

Figure 2.2 shows some of the causes of undernutrition.[18] The effects of malnutrition are being intensively investigated in animals and the studies replicated in man where possible. Animal studies[19] demonstrate that malnutrition early in life is associated with defects in the central nervous system and with impaired behavioral responses. More recently, observations of malnourished children

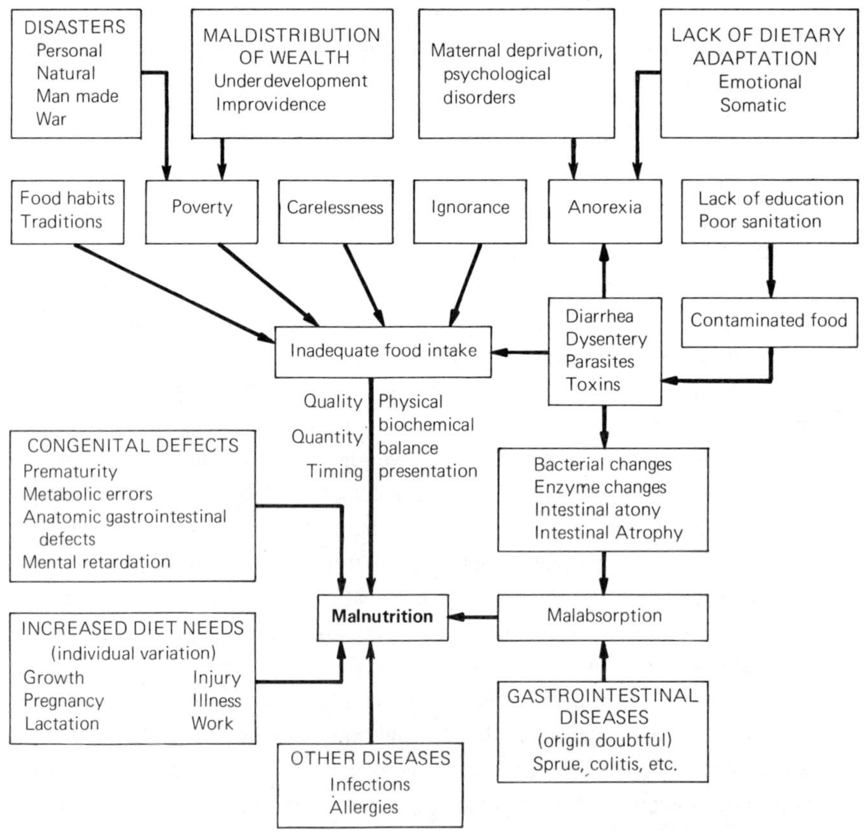

Figure 2.2: *The multiple etiology of malnutrition. (Adapted from Williams: Malnutrition. Lancet 2:342, 1962. Reprinted from Williams: Nutrition and Diet Therapy. St. Louis, Mosby, 1977, with permission.)*

suggest the same reaction.[20] The long-term consequences of malnutrition appear to depend on the stage of cellular growth during which it occurs. Malnutrition during cell division causes permanent growth retardation whereas that occurring later causes reduced cell size that can be corrected by proper feeding.

Malnutrition has been implicated in the causation of impaired T-cell function in the immune response.[21] If malnutrition occurs at a critical time during early postnatal development, there may be a long-lasting effect on cellular immunity. This area needs more study because the conclusions are indefinite. All of the above findings place the pregnant mother and the neonate in a high-risk state.

During times of physical or emotional stress, good nutrition is vital. The response of the body to any threat may be delayed in case of nutritional deficiencies.

Overnutrition is the most common form of malnutrition in this country. Most energy is expended in "simply moving the body around. With a fixed amount of activity—number, extent, speed and force of movements—energy expenditure tends to be directly proportional to gross body weight."[22] Studies have reported that overweight and obese persons are less active than persons of ideal weight. Their consumption of food may be the same or even less than that of persons with ideal weight.[23] When they do move about more energy is required to move the greater body mass and may impose an unhealthy strain on some part of the body.

Obesity can be classified according to its etiology or its pathogenesis. Mayer classifies the etiology of obesity as genetic; of hypothalamic origin; of central nervous system origin; of endocrine origin; or otherwise as induced by immobilization in adults and in children caused by psychic disturbances and by social and cultural pressure. He classifies the pathogenesis of obesity in terms of regulatory functions. This means that something is wrong with the central mechanism regulating food intake, similar to the cause of immobilization or sedentary life-style mentioned above. Or, the pathogenesis may be metabolic—there is an abnormality in the metabolism of fats and carbohydrates.[24] Some distinguish obesity into, first, the type with onset in childhood, a hyperplastic type in which there is an increased number of adipose cells. This tends to be more refractory to treatment. The other type is adult onset obesity in which the fat cells are not increased in number but they hypertrophy.[25]

Regardless of type, obesity is a serious health problem and should be respected as such. There is a tendency to stereotype obese persons as slovenly with little will power or concern about their own problem. Not only observers but the obese person himself may also have this attitude. Obese children or persons with onset of obesity in childhood are likely to be obsessively concerned with their image. They may become passive, possibly withdrawing and expecting rejection. All of this leads to unhappiness, social isolation, and inactivity, and perpetuates their obesity.

In assessing the obese individual it is important to obtain the age at onset and ask questions about its course. Was there some sort of stress associated with its inception? What efforts have been taken to reduce weight and with what success? How does the client feel about his obesity? Have his relationships with family and friends changed? What is the psychologic effect of obesity on the individual?

Dietary habits must be studied to understand food and eating patterns: At what times of the day is the client hungry and how does he satisfy that hunger? Is there a social and cultural basis supporting the overeating within the family relationship? Does the cook fix large meals of potatoes, pasta, desserts, etc., and expect everyone to eat them? What is the economic picture—can he afford a variety of foods, especially meats and fresh produce?

Does the client exercise regularly? It is important to know the amount of exercise and how strenuously it is performed. Playing a lazy game of tennis or riding a golf cart is not strenuous.

The risk factors of obesity are well known. The client should be checked for hypertension, diabetes mellitus, and iron deficiency anemia. At the same time, physiologic causes of obesity such as endocrine factors should be ruled out.

Establishing psychogenic causes of obesity is difficult. Gillis and Allyn state that "obesity is a state of disequilibrium in which the individual has effected some sort of compromise between his needs and need-gratification."[26] As was stated earlier, eating may not be satisfying hunger or the need for nutrition. It may be more intimately connected with safety, security, and love needs. If, indeed, overeating is a means of coping, then dieting to reduce may be interfering with this defense mechanism and causing more trauma. In assessing the client the nurse must be cognizant of these possibilities. To manage one problem and not the other may be ineffectual and also may be detrimental to the well-being of the client. If severe problems are encountered, then psychotherapy should be advised.

• *Client Situation*

Joan H. came in for her yearly health checkup. Physical findings showed the following:

Age *45* Height *157 cm (5'2")* Weight *61 kg (130 lb)*
Triceps Skinfold *22 mm* Pulse *68* B/P *114/80*

General appearance is that of a moderately overweight individual. Other physical findings were essentially normal. She had no significant past history of illness. Based on this data Joan was diagnosed as being overweight for height and age. To plan nursing intervention it was necessary to do further assessment of diet and exercise and other factors influencing nutrition.

The "nursing process" as defined by Yura and Walsh "is an orderly, systematic manner of determining the client's problems, making plans to solve them, initiating the plan or assigning others to implement it, and evaluating the extent to which the plan was effective in resolving the problems identified."[27] Different models have been proposed that incorporate the nursing process; one of these is Roy's adaptation model.[28] Using this model the nurse assesses the client's behavior, determines if it is adaptive or maladaptive and plans care that will support or promote adaptation. Elements of this model as shown in the following list will be used in discussing the situation of Joan H.

Client behavior (four systems are assessed): physiologic, self-concept, role function, and interdependence.

Adaptive (A) or maladaptive (M)

Influencing factors:

Focal stimuli: the immediate cause of the behavior

Contextual stimuli: other factors in the situation that may be contributing to the behavior

Residual stimuli: other factors in the background that may contribute but are difficult to validate or influence

Nursing diagnosis: client problem amenable to nursing intervention

Client goals: expected outcomes in terms of client behavior

Intervention: nursing action to assist client to reach goal

In this case the focal stimuli or the immediate cause of Joan's overweight is caloric intake in excess of caloric expenditure. Joan filled out questionnaires as described under dietary assessment. On 24-hour recall it was found that she typically arises at 6:00A.M., eats breakfast with her husband at 6:30A.M., and is at work at 8:30A.M. She has a midmorning cup of coffee and a snack, takes a bag lunch to work that she eats at noon alone if she is busy; otherwise she eats with coworkers. She has an afternoon cup of coffee with cookies, returns home by 5:00 or 5:30P.M. and has dinner with her husband and three children at 6:30. She has a glass of wine and a cube of cheese before retiring at 11:00P.M. She described this as a typical day. The following is her record of intake with their assigned caloric values.

	*Calories**	*Exchanges*
Breakfast		
Orange juice, 4 oz., frozen	55	1 Fruit
Bacon, 2 slices, fried	85	2 Fat
Egg, 1 large, fried	100	1 Meat, 1 Fat
Toast, white, 1 slice	70	1 Bread
Margarine, 1 pat	35	1 Fat
Milk, half glass, whole	80	½ Milk
Coffee 1 cup	–	
with 1 tsp. sugar	14	1 Sugar
Total, breakfast	440	
Midmorning Snack		
Coffee, 1 cup	–	
with 1 tsp. sugar	15	1 Sugar
Cookies, 2	100	1 Bread, 1 Fat
Total, midmorning snack	115	

*Calorie values from Calories and Weight, The USDA Pocket Guide, Agriculture Information Bulletin No. 364, US Department of Agriculture, Washington, DC, 1974.[29]

Lunch		
Sandwich	140	2 Bread
Bread, white, 2 slices	105	1 Meat
Cheese, 1 slice, American	66	1 Meat
Boiled ham, 1 slice	35	1 Fat
Margarine, 1 pat	80	2 Fruit
Apple, 1 medium	80	½ Milk
Milk, ½ glass, whole		
Total, lunch	506	
Afternoon Snack		
Coffee, 1 cup	–	
with 1 tsp. sugar	15	1 Sugar
Cookies, 2	100	1 Bread, 1 Fat
Total, afternoon snack	115	
Dinner		
Potatoes, mashed, 1 cup	140	2 Bread
Gravy, ½ cup	140	1 Fat, 1 Bread
Meat, roast beef, 2 slices (6 oz.)	440	6 Meat
Green beans, ½ cup	15	1 Vegetable, A
Tossed salad, lettuce, onion, tomatoes,	20	1 Vegetable, A
Croutons and	20	1 Bread
Salad dressing, 2 tblsp., Italian	160	3 Fat
Ice cream, 1 cup	260	2 Bread, 2 Fat
Milk, ½ glass, whole	80	½ Milk
Coffee, 1 cup	–	
with 1 tsp. sugar	15	1 Sugar
Total, dinner	1290	
Bedtime Snack		
Wine, 1 glass	85	2 Fat
Cheese, 2 inch cube	130	2 Meat
Total, betime snack	215	
Total for all meals	2681	

The dietary questionnaire used to establish her food pattern over time indicated that Joan ate a variety of foods, had an adequate intake of nutrients, and needed no supplements. She has a good appetite, no particular dislikes, and no unusual eating habits. She does her own grocery shopping and cooking, and has adequate food storage and cooking facilities.

Joan is 45 years of age, married, has a husband and three children, ages 19, 18, and 16, at home. She is employed fulltime, teaching junior high level students in the county school system. Joan had been working only as a substitute teacher until two years ago. She associates a gradual increase in weight with her return to fulltime work.

Joan partakes of no planned daily exercise. She drives to work and to the store, her "longest walk is through the school halls, most strenuous activity is pushing the vacuum cleaner or climbing stairs." Most of her time is spent walking about the classroom and sitting behind the desk. In the evening when she comes home she does some light housework, schoolwork, (grading papers, preparing classes) and watches television. On the weekends she grocery shops and cleans house. She may go for a walk or go swimming but with no regularity.

Based on the desirable weight table Joan should weigh 107 to 119 lb, or 49 to 54 kg. Because she weighs 130 lb and is mildly active her caloric requirement for maintenance is 1820 calories, based on Table 2.11.[30] Joan is consuming 2681 calories, or, according to these statistics, 860 calories daily in excess of her expenditure. This excess has been deposited as fat and adds up to her being overweight.

At this time this information was shared with Joan and it was recommended that she reduce her intake and try to exercise more. Joan understood and agreed that she desired to lose weight.

One year later Joan was again examined. This time she was quite excited: she had lost weight and was now maintaining her weight between 110 to 115 lb. She had gone on a popular high fat, low carbohydrate diet for reducing and said she had never felt better. Six months later Joan was weighing 120 lb but blamed that on some "nervous bouts of eating" and said she would lose this by resuming the diet more energetically.

Exactly two years after she had achieved the weight loss and was down to 110 to 115 lb, Joan returned to clinic weighing 135 lb. This time she was discouraged. She had gained up to 140 lb; she had been able to lose 5 lb on the high fat diet but now was unable to lose more. She could not maintain a desirable weight. She objected to being denied carbohydrates, especially fresh fruits. She understood that she needed to supplement her high fat, low carbohydrate diet with vitamins and she was tired of buying expensive vitamins. "Vitamin E is very expensive and what exactly does it do?" This time she said, "Alright, I'm ready for help; there does not seem to be an easy, get thin quick formula that works."

Joan was again interviewed and her diet was reassessed. She had made changes in her eating pattern as indicated by her 24-hour recall which she stated represented a typical day. The nurse analyzed the diet, calculating the

Table 2.11 *Activity and Caloric Requirements*

	Inactive	Mildly Active	Medium Active	Active	Very Active
			Multiply your weight by:		
Weight:	*12*	*14*	*16*	*18*	*20*
95	1140	1330	1520	1710	1900
98	1176	1372	1568	1764	1960
101	1212	1414	1616	1818	2020
105	1260	1470	1680	1890	2100
110	1320	1540	1760	1980	2200
115	1380	1615	1840	2070	2300
120	1440	1680	1920	2160	2400
125	1500	1750	2000	2250	2500
130	1560	1820	2080	2340	2600
135	1620	1890	2160	2430	2700
140	1680	1960	2240	2520	2800
145	1740	2030	2320	2610	2900
150	1800	2100	2400	2700	3000
155	1860	2170	2480	2790	3100
160	1920	2240	2560	2880	3200
165	1980	2310	2640	2970	3300
175	2100	2450	2800	3150	3500
185	2220	2590	2960	3330	3700
195	2340	2730	3120	3510	3900
200	2400	2800	3200	3600	4000
210	2520	2940	3360	3780	4200
220	2640	3080	3520	3960	4400

Inactive: does nothing actively.
Mildly active: rides to work, sits at work.
Medium active: teacher, mother of small children.
Active: on the move most of the time.
Very active: physical worker plus extra exercise.

calorie values and identifying the food exchanges being used. The analysis is demonstrated in the following list.

Joan was using the following food exchanges: 4 of vegetable A, 1 ½ of bread, 16 of meat and 12 ½ of fat. According to Church[31] a recommended proportion would have been: 2 milk, 1 vegetable A, 1 vegetable B, 6 fruit, 6 bread, 4 meat, and 4 fat. It was obvious that Joan had deficiencies in essential nutrients, especially those supplied by fruits and milk. She was consuming heavily in the meat and fat groups, which was increasing her caloric intake.

Joan desired to weigh 120 lb. To do so she had to lose 15 lb. Each pound of body fat equals 3500 calories. To lose adipose tissue effectively it is advisable to lose at rates of 1 to 2 lb a week. Greater amounts are likely to be losses of fluid and will not be maintained. Therefore, to lose two pounds a week a person would have to cut his intake by 1000 calories a day (7000 calories a week). Diets of less

	Caloric Value	*Food Exchange*
Breakfast		
V-8 juice, 4 oz.	25	1 Vegetable A
Egg, 1 large, fried	100	1 Meat, 1 Fat
Toast, whole wheat, 1 slice	60	1 Bread
Margarine, 1 pat	35	1 Fat
Coffee	–	
Total, breakfast	220	
Midmorning Snack		
Coffee, 1 cup	–	
Cheese, American, 2 inch cube	130	2 Meat
Total, midmorning snack	130	
Lunch		
Tossed salad–lettuce, onion,	20	1 Vegetable A
salad dressing, 2 tblsp., Italian	160	3 Fat
Ham, 2 slices	132	2 Meat
Cheese, 2 slices, roll-up	210	2 Meat
Total, lunch	522	
Afternoon Snack		
Fresca drink	–	
Cheese, 1 slice	105	1 Meat
Dill pickle	–	
Total, afternoon snack	105	
Dinner		
Meat, roast beef, 2 slices	440	6 Meat
with gravy, ¼ cup	70	½ Bread, ½ Fat
Green beans, ½ cup	15	1 Vegetable A
Tossed salad	20	1 Vegetable A
with 2 tblsp. Italian salad dressing	160	3 Fat
Wine, 3½ oz. glass	85	2 Fat
Coffee, 1 cup	–	
Total, dinner	690	
Bedtime Snack		
Wine, 3½ oz. glass	85	2 Fat
Cheese, 2 inch cube	130	2 Meat
Total, bedtime snack	215	
Total for all meals	1882	

than 1200 calories are not so palatable, more difficult to adhere to, and may lack nutrients so they are not highly recommended. Joan is presently taking in 1882, or roughly 1900, calories daily. She can reduce her intake to 1200 and so decrease her daily caloric intake by 700 calories. This equals 4900 calories or an equivalent of 1.4 lb per week (4900÷ 3500).

Caloric intake and caloric output are the two variables that make up body weight. When the caloric intake cannot be decreased further, then the caloric output must be increased. Types of activity and their caloric expenditure are given below.[32]

Type of Activity	*Calories per Hour*
Sedentary activities, such as: Reading; writing; eating; watching television or movies; listening to the radio; sewing; playing cards; and typing, officework, and other activities done while sitting that require little or no arm movement.	80 to 100
Light activities, such as: Preparing and cooking food; doing dishes; dusting; handwashing small articles of clothing; ironing; walking slowly; personal care; officework and other activities done while standing that require some arm movement; and rapid typing and other activities done while sitting that are more strenuous.	110 to 160
Moderate activities, such as: Making beds, mopping and scrubbing; sweeping; light polishing and waxing; laundering by machine; light gardening and carpentry work; walking moderately fast; other activities done while standing that require moderate arm movement; and activities done while sitting that require more vigorous arm movement.	170 to 240
Vigorous activities, such as: Heavy scrubbing and waxing; handwashing large articles of clothing; hanging out clothes; stripping beds; walking fast; bowling; golfing; and gardening.	250 to 350
Strenuous activities, such as: Swimming; playing tennis; running; bicycling; dancing; skiing; and playing football.	350 or more

Joan needs to increase her caloric expenditure by 2100 calories to lose 7000 calories or 2 pounds a week (7000−4900=2100). She must engage in some exercise that will help her burn up 300 calories a day.

Joan was presented with all of this information, which she grasped readily. Together she and the nurse decided on a conventional 1200 calorie diet.

Dickie[33] and Williams[34] also describe a 1200 calorie reducing diet by Gordon[35] that may be used by overweight people who cannot lose by conventional methods, who have metabolic rather than regulatory obesity. Joan stated that she had the *Calories and Weight* USDA Pocket Guide[29] and Better Homes and Garden's *Eat and Stay Slim*.[36] The latter had food exchange lists, diet guides and menu suggestions that she could use.

Different authors distribute the food exchanges differently in the 1200 calorie diet. The diet decided on must contain adequate nutrients; to do so it must have variety. It must take into account food patterns, likes and dislikes of the client, and be economically and commercially available. Following loss of weight the diet must be alterable into a lifelong maintenance diet.

Tables 2.12 and 2.13 show the composition of foods within the exchange groups and application to the 1200 calorie conventional diets as determined for Joan.

Sugar and alcohol are not included in this diet. Both of these are empty calories, that is, they provide no essential nutrients, only calories. On a reducing diet each bite should count, both with respect to calories and nutrients. This diet did allow Joan more meat exchanges than others.

Up to this point Joan had appeared eager; now she drew back from the table, stopped smiling, and appeared more pensive. The nurse commented, "Is something wrong, you appear thoughtful, perhaps troubled?" Joan responded that she did not see how she could possibly get in all of that exercise and she did not like to give up her wine with meals and at bedtime. "I relax with a glass of wine and talk to my husband; it's a time I enjoy."

Up to this point only an assessment of focal factors or immediate causes of the problem had been done. To interpret Joan's present attitude and to plan intervention, more knowledge and understanding of the contextual and residual stimuli or other factors influencing the situation was necessary. Roy[37] states that contextual stimuli include genetic makeup, sex, developmental stage, drugs, alcohol, tobacco, self-concept, role functions, interdependence, social interaction patterns, coping mechanisms and styles, physical and emotional stress, cultural orientation, religion, and environment. Some of these may also be categorized as residual stimuli that are difficult to validate or to influence. It is important when assessing to identify both positive and negative, or adaptive and maladaptive fac-

Table 2.12 *Food Exchange Values*

Food Exchange	Approximate Measure	Carbo-hydrate (gm)	Protein (gm)	Fat (gm)	Calories
Meat	1 oz.	—	7	5	75
Bread	1 slice	15	2	—	70
Vegetable A	as desired	—	—	—	—
Vegetable B	½ cup	7	2	—	40
Fruit	Varies	10	—	—	40
Milk	1 cup	12	8	10	170 (skimmed = 80)
Fat	1 tsp.	—	—	5	45

Table 2.13 *Joan's 1200 Calorie Diet*

Food Exchange	No. of Exchanges	Carbo-hydrate (gm)	Protein (gm)	Fat (gm)	Calories
Meat	7	—	49	35	525
Bread	3	45	6	—	210
Vegetable A	as desired	—	—	—	—
Vegetable B	1	7	2	—	40
Fruit	3	30	—	—	120
Milk	2 (skimmed)	24	16	—	160
Fat	3	—	—	15	135
Total		106	73	50	1190

tors. The nurse must identify not only ineffective and destructive systems but effective support systems.

The following contains statements from the interview with Joan:

Q: Were any of the members of your family obese?
A: My family on my father's side was short and tended to be stout but not fat; on my mother's side they were thinner. I have no brothers and sisters.
Q: Did anyone have diabetes, heart trouble, or high blood pressure?
A: No, not that I know of.
Q: Were you overweight as a child or as a teenager?
A: No.
Q: When did you first start putting on additional weight?
A: After the children were born, after I went back to work, probably when I was around 30 to 35.
Q: Did you gain a lot at first or was it gradual?
A: It was gradual—it seemed as though every couple of years I put on a pound or two that just stayed. A year ago my menstrual periods stopped and it seems as though it's harder to lose weight now.

Q: You associate some of your problem with menopause?
A: Yes.
Q: What did you weigh when you were 25 years old?
A: Between 115 to 120.
Q: Did you feel better then?
A: Yes.
Q: Do you think you looked better?
A: Oh, yes.
Q: Tell me, is your husband overweight?
A: Oh, no, he's thin; he's an exercise nut. He used to run competitively in high school and so he still likes to run.
Q: Do you run with him?
A: No, I can't keep up with him and I don't have the time. I get home from work and have to fix dinner for the children. After dinner I usually have schoolwork to do.
Q: How about the children—I see you have three, all teenage, are any of them overweight?
A: No, if anything they tend to be thin.
Q: What does your husband say about your being overweight?
A: Oh, he says he loves me anyway; I'm still physically attractive to him. He does say that I should get more exercise. He thinks I should take the time to do it, let something else go, or just tell them to wait.
Q: How do you feel about that?
A: That's a lot easier to say than to do. I guess I would feel guilty not getting the kids' dinner on time or not doing my work.

Similar questions were asked about the children's reaction to their mother's overweight with similar responses. Joan was then asked about her job.

Q: Do you like your job?
A: Yes.
Q: You have stated that you work long hours—is this a part of the job, do the other teachers do this also?
A: I think some do. I have some administrative responsibilities that the others do not have; maybe that's why I work longer.
Q: Do you think you owe yourself more time to do something for yourself?
A: Probably, but it's hard to do.
Q: You mentioned that you had nervous bouts of eating. Could you tell me about these?
A: Sometimes when I'm under pressure with a deadline to meet, or so many things to do all at once, I sit at my desk with a cup of coffee and I get up and go to the refrigerator for something to nibble. It seems to let off steam.
Q: Does this happen often?
A: Fairly often; actually it's like that most of the time during the school year.
Q: During the school year, do you do differently during the summer?
A: That's when I try to lose weight to get ahead for the school year.

Questions about religious and cultural influences revealed that Joan was Protestant, a WASP, with no particular religious or cultural practices affecting her diet.

Economically Joan's family is middle class. They live comfortably and finances do not present a problem in buying adequate food or in providing necessities and some luxuries for the family. Joan does buy convenience foods. She keeps a supply of TV dinners on hand in case some of the children need to eat before she has dinner ready. She also uses some packaged meat products. The family does not eat desserts except on special occasions. Joan does worry that her children do not always eat a balanced diet.

The nurse sorted the data she had collected into the following categories.

Assessment

Self concept Joan recognizes that she is overweight and that this is a health problem. Her husband and children both support her: her being overweight has not decreased her value in their eyes. This is adaptive behavior related to Joan's body image or physical self. She really does have a problem and she wants to correct it.

Joan recognizes that she is placing unreasonable demands on herself—spending all of her time working, worrying about getting the job done, cooking dinner on time, etc. Her problem is one of guilt: she has established some sort of norm for herself and she is not sure she is meeting that norm. She also expresses some powerlessness in not knowing what to do to achieve more realistic goals. Recognizing her behavior and being able to discuss it categorizes it as adaptive behavior. Adaptive behavior helps the person to cope with the changing environment in an attempt to maintain his integrity, in the above case the integrity of the self-concept.

Role function Joan's mastery of role function is related to her self-concept. As far as her family is concerned she is performing adequately in her roles of wife and mother. She is probably performing alright as a teacher. Joan's expectations of herself are creating conflict within herself.

Interdependence Interdependence relates to the use of both independent and dependent behaviors in relating to others and coping with the environment. The coping style may be called balanced (interdependent), dependent, or independent depending upon the predominant style used. Each style is adaptive so long as it meets the person's needs for integrity. Joan was going beyond what was expected of her in terms of working long hours, trying to do all of the work herself, and in still trying to manage her home as she had before returning to work. The nurse perceived that Joan had a problem with dysfunctional independence, the use of independent behaviors to the point where she was not taking care of her own health needs. In Joan's situation the nurse felt that there were perhaps some less obvious inner conflicts giving rise to Joan's behavior as evidenced by her aggressive drive for overachievement. If necessary these could be explored later. At the time of Joan's last visit the nurse's assessment appeared as follows:

Behavior	*Adaptation Status**	*Influencing Factors Focal Stimuli*
1. Joan: Female, age 48 Height: 5'2" (157 cm) Weight: 130 lb (61 kg) Triceps skinfold 24 mm	M	1. Eating too much for present caloric requirements
2. Dietary intake: 1882 calories, no milk and only one fruit, high in meats and fats	M	
3. Sedentary behavior, very little exercise	M	
4. Desire to lose weight	A	

*A = Adaptive; M = Maladaptive

Contextual Stimuli	*Residual Stimuli*	*Nursing Diagnosis*
1. Age 48 (decreased metabolic need) 2. Menopause 3. Insufficient knowledge of nutrition 4. Nervious eating bouts 5. Relaxing with glass of wine (also serves need of interpersonal relationship with husband) 6. Spends all of time working – places high value on doing homework as she did before becoming a teacher (feelings of guilt and powerless to change) 7. Spends long hours on school work – no time on herself (dysfunctional independence) 8. Value placed on health care for self less than that placed on work 9. Recognizes that her	1. No history of obesity in family 2. No history of obesity related illnesses 3. History of gradual increase in weight 4. Probably eats larger portions than she is aware of 5. Tried high protein, high fat, low carbohydrate diet and lost weight in past 6. Full-time school teacher, also mother of 3 teenage children and wife, homemaker 7. No pattern of regular exercise in the past	Overweight (overnutrition) due to caloric intake in excess of caloric expenditure

appearance would be improved by loss of weight
10. Expresses disgust and discouragement with attempts to lose weight on fad diet
11. Support of husband and children
12. Recognizes that she needs more regular exercise

Client Goal

1. Lose 10 to 15 lb, desired weight 118 to 120 lb
2. Decrease caloric intake 700 calories/day
3. Eat diet containing adequate nutrients in all food groups
4. Partake of regular exercise (to lose desired weight she must increase caloric expenditure by 300 calories/day)

Nursing Intervention

1. Provide Joan with 1200 calorie conventional diet and necessary health teaching to understand how to follow it. (Calorie Pocket Guide and Menu suggestions re: Better Homes and Gardens, Eat and Stay Slim)
2. Explore Joan's knowledge of food exchange system; be sure she understands getting adequate intake from each group
3. Set up plan of regular exercise (see text)
4. Hold conference with family to enlist aid and understanding of plan, effects it will have on them
5. Institute behavioral modification techniques (see text)
6. Set up plan for regular evaluation and followup

Having outlined exactly what was necessary in terms of caloric intake and expenditure for Joan to lose weight and for her to understand it was only one part of the problem. Joan had been an on-again, off-again dieter. To lose weight and maintain it requires a change in lifetime habits. The nurse decided to employ some techniques of behavior modification.

Behavioral modification is based on principles of learning. Given a certain behavior that you want to occur, reinforcement of that behavior increases its probability of recurrence. Likewise, if it is not reinforced the probability that it will be eliminated is increased. A functional analysis of the behavior needs to be done to see what its antecedents are. What cues the behavior, what is its trigger? Identify the nature of the behavior, what happens, how frequently, and what is the pattern. Finally, what are the consequences of the behavior: what happens after the behavior that reinforces it?

In the case of overnutrition the target behaviors are overeating and lack of exercise. What are their antecedents? Levitz[38] states that obese people tend to eat in many places (kitchen, dining room, television room, office, car, theatre, etc.) and at different times. These times and places become signals and discriminative stimuli for eating. "I always put on the coffee pot as soon as I get to work," "I like a coke between meetings," and "Potato chips and beer go with watching football." Many situations can be responded to by overeating. Quite often the situation is a stress- or tension-producing one and the person eats to "let off steam, as a relief valve." Thus the consequence of the behavior may be an emotional release and this serves as reinforcement. But is eating the behavior necessary to get release—might not some other behavior serve as well? Normal or undernourished people do not respond to stress by eating, so the behavior is not normal or necessary.

To effect behavior modification it is not necessary to alter the antecedent cue, although it may be desirable to do so. The person who overeats in response to stress may alter that behavior by finding some activity other than eating that is appealing, engrossing, and readily available. A certain time and place should be identified with eating. This does not rule out midmorning and midafternoon meals if they are part of the diet prescription, but they should be made distinctive. The client should be told to go to the dining area, make the eating the only activity, not an accompaniment to work, television, reading, etc. Other means to alter the response or eating behavior include eating slowly, savoring each bite, putting the utensil down between bites, and not hesitating to push the plate away with food on it. These techniques are designed to get the satiety center to signal full with the least amount of food in the stomach. If the pattern of overeating includes certain foods that are tempting the client should not have them available. It helps to eat with someone who can offer praise for adherence to the diet.

This leads to a discussion of self management and the use of reinforcers. With obesity the client will be responsible for managing his own behavior. He may make a contract with himself in which he rewards desirable behaviors. He can chalk up so many points for skipping the snack with coffee, for not eating while watching television, etc. When a certain number of points are accumulated he can treat himself with something valued.

All of these same techniques apply to energy expenditure. Compare the procedure to programmed learning. Each frame needs reinforcement, each step needs reward and each one helps to shape behavior into a desired lifestyle.

In Joan's situation lack of exercise was the main problem in maintaining a desired weight. She felt that she did not have enough time and she did not like to do exercise by herself. She knew that some of her fellow teachers had similar problems. The nurse encouraged her to discuss it with them and to develop an exercise plan.

The nurse also held a conference with Joan's family. They discussed the fact that Joan felt guilty if she did not always have dinner ready at an early hour for the children. When actually confronted with the issue the children indicated that it was not all that important to them. They wanted to have a reasonable idea of what time the dinner would be served so that they could arrange their activities around it, not that it had to be early. Also during open discussions of the issue the children volunteered more activity in helping prepare the evening meal. Because in so many instances they had not been asked, the problem had not been shared with them, and so they were not aware of its magnitude. Later they gave Joan some of her most positive reinforcement by their praise of her changed appearance.

The nurse asked Joan's husband if there was any way that Joan could join him for some of her exercise. He stated that he could alter his routine at the track and she could join him there. This plan might give them more time to talk with each other and to have something more in common. This may decrease the desire for wine with her husband that primarily served the need for an interpersonal relationship.

Joan did talk with two other teachers and now they go to the school exercise room at the end of the day where they participate in an exercise routine based on the Air Force exercises. At least three times a week she goes to the track with her husband and walks at a rapid pace for half an hour. She plans to increase this to one hour. Every Friday the three teachers eat lunch together and compare their daily logs to see how they are managing. Once a month they go shopping or take in a show and splurge a little. If any one of them does not meet her goals then the three cannot go.

One of the teachers has a friend in TOPS (Take Off Pounds Sensibly) and they are considering joining that group. It has been reported that organized self-help groups are of benefit in the modification treatment for obesity.[39]

In setting up the plan of treatment for Joan the nurse included a regular schedule for evaluation. Joan was to call the nurse every Friday and to return in one month's time. These occasions would be used to measure the observable changes and to record progress toward the goals. Since the program is very much do-it-yourself the client needs much encouragement and support. Praise for small gains is important as well as avoidance of any negative comments if progress is not going well. Analysis of what is adaptive and what is maladaptive behavior should continue, with support of adaptive behavior and elimination of that which is maladaptive.

In terms of looking ahead toward maintenance, as Joan loses the weight she can gradually add back items and increase her intake back to 1900 calories. Joan has already expressed that she still enjoys a glass of wine at bedtime. This would count as two fat exchanges and may be added. She said occasionally that she would like some dessert, maybe once a week. It is important that she is gaining the understanding of caloric balance. Currently she is marking her intake of exchanges on a daily record and recording her exercise. Gradually this will become automatic and recording will not be necessary. Observing her weight pattern will be enough to keep her aware of her caloric needs.

Undernutrition–Anorexia Nervosa

The example given of overnutrition due to overeating can be contrasted with an example of undernutrition due to undereating. This is the case of anorexia nervosa, a form of malnutrition characterized by self-starvation, which now appears to be increasing. Again, this problem occurs more in developed countries and often in well-to-do families. A young girl becomes obsessively concerned about her image, equating thinness with beauty and desirability, and resorts to different methods to reduce her caloric intake so that she will lose weight. Statistically, anorexia nervosa usually occurs in female Caucasians between the ages of 13 and 30; only 4 to 6 percent of the victims are male, and 15 to 21 percent of all victims die of starvation and complications.[40] Incidence varies, some cases of course not being recognized and treated and some not reported. One statistic states that one in 100,000 females has the disease, another that it may be as high as one in 300 in some groups.[41]

The cause of the disease is not really known; however, five diagnostic criteria have been identified: (1) onset of symptoms before 25 years; (2) loss of at least 25 percent of original body weight, leading to emaciation; (3) a negative attitude toward eating, food, and weight that cannot be overcome by hunger, threats, or reassurance that the person is not fat; (4) no other physiologic or psychologic problem that can explain the weight loss; and (5) any four of the following: periods of hyperactivity, such as overindulgence in exercise; self-induced vomiting or excessive use of laxatives; belief that the thin appearance is acceptable and desirable; a history of having been overweight; cessation of menstrual periods (as a result of the disease); abnormal reactions (not tired after exercise, not hungry although not eating); and a preoccupation with diets and occasional bouts of excessive eating usually followed by self-induced vomiting.[42]

The anorectic lacks a fatty layer and always feels chilly. He is usually severely constipated. Skin changes will be noted, with skin appearing dark and dirty with a roughened texture (follicular hyperkeratosis). He may develop long silken hairs over his body and lose scalp hair.

At the time of adolescence there is an increased need for calories and nitrogen in the diet. In girls this correlates with the onset of menarche and in boys with the growth spurt. If these needs are not met, especially the protein need, there is a loss of resistance to infection. If the caloric need is not met the individual is likely to become less active so that the caloric expenditure is decreased. It is important that adolescents understand these needs. However, in anorectics, knowledge of nutritional needs is not enough. Although exceptionally thin they think they are fat and feel bloated after eating a small amount.

As in the situation of the obese and overweight individuals, behavior modification is one method of treatment. The goal here of course is to increase the caloric intake, to gain weight, and to consume recommended amounts of all the nutrients. The family should be included in the treatment plans both to aid the victim and to take into account the changes the disease has had on the family and the effect its treatment will have. Psychotherapy may be necessary. Again, a long-term change in eating habits must be effected and the individual must be helped to form a healthy body image. Shaping by proceeding in small steps with positive reinforcement (praise not punishment) at each step is necessary.

Fluid and Electrolyte Balance, Elimination

Problems of fluid and electrolyte balance and elimination have not specifically been referred to up to this point. Some authors consider these as separate from the concept of nutrition. If one considers man's nutritional state to be the balance between all that is ingested, its metabolism, and its output, then fluids and electrolytes as well as elimination become a part of nutrition. The assessment tools already given take these processes into consideration.

The following example is one being encountered more frequently today: that of the client in the end stage renal failure. Because the federal government is now paying for the care of these patients more are surviving for longer periods of time and are being treated by hemodialysis and renal transplant. Portions of the situation given are excerpted from a paper presented by students.[43]

John G. is a 48-year-old black male with a history of end stage renal failure. An operation was performed to provide him with his third renal transplant. Subsequently the transplant was acutely rejected. During the postoperative transplant nephrectomy period the following care plan was derived.

A first level assessment of John's behavior in the physiologic, self-concept, role, and interdependence systems was done. It should be realized that throughout the nursing process priorities are set on the behaviors assessed. A decision is made about which of them require's further assessment to determine influencing factors, and then which problems have priority for nursing intervention. Bower[44] defines criteria for setting priorities in this order: (1) those threatening the life or integrity of the client; (2) those threatening severe, drastic change to the client; and (3) those affecting the client's normal growth and development.

When collecting data it is important to do it systematically, both in history taking and in physical assessment. Some of the behaviors reported for John are from direct observation, some from interview, and some from laboratory reports in the client record. After collecting the data it can be sorted and organized into similar categories. The following plan for John presents the significant data found utilizing the nutritional assessment tool in the beginning of the chapter. The data have been organized into problems with similar focal stimuli. Since the individual functions as a unified whole, behavior in one system influences another. Table 2.14 gives a plan for some of John's first-level assessment behavior in the self-concept, role, and interdependence modes which presented as contextual and residual stimuli or influencing factors for his nutritional behaviors. The plan that is presented focuses on the nutritive status and therefore the total assessment and plan for all physiologic needs and the other systems is not included.

Dietary Goals for the United States

This chapter has focused primarily on the *assessment* of nutrition. As the world population has increased and as we have become more developed and civilized our nutritional patterns have changed and therefore our problems have changed. Community and nationwide surveys are being encouraged to identify these community and national patterns. In addition to collecting and grouping such data about individuals as has already been outlined, these surveys include agriculture data and food balance sheets (crop production, surplus, export, import, etc.); socioeconomic data and information on marketing, distribution and storage; vital health statistics; and medical surveys of prevalent disease patterns.[45]

The Select Committee on Nutrition and Human Needs of the United States

Table 2.14 *Assessment of John G's Nutritional Status and Influencing Factors*

Behavior	Adaptation Status*	Influencing Factors: Focal	Influencing Factors: Contextual	Influencing Factors: Residual
Nutrition Well-developed black male; attentive, interested, responding appropriately to questions	A			48 years old, mature adult in developmental stage of generativity
Ht. 6′ 1″. Wt. pattern fluctuates with dialysis. Has fluctuated as much as 10½ lb between dialyses (3 X wk). Range of wts.: 3/4—171½ lb; 3/25—193 lb	M	End stage renal failure resulting in inadequate urinary output with fluid retention	Has knowledge of process of renal failure—problem diagnosed 5 years ago Has hemodialysis 3 times a week. Previous to hospitalization went to metropolitan dialysis center	11th grade education
Skin — edema present in periorbital, scrotal, and ankle areas. Abdomen slightly distended. Mucous membranes moist	M A		Decreased mobility — recovering from acute rejection of transplant (2 weeks post transplant) and removal (nephrectomy) of the transplant	Married, lives with wife and 3 teenage children (roles of husband, father, breadwinner)
Urinary output less than 20 cc/day	M		Knowledge that excess fluids and wastes removed in dialysis	Sick roles, of both acutely ill and chronically ill person
Breath sounds normal in left lung and diminished in right lower lobe. Resp. rate 20/min, regular and unlabored	Adapting		Had pleural effusion and pneumonia postoperatively, now resolving	
Heart rate 100 to 108. NSR. B/P 150/88 to 200/110. Presence of fistula in left arm. Thrill palpable	M Adaptive to disease process		History of hypertension. Treated with apresoline in past but receiving no antihypertensive now	
Alert and oriented	A		Has been dizzy sometimes after dialysis	

*A = Adaptive; M = Maladaptive

(cont.)

Table 2.14 *Assessment of John G's Nutritional Status and Influencing Factors (cont.)*

Nursing Diagnosis	Client Goal	Nursing Intervention
Fluid volume overload due to fluid retention, 2° end stage renal failure	Wt. gain between dialyses of 1 lb per day with no signs of overhydration	1. Reinforce instruction about disease process and treatment, validate client's knowledge. A. Be alert for readiness on John's part to accept information. B. Provide for short spaced periods of information. C. Expect periods of frustration, hostility, recalcitrance as part of normal process.
	Ability to discuss changes in lifestyle occasioned by disease process, to talk realistically about future on hemodialysis, possibility of any future transplant	2. Encourage John to express his thoughts and feelings, e.g., when instructing in hemodialysis, ask him how he expects to get to the center, will this cause any problem at home, etc. Be alert for cues to follow-up. 3. Do not be judgmental in approach. 4. Focus on positive assets; support of wife and children; ability to do self-care.
		5. Accurate measurement and recording of fluid intake (all channels) and fluid output (all channels). A. Record estimates or descriptions of abnormal amounts of fluid lost from (1) the skin, (2) the GI tract (vomiting and diarrhea), (3) wounds and dressings. B. Since John measures own intake praise him for accurate recording, help him to realize importance of this activity. (Gives him sense of responsibility for own care—helps satisfy need for independence, creates self-esteem.) 6. Record daily weight.

(cont.)

Table 2.14 *Assessment of John G's Nutritional Status and Influencing Factors (cont.)*

Behavior	Adaptation Status*	Influencing Factors		
		Focal	*Contextual*	*Residual*
Dietary: Fuild restriction of 1500 cc/day Likes coca-cola and admits to exceeding restriction.	M	Fluid intake greater than fluid output	Availability of fluids Restriction is monitored by client. Accurate intake questionable	Values independence
Says he "gets back at the machine by going off restriction."	M		Role conflict — recognizes necessity to adhere to restrictions but also desires to lead normal life	
2 gm Na diet. Eats all of diet — "used to it — no complaints"	A			
			Feels that nurses exaggerate need for fluid restriction	Attitudes toward sexuality — being told what to do by females
			Motivation to adhere to regime decreases as the probability of getting a functioning allograft decreases	
			Realizes that lifeline is the machine. Thinks that transplant would enable him to perform roles as he desires. Problem of powerlessness with respect to his self-ideal and expectancy.	Formerly employed as truck driver for floral company Unskilled laborer
			Boredom, time on his hands lying in bed, etc.	
			Does adhere to diet	
"I have diabetes and take insulin—the doctors say got it from the steroids." Blood glucose 122	Adapted to disease process		Wife supportive — encourages him. Prepares proper diet for John when at home.	

*A = Adaptive; M = Maladaptive

(cont.)

Table 2.14 *Assessment of John G's Nutritional Status and Influencing Factors (cont.)*

Nursing Diagnosis	Client Goal	Nursing Intervention
	Maintain fluid restriction	7. Discuss fluid restriction with John. Establish preferences and usual drinking patterns, coordinate this pattern with drinks delivered by dietary department and fluids from the floor.
	Verbalize understanding for and acceptance of need for limitations in fluid and diet	8. Give positive reinforcement for John's efforts to maintain restriction. Do not punish.
		9. Provide activities to decrease boredom. A. Plan regular visits with John just to talk. B. Find out if John has "favorite" in staff—give this person time to be with John. C. Contact occupational rehabilitation. D. Encourage wife, family to visit.

(cont.)

Table 2.14 *Assessment of John G's Nutritional Status and Influencing Factors (cont.)*

Behavior	**Adaptation Status***	**Influencing Factors** *Focal*	*Contextual*	*Residual*
Laboratory values, signs and symptoms				
A. Complains of muscular cramps and weakness. Diarrhea.	M	Serum Na decrease due to its shift into edema fluid, some loss to diarrhea	Sodium restricted diet	
Na = 134 mEq/liter	M			
B. Cl = 99 mEq/liter K = 4.4 mEq/liter CO_2 = 26 mEq/liter	A			
C. Ca = 8.0 mgm % PO_4 = 8.4 mgm %	M	Ca and PO_4 have inverse relationship. Inability of kidney to secrete PO_4, PO_4 ↑ and Ca ↓		
D. BUN = 145 mgm % Cr = 19 mgm %	M	Retention of nitrogenous wastes because of renal failure		
States sleep pattern is sometimes disrupted in hospital	M	Sound sleep pattern not established due to mental activity, worry, etc. and also lack of physical exercise	Lack of usual environmental routines contributing to sleep	
"Sometimes I get upset because the doctors give me different stories."	A (normal behavior for acutely ill hospitalized person)		Grieving process over rejection of 3rd allograft. Present hospitalization viewed as another failure	

*A = Adaptive; M = Maladaptive

(cont.)

Table 2.14 *Assessment of John G's Nutritional Status and Influencing Factors (cont.)*

Nursing Diagnosis	Client Goal	Nursing Intervention
Hyponatremia due to displacement in edema, possible diarrhea, 2° renal failure	Relief from muscle cramps and weakness Normal serum Na	1. Report to doctor for possible medical treatment, dietary changes. 2. Observe for behavioral changes or neurologic signs indicating more severe hyponatremia. 3. Continue fluid restriction. 4. Record I and O.
		1. Adaptive behavior – continue to observe for signs and symptoms of excesses or deficiencies of electrolytes: primarily changes in muscle tone of any or all muscle groups (weakness, flaccidity, ileus, fatigue, cramps, spasms) and changes in neurologic state (anxiety, restlessness, apathy, mental confusion, paresthesias).
Hypocalcemia, hyperphophatemia 2° renal failure	Normal serum Ca and PO_4	1. Observe for manifestations of Ca deficiency: numbness in extremities, excessive irritability, muscle twitchings, tetany, convulsion.
Azotemia 2° renal failure.	Normal BUN and Cr	1. Observe for neurologic signs and symptoms. 2. Avoid breakdown of tissue, releasing more protein. 3. Avoid infections.
Lack of adequate sleep due to changes in habit patterns and stress associated with illness	Obtaining good night's sleep – waking refreshed	1. Coordinate John's sleep and activity pattern with that of hospital insofar as possible.
(Problems of grieving, guilt, etc., treated in greater depth in areas of self-concept and role)	Increased ability to cope with stress of disease as evidenced by: ability to discuss wife's role in household support and discipline of	2. Provide privacy and minimize number of intrusions during night. 3. Minimize environmental noise and lights.

(cont.)

Table 2.14 *Assessment of John G's Nutritional Status and Influencing Factors (cont.)*

Behavior	Adaptation Status*	Influencing Factors		
		Focal	*Contextual*	*Residual*
"I worry about my kids."	A		Guilt feelings over wife's having to support household.	Strong belief that man's role is to support family; wife at home
"I don't know how my wife is making out at home."	A	(Also related to problems of F and E imbalance)	Attends vocational rehabilitation school.	Unable to hold job last 2 yrs.
			Visited by brother 3 times/week who checks on household for John	Belief that father is disciplinarian
Impotent	M	Neuropathy 2° chronic renal failure	? Denial of problems with sexual performance	Attitude toward sexual prowess, manliness, ability to satisfy mate
States, "My wife and I have no problems with sex."			Threat of rejection by wife	"Don't talk about that to women."
			Role conflict	
			Visited regularly by wife	
Stools: 2 to 3/day, dark brown semiliquid, "diarrhea"	M	Loose stools likely due to fluctuating F and E balance	Had period of ileus postoperative nephrectomy, now followed by diarrhea type stool	
States he has intermittent lower abdominal pain not requiring medication			Chronic illness and decreased mobility. Na deficiency	
Normal bowel sounds at this time	A			
2 wound drains in place at nephrostomy site—drains 100 to 200 cc serous fluid/day. Reported to be lymph fluid	Adapting		Postoperative nephrectomy, acute rejection. Increase in WBC to counteract infection—adaptive response	

*A = Adaptive; M = Maladaptive

(cont.)

Table 2.14 *Assessment of John G's Nutritional Status and Influencing Factors (cont.)*

Nursing Diagnosis	Client Goal	Nursing Intervention
	children in positive fashion, without guilt; ability to express frustrations and to judge them realistically, not placing "blame" on self or others; positive expressions in form of ways he can help or things he can do to improve situation, asking for assistance	4. Provide physical and recreational activities, find out how John relaxes at home before going to bed. 5. Give medication as ordered, Dalmane 30 mgm p.o. hs. 6. Have conference with health team, wife and client to discuss these problems and investigate alternative solutions. 7. Encourage attendance at vocational rehab.
Impotence 2° renal failure	Ability to discuss problem of impotence with nurse or doctor, and wife	1. Discuss problem with John. If he refuses suggest a male figure who he might talk to – perhaps another renal patient. 2. Discuss problem with wife.
Diarrhea due to changes in F and E balance, 2° to end stage renal failure	Cessation of diarrhea as evidenced by decrease in frequency of stools and return to stools of normal character	1. Observe and record frequency and nature of stools. 2. Estimate amount of fluid loss. 3. Report to M.D. for possible medical treatment.
Nephrostomy wound healing appropriately		1. Continue sterile wound care, observe character of drainage, report output.

(cont.)

Table 2.14 *Assessment of John G's Nutritional Status and Influencing Factors (cont.)*

		Influencing Factors		
Behavior	**Adaptation Status***	*Focal*	*Contextual*	*Residual*
WBC 10,500				
Hct 19.1; Hgb 10 gm %; Platelets 95,000	M	Lack of erythropoeitin	History of anemia with renal disease	
No complaints of dyspnea or angina		Depressed bone marrow	Has had oozing from needle puncture sites after dialysis (fistula), from nephrectomy wound site, and scrotal bleeding	
		Shortened life span of blood cells	Use of heparin during dialysis	
			Receiving halotestin 10 mgm q.i.d. for anemia	
Reddened area present on sacrum	M	Prolonged pressure on sacral prominence with decreased circulation to site	Immobility, lies in bed on back most of time	Concept of sick role
			Uses wheelchair for transport	
			Shares semi-private room with another client	Sense of privacy related to physical exposure
			Tissue edema interferes with tissue nutrition	
			General deteriorating condition—imbalance in anabolism and catabolism	
			Edematous tissue subject to breakdown	

*A = Adaptive; M = Maladaptive

(cont.)

Table 2.14 *Assessment of John G's Nutritional Status and Influencing Factors (cont.)*

Nursing Diagnosis	Client Goal	Nursing Intervention
Anemia due to lack of erythropoeitin 2° renal failure	Hgb and Hct within or near normal limits (Renal patients adapt to decrease)	1. Keep pressure bandage supplies at bedside—apply direct pressure over needle puncture site of fistula or bleeding.
Potential bleeding from all sites	No signs or symptoms of bleeding tarry stools hematemesis ecchymosis neurologic changes change in vital signs	2. Elevate scrotum, prevent friction to decrease skin breakdown.
		3. Observe for signs and symptoms of bleeding, change in sensorium, weakness, fatigue, pallor.
		4. Check Hgb and Hct result daily.
First stage decubitus ulcer due to immobility and decreased circulation	Absence of signs of decubitus ulcer: no redness no irritation healthy pink color tissue integrity	1. Encourage John to get out of bed, to walk at least 4 times day.
		2. Full ROM while in bed, turning side to side, avoid long periods on bony prominences.
		3. Keep skin clean and dry.
		4. Use lotion and apply circular massage to bony prominences at least every eight hours.
		5. Keep linen clean, dry and free of wrinkles.
		6. Check with nutritionist on dietary needs to obtain adequate protein for anabolism. (Protein may be decreased due to renal failure).
		7. Examine skin for any redness, discoloration, or blistering at bony prominences every eight hours.
		8. Discuss with John the relative values of frequent turning and movement and to examine own skin on daily basis.

Senate has conducted hearings on the nutritional status of the people of the United States. They found as a result of their study that the dietary patterns of our people have changed drastically in this century. Formerly complex carbohydrates—fruits, vegetables, and grain—were the mainstay of the diet; they now have a minor role. We have increased our fat and sugar consumption by 50 percent since the 1900s. They now account for 60 percent of the total caloric intake.[46] Heart disease, cancer, cerebrovascular disease, diabetes, arteriosclerosis, and cirrhosis of the liver are six of the ten leading causes of death; these have been linked to an increase in fat intake, especially saturated fats. Cholesterol, sugar, salt and alcohol have all been implicated in the evolution of these diseases and their consumption by Americans is on the increase. Ironically, in the presence of plenty these dietary changes are contributing to an increase in malnutrition. People are not consuming enough of the foods that contain vitamins and minerals, the micronutrients. Sugar and alcohol provide empty calories. In the same hearings Dr. Theodore Cooper, Assistant Secretary for Health, "estimated that about 20 percent of all Americans were overweight to a degree that may interfere with optimal health and longevity."[47] Improved nutrition might decrease the amount of the nation's health bill by one-third.[48]

As a result of these studies the committee has outlined the following goals[49]:

1. Increase carbohydrate consumption to account for 55 to 60 percent of the energy (caloric) intake.
2. Reduce overall fat consumption from approximately 40 to 30 percent of energy intake.
3. Reduce saturated fat consumption to account for about 10 percent of total energy intake; balance that with polyunsaturated and monounsaturated fats, which should account for about 10 percent of energy intake each.
4. Reduce cholesterol consumption to about 300 mg per day.
5. Reduce sugar consumption by about 40 percent to account for about 15 percent of total energy intake.
6. Reduce salt consumption by about 50 to 85 percent to approximately 3 g per day.

Convincing arguments are presented with epidemiologic evidence to support these goals. Nevertheless, the committee views changing the nutritional habits as a difficult task. The public is heavily influenced by television and advertising; producers gain little by advertising natural foods. The dramatic increase in consumption of soft drinks is one example. "Beverages now comprise the largest single industry use of refined sugar."[50]

To achieve their goals, the committee has made recommendations based on this report. Among these recommendations, health and nutrition education is first and foremost and has the greatest implication for nursing. As nurses move into expanded roles and primary health care, and the nation moves toward national health insurance and prevention, nursing must assume a more active role in nutritional assessment and care.

References

1. Carrel A: Man the Unknown. New York, Harper & Row, 1935, p 88
2. Webster's New World Dictionary. New York, Collins & World, 1975, p 412
3. Maslow AH: Motivation and Personality. New York, Harper & Row, 1970
4. Bettelheim B: Food to nurture the mind. School Rev 83, May, 1975
5. Jelliffe DB: The Assessment of the Nutritional Status of the Community. WHO Monograph No. 53, Geneva, 1966
6. Christakis G (ed): Nutritional assessment in health programs. American Public Health Assoc., Wash. DC, 1973. Reprinted from Am J Public Health 63: (Suppl), November, 1963. (Available from American Public Health Assoc. Inc., 1015 Eighteenth St., NW; Washington, DC 20036)
7. Fomon SJ: Nutritional disorders of children: Prevention, screening, and followup. US Dept. of HEW, 1976. (DHEW Publication No. HSA 76-5612)
8. Whitehead FE: Nutrition teaching. Food Nutr News 34:9:1, June, 1963
9. Recommended dietary allowances, 8th rev. ed. Food and Nutrition Board, National Research Council, National Academy of Sciences, Washington, DC, 1974. (Available from Printing and Publishing Office, National Academy of Sciences, 2101 Constitution Ave, Washington, DC 20418)
10. Adams CF: Nutritive value of American foods in common units. Agriculture Handbook No. 456. United States Department of Agriculture, Washington, DC, 1975. (Available from Government Printing Office, Washington, DC 20402)
11. Christakis G[6]: p 21
12. McLaren DS (ed): Nutrition in the Community. New York, Wiley, 1976, p 63
13. Christakis G[6]: pp 38–75
14. Screening children for nutritional status: suggestions for child health programs. US DHEW, PHS, Pub. No. 2158, 1971
15. Scrimshaw NS, Taylor CE, Gordon JE: Interactions of Nutrition and Infection. Geneva, WHO (in press), cited in Jelliffe, DB, 1966, p 8
16. Robinson CH, Lawler MR: Normal and Therapeutic Nutrition, 15th ed. New York, Macmillan, 1977, p 406
17. McLaren DS[12]: p 114
18. Williams CD: Malnutrition. Lancet 2:342, 1962. Adapted in Williams SR: Nutrition and Diet Therapy. St. Louis, Mosby, 1977, p 341
19. Pike RL, Brown ML: Nutrition: An Integrated Approach, 2nd ed. New York, Wiley, 1975, p 756
20. Ibid, p 756

21. Immune Response of the Malnourished Child. A position paper of the Food and Nutrition Board, National Research Council, National Academy of Sciences, Washington, DC, 1976, pp 10–13
22. Keys A, Grande F: Body weight, body composition, and calorie status. In Goodhart RS, Shils ME (eds), Modern Nutrition in Health and Disease. Philadelphia, Lea & Febiger, 1973, p 1
23. Mayer J: Obesity. In Goodhart RS, Shils ME (eds), Modern Nutrition in Health and Disease. Philadelphia, Lea & Febiger, 1973, p 634
24. Ibid, p 634
25. Robinson et al.[16]: p 406
26. Gillies DE, Alyn IB: Patient Assessment and Management by the Nurse Practitioner. Philadelphia, Saunders, 1976, p 201
27. Yura H, Walsh MB: The Nursing Process. New York, Appleton Century Crofts, 1973, p 23
28. Roy Sr. C: Introduction to Nursing: An Adaptation Model. Englewood Cliffs, N.J., Prentice-Hall, 1976
29. Calories and Weight, the USDA pocket guide. Agriculture Information Bulletin No. 364. US Department of Agriculture, Washington, DC, 1974
30. The fat American. Washington Post, March 1, 1977, p A10
31. Church CF, Church HN: Food Values of Portions Commonly Used. Philadelphia, Lippincott, 1970, p 172
32. Page L, Roper N: Food and your weight. US Department of Agriculture, Home and Garden Bulletin No. 74, July 1973, p 4
33. Dickie RS: Diet in Health and Disease. Springfield, Illinois, Charles C. Thomas, 1974, pp 96–97
34. Williams SR: Nutrition and Diet Therapy, 7th ed. St. Louis, Mosby, 1977, p 507
35. Gordon ES et al: A new concept in the treatment of obesity. JAMA, 186:50, 1963
36. Better Homes and Gardens: Eat and stay slim. New York, Meredith, 1968
37. Roy Sr.C[28]: p 32
38. Levitz LS: Behavior therapy in treating obesity. J Am Diet Assoc 62: 23, January, 1973
39. Jordan HA, Levitz LS: Behavior modification in a self-help group. J Am Diet Assoc 62: 27–29 January, 1973
40. Whitaker JD: Dieting gone berserk. The Washington Post, March 2, 1977, p A1
41. Ibid, p A6
42. Nolen WA: Anorexia nervosa: the dieting disease. McCall's, CIV (No. 9):72, June, 1977
43, Aronson J, Hurd S, Kunkel B, Reilly, J, Cecile Sr. M: Application of the Roy adaption model to a patient with chronic renal failure. Unpublished paper, School of Nursing, Catholic University of America, Washington, DC, April 1977
44. Bower JL: The Process of Planning Nursing Care, 2nd ed. St. Louis, Mosby, 1977, pp 16–17
45. McLauren DS[12]: p 59
46. Senate Select Committee on Nutrition and Human Needs: Dietary Goals for the United States. Washington, DC, US Government Printing Office, 1977, p 9
47. Ibid, p 9

48. Ibid, p 9
49. Ibid, p 12
50. Ibid, p 43: quotation from Page L and Friend B: Sugars and Nutrition. Nutrition Foundation.

Supplementary References

Diekelmann, N: Primary Health Care of the Well Adult. New York, McGraw-Hill, 1977

Lowenberg ME et al: Food and Man, 2nd ed. New York, Wiley, 1974. (Good source on food customs and the influence of culture and religion)

Taylor CM, Riddle KP: An annotated International Bibliography of Nutrition Education, Materials, Resource Personnel, and Agencies. Teacher's College Press, Teacher's College, Columbia University, New York, N.Y., 1971

Chapter Three •

The Need for Territoriality

Lynne Oland

Human behavior is strongly molded by a territorial drive. Territorial behavior provides people with a mechanism for meeting, to different degrees, the needs of privacy, security, autonomy, and identity. Satisfaction of each is necessary for stable self-system functioning. In developing an understanding of the concept of territoriality, we begin to discern one aspect of the relationship between a person and space.

We will first explore the phenomenon of territoriality, then discuss how nurses may apply their knowledge of spatial behavior to support territorial expression by their clients. Finally, we will consider situations in which there is territorial dysfunction, with the purpose of instigating creative thought about the range of nursing strategies that can be implemented to reduce the stress of that dysfunction. Territoriality is a vital and basic force that must be recognized in the practice of nursing.

Despite the proliferation of studies on human territoriality, which includes the concept of personal space, the data produced afford us the means for only a beginning appreciation of the nature of territoriality. Most of the studies have used an observation technique based on parameters that are defined in different ways and that have little theoretical structure. This has produced a large amount of data about how close we will come to each other in different situations, how much status a certain amount of territory conveys, and how we mark out our territory, but only a few hypotheses about the cognitive basis of territorial behavior. Relationships among the hypotheses are still tentative so that at best we can construct only a basic conceptual structure of a very complex phenomenon. Even the quest for an acceptable definition continues.

Territoriality is a concept that has been evolving since the 1920s, but was addressed mainly in ethologic literature before the 1960s.[1] Ethologists described a pattern of territorial behavior that, with minor variations, is nearly ubiquitous throughout the animal hierarchy and began to suspect that humans would also display territoriality. Ardrey reviewed the known animal manifestation of territoriality and defined territory as an area defended by an animal from other members of his own species.[2] He argued that man shares the territorial drive.

Subsequent efforts regularly equated human and animal behavior in an effort to establish the existence of a strictly analogous genetically based pattern. However, as studies began to focus less on animal patterns and more on the human phenomenon, the disparity of behavior belied direct analogy. Although humans distinctly display territorial behavior, a similarity to animal behavior lies only in the basic pattern. Humans and animals clearly establish territories and will defend them. For both, territories define acceptable interaction distance and insure adequate space for individuals. Unlike animals, humans use space in a highly diversified manner, express territoriality in the service of a large variety of purposes, and may establish discontinuous territories.[3] The concept of territoriality began to include the idea of psychologic defense of a space that some individual (or group) claimed as belonging to him.[4]

The latest stage in the process of defining territoriality has resulted in a broad expansion of the concept. Some authors now propose that in addition to physical territories, people establish psychologic territories such as areas of expertise, skills, or social positions that are recognized by the central nervous system in the same manner as geographic territories.[5] Thus, territoriality includes "perceptions and use and defenses of places, people, objects, and ideas . . . in response to the actual or implied presence of others and in response to the properties of the environment" in order to satisfy certain needs.[6] Clearly, the range of behavior is extensive, especially when ideas are also considered to be objects of territorial behavior.

Some examples may clarify the type of behavior under discussion. Territoriality in humans is not the sole province of individuals, but is also observed in groups ranging from dyads to communities and nations.

Mr. S. buys a new home and installs a fence, lines it with evergreens and posts a "No Trespassing" sign. He has established legal possession of the land and clearly marked its borders. He intends to prevent invasion onto his territory by perimeter defenses and by the more symbolic sign.

Mrs. R., who lives in a hotel for senior citizens, habitually uses a rocker in a corner of a back porch. Even when she is not present, fellow residents will warn potential invaders that the space belongs to Mrs. R. She has established a territory by virtue of frequent and consistent use. Others identify the chair with Mrs. R. and defend it in her absence.

The A.'s spread a blanket on the beach and leave a picnic basket on a nearby table. Although the space so marked is definitely public, the table is left unoccupied and space is left around the blanket. Were the beach actually a very small cove, the A.'s could reduce the possibility of others using the remaining beach space by spreading their blanket in the middle of the available area.

Mr. H. is riding home from work in a crowded bus. Bodies surround him and there is frequent physical contact. He avoids eye contact with other passengers, keeps his arm close to his body, and seems out of contact. Lacking a means to maintain an acceptable distance from the strangers around him, Mr. H. retreats to the center of the space left to him, the space his body is occupying. He retains his privacy by using nonverbal body cues to defend against intrusion.

Mrs. M., a nurse who has specialized in orthopedic nursing for seven years, is working with a client who insists on telling her how to set up the traction equipment. Mrs. M. feels herself becoming annoyed and thinks "who is he to be telling me about traction?" She has established an area of expertise, a territory of knowledge, and responds defensively to a challenge to her control over that territory.

Congress is to be reorganized to reduce expensive overlap in committee function. In principle, all agree. In final vote, the chairpersons fight to retain their committees, which convey to them power and recognition.

Finally, national boundaries, wars over use of resources, and defense systems are examples of territorial behavior at the national level.

Territorial behavior may be explored as a manifestation of the function of the aggressive–protective behavioral system, one of the eight systems defined by Johnson.[7] The behavioral responses of this subsystem preclude excessive or unwanted closeness, and protect the self, significant others, or property from threat to the total system. Territoriality permits the individual to establish a comfortable degree of interaction with the people and objects in his environment. Stated another way, it assures a balance between privacy and community that minimizes physical or psychologic threat to the self while the individual pursues a course of action designed to satisfy his social needs such as affiliation, dependency, and love. Successful maintenance of territory insures a sense of safety or security, a second priority need in Maslow's formulation.[8]

Because all of the eight behavioral systems Johnson describes* are interrelated, a dysfunctional territorial response in the aggressive–protective subsystem will produce a secondary response in the other subsystems. Evidence of this dysfunction is most likely to occur in the dependency, affiliative, achievement, and restorative subsystems.

Consider a situation of frequent territorial invasion or territorial loss. Achievement goals are usually facilitated by a secure environment. An invasion, threatening security, activates protective responses that divert energy away from achievement to the more basic need of territorial maintenance. Similarly, the lack of security produces a more vulnerable individual who may choose withdrawal and isolation as a means of avoiding threat. He will limit affiliative behaviors that require some degree of closeness and trust.

Invasion or loss of territory reduces a person's autonomy, which is derived from control or power over a territory. The individual may respond with excessive dependency on another to provide or supplement the lost control. He may isolate himself from others or may develop a self-deluding facade of autonomy over a territory while being aware, at some level, of the inherent vulnerability of this position. His independent behavior is at this point dysfunctional.

Finally, anticipation of invasion or unfamiliar territory intensifies vigilance in the effort to protect oneself. The rise in tension parallels energy expenditure, which in turn depletes energy available for the function of other subsystems. Heightened tension is inconducive to rest so that the restorative goal is not reached, and the entire self-system suffers further decline in available energy.

Characteristics of Territories

A territory is the area of space or knowledge that an individual (or a group) denotes as his and over which he maintains control, defending it if necessary. A territory is identified with a person (or a group) and this identification is recognized by others. Professors are accorded the right to speak authoritatively in their

*According to Johnson, a behavioral system is a "complex of observable features or actions which determines and limits the interaction of an individual and his environment and that establishes the relation of the person to the objective events and situation in his environment." There are eight subsystems universally characteristic of human beings: ingestive, eliminative, dependency, sexual, affiliative, aggressive, protective, achievement, and restorative subsystems. Each subsystem has a goal, and is characterized by a particular set or pattern of behavior from which individuals choose. The behavior we observe is a function of that choice. All of the subsystems are interrelated, energy distributed among them. They may be examined according to the general systems approach.[7]

area of expertise. A homeowner's right to establish rules governing behavior on his property is rarely questioned. Although a specific territory is probably most real to its owner, territoriality is an effective general behavior pattern because we mutually acknowledge possession of territory.

Territories are roughly divided into central and peripheral components. The latter is bounded by a border with varying degrees of permeability and is contiguous with other territories or with neutral or public areas. The peripheral area serves as a buffer zone, protecting the more central region from invasion so that the individual residing therein is relatively secure and enjoys some degree of privacy. The central portions of a territory are highly cathected areas, that is, the individual invests them with particular significance and is willing to maintain them using an amount of energy proportional to the importance and centrality he attaches to them. The central zones are more closely tied to an individual's identity and are marked with more personal objects or symbols. The home as opposed to the surrounding grounds, the desk at an office or schoolroom, the specialty area, and the body or the internal psychologic self in contrast to the closely enveloping space are all examples of central zones of a territory.

The orthopedic nurse described earlier controls the geographic space of a unit that is hers relative to that of the client. She also maintains and develops an area of knowledge, nursing, which may be viewed as a knowledge component of psychologic territory. Orthopedic nursing as her area of expertise forms the central zone of her territory. Were she to be asked to care for gynecologic clients, she could function using basic principles of nursing, but would be less likely to defend her actions or initiate care requiring specific knowledge about nursing of clients with a gynecologic problem. She would then be operating in the peripheral zone of her knowledge territory. Her total nursing territory is contiguous with those of other health workers, is a boundary under constant dispute, and varies with a great number of situational conditions.

Ethologists have observed that animals seem to possess more energy and strength when they are lodged in their own territory, especially near the central zone. Invaders are almost automatically placed at a disadvantage and most likely will be routed. Most animals avoid territorial encroachment unless a weakness is perceived in the owner.[9]

Human behavior resembles this pattern. Whereas outside the home or other personally identified territory, a person maintains a dominant position only in relation to his social status, his position of dominance is usually unquestioned inside his territory,[10] except by those with whom he shares a common territory. In this case, other factors such as sex, role, or social position determine dominance. He is secure and in control of that territory. Coleman described a patient who had been agitated and defensive in a hospital setting, but who was calm and self-assured in his home.[11]

Types of Territories

Using the individual as a point of reference, we may describe several human territories that extend outward from the self. Four basic territories will be explored: psychologic, body, public, and home. Because interaction distance involves movement within territories, these too are discussed as they relate to the types of territories.

The first is a very abstract unmeasurable kind of territory that can be called a psychologic territory, or the internal territory of the self. Self in this context means the individual's experience of himself as a real unity of mind and body with a specific identity. It includes knowledge about the self, and how it functions, attitudes, beliefs, values, memories, social position, and both general and specific knowledge about the external environment. Not all of it is conscious or available to the individual by introspection. One of the functions of territorial behavior is defense against loss, violation, or devaluation of the self. The self seeks to maintain his integrity and his control, thus preserving his personal privacy and individual freedom.

A second territory has the physical body as its core and is designated as body territory, or personal space. This territory varies greatly in size and shape and is not fixed to any geographic space. Researchers have studied the usual conformation of this space as it is perceived around an individual, subject to sociocultural variations. Generally, the space takes the shape of an egg, with the person's back paralleling the broad end, the sides having a moderate area beside them and the largest area being in front.[12,12a] An area circumscribing a line of vision to a relatively close person or object extends body territory. The borders of the body territory exist in a dynamic state, shifting with change in contextual factors such as the relationship between interacting individuals, the purpose of the interaction, and the setting itself. Others may be more aware of the configuration of the territory than the individual himself.

An image of the body is formed as the central nervous system slowly develops a schema from the sensory data it receives from the body itself and from the physical environment, overlaid by input it receives from interaction with other people. Although the image constantly changes, it attains relative stability and completeness by early adulthood.[13] Awareness of one's body territory is established as part of the process of defining the self as a distinct and separate entity. Body territory, with its apparently nonphysical boundary, is part of the acquired body image, an internalized projection of the body's boundaries beyond the physical mass.[14] The body, with its territory, is eventually understood as a conceptual whole although the environment may be repeatedly and variably subdivided. Space is defined according to its meaning, use, or our relationship to it. For example, space is designated as familiar or unfamiliar, living or eating space, my space or yours, or public space.

An image of body territory may be developed from operation of superficial sensory receptors that detect thermal, kinetic, chemical, and pressure changes in the nearby environment.[15] Alternately, if we view man as an electrodynamic field with the visible body as a concentrated energy reservoir, the area immediately outside the body is interpreted as a less dense and therefore less visible field. The boundaries of the body would thus exist outside those traditionally recognized and be marked at some distance at which the energy concentration is still high enough to be sensed. These boundaries and their permeability would vary depending on the dynamic state of the field. This model accounts for the apparent physical discontinuity, but functional holism, of the body and the space immediately around it.

Body territory may simply be a psychologic extension of the self, an extension slightly beyond the visible physical boundaries of the body. It is a zone of heightened awareness, a product of physiologic processes and psychic energy investment that demarcates that space as belonging to the self and as distinct from the rest of extracorporeal space. Others respect the space as personal and refrain from intrusion by using acceptable interaction distances as defined by an individual's particular culture.

In the course of some interactions, the involved people are spaced within the area recognized as body territory. Hall has described two close interaction distances, an intimate distance in which individuals are touching or separated by up to 18 inches and a personal distance that separates individuals by 1.5 to approximately 4 feet.[16] At intimate distances, sensory awareness of the other person is intensified. Touch is frequent and voice tones are low. Visual distortion occurs, with small details brought into focus and parts seeming larger than normal. Except under certain conditions in which permission for approach to the intimate distance is granted or implied, the distance is reserved for interaction with trusted and very familiar people. Uninvited closeness that is not a function of impersonal crowding is usually threatening because in this culture it may indicate either an aggressive or a sexual intent.[17] At the very least, it decreases the individual's options for action because it physically bars movement in certain directions. Children are particularly demonstrative in this regard. They will openly display displeasure if another person is taking the liberty of holding them or patting them against their will. The child shakes his head as if to remove the offending touch, runs behind a protective parent, or squirms to get away. An adult may realize that on some days he seems to need more operating space and will modify his behavior to achieve more space. He may sit at farther distances from others. find a secluded space, or avoid interactions requiring closeness.

Spacing at a personal distance permits use of touch or simply visual/verbal interaction without a sense of overwhelming closeness. Visual distortion is absent although details are still clear. Voice tone may be moderate. Conversations between individuals at this distance are private and may be confidential. Others avoid contact with their shared personal space, preferring to skirt it rather than move through it, however quickly.

The interactional distances established between individuals are a function of all of the variables operating within the field at a particular space/time locus.[18] The distance is both determined by and shapes the nature of the interaction although the decision and interpretation may be made unconsciously. In the previous example of the adult needing space, the person established greater than normal interaction distances. His intent would be signalled to others by use of both verbal and nonverbal cues. The other individuals would perceive the cues, avoid close spacing with him, and would generally limit conversation to more casual, noninvolving topics. On the other hand, if one of these other people wished to convey information about a private business matter, for instance, he would decrease the interaction distance. The situation notwithstanding, individuals tend to observe a characteristic pattern of spacing based on their personal preference and experience.

Internal space and body territory differ from other territories controlled by a person by virtue of their inseparability from the physical body.* They are therefore not fixed in space but move with the individual. The person operates within a space/time environment that is subdivided into territories designated as public territory or as his or others' private territories that are usually more or less permanent.

Public territory is space open to use, within the bounds of social norms, by anyone. Within a public or neutral territory, an individual may establish a temporary territory that he personalizes, marks, and that others recognize as his within certain limitations. As more people attempt to use public space, obvious and recent occupation must be evident to avoid loss of the temporary territory. Only rarely will marked territory be invaded and then almost always by males.[19] We seem to establish temporary territories out of a desire to minimize intrusion of our body territory.[20] Because others generally acknowledge an individual's possession of a space and will avoid invading it, the person who has established a temporary territory has set boundaries that determine interaction distance. Temporary territories usually offer little in the way of sustained privacy.

*Although researchers are currently studying techniques of mental projection or apparent psychic separation of mind and body, the origination and control of the projection resides in the neural processes occurring within the self, whose locus is the body.

Home territory is the physical space that an individual regards as his own by legal right, by social or occupational position, or by frequent and intensive use. Establishing a home territory creates a predictable, fairly structured, familiar, and therefore safe, environment. Affiliated individuals such as family, organizational, or community groups may share home territories. Unfortunately, the idea of home territory can be broadly extended so that the designation of a territory as home territory becomes less meaningful. For example, speaking to a friend or neighbor, we might point out a piece of property including a house as our home territory. Meeting a stranger on a train, we might identify home territory as a town or even a state. In the context of this discussion, the term home territory will mean the individual's used and familiar space, the area over which he maintains control, defends, and identifies as his own. There may be several such territories separated physically, but "owned" by a single individual. Access to home territories is limited by the claimant who will respond to others from a dominant position while on home ground. In some cases, status or recognition may accompany possession of a particular territory. Within his territory a person is relatively autonomous, can limit or determine social interaction, and thus achieves some degree of freedom of choice and privacy.[21]

Although the reason for a meeting and the type of relationship between individuals are primary determinants of interaction distance, social and public distances are more commonly used in home and public territories. At social distances, interactions are primarily verbal and visual because they occur across a space of 4 to 12 feet. Visual detail is less evident and speaking volume is normal to slightly enhanced. Encounters at a social distance tend to be casual or to be used for completion of business transactions. Involvement between individuals is minimal, allowing privacy through anonymity, superficial knowledge of the other, and decreased feasibility of personal and physical domination.[22]

Public distances minimize social interaction by increasing the difficulty of such interaction. The voice must be raised, gestures broadened, and attention specifically directed toward the other person. Details tend to be obscured. A sense of separateness and anonymity is heightened.[23]

Territorial Determinants

Territorial behavior is instrumental in the procurement of privacy, security, and autonomy, and supports the preservation of identity. Some suggest that the desire to maintain or achieve privacy is the primary determinant of territorial behavior.[24] However, each of the above needs are prerequisites for continuing adaptive functioning of the self. Together they constitute the determinants of territorial behavior.

Privacy is a personal and internal state of being in which the affairs of the self are conducted. Privacy is equated with physical seclusion, freedom from interruption of thought, freedom from noise or visual intrusion into our space, and absence of unwanted physical closeness. In the absence of others or with chosen intimates, we achieve a freedom from the constraints of role expectation and the constant surveillance of others. We may relax our vigilance somewhat. Privacy permits a release of tension in ways or intensity usually unacceptable in public.[25] We explore the structure and processes of our innermost selves in private and decide what must remain within the depths of our internal territory. Those who delve into those depths invade our privacy. They try to reach into the guarded areas. Privacy is maintained when individuals select the type and amount of information about themselves that they wish to divulge, determine who shall receive that information, and are successful in their efforts.

However, privacy does not necessarily imply that one is physically secluded from others; nor does it mean only guarding secrets. Privacy may be viewed as a state in which the self and an object of consciousness are experienced as a unity with little regard to time or space or attention to the outside world.[26] The person is immerged in a sometimes fragile, sometimes strong relationship with the idea or object of focus. Fantasy, creative thought, meaningful self-evaluation or integration of experiences are the products of the private being whose attention is not diverted by a barrage of unrelated stimuli. There is a sense of personal autonomy in this experience or state of privacy. Such privacy is necessary for growth of the individual self and for maintenance of total system integrity. Some persons are capable of achieving this state without physical seclusion; others require separation.

There are many modes of privacy: solitude or physical seclusion is one, anonymity another, and the creation of psychologic barriers or withdrawal of the self is a third. As long as none of these modes becomes dominant to the exclusion of behaviors necessary to meet social needs, they are adaptive behaviors. By maintaining physical and psychologic territories, the individual can adjust interaction distances or use his territory as a secure and private retreat.

Earlier in this discussion, the relationship between territoriality and security was partially explained. Security is in part a function of predictability. Familiar territory is safe because the individual is operating with knowledge of the dimensions and characteristics of the space that are less well understood by invaders. Central territory is further protected by the surrounding peripheral zones. In addition, we increase the predictability of interaction by means of territorial behavior. Although the exact nature of the relationship between territory and human social order has not been clearly established, territoriality probably influences social role dominance patterns and status. The social relationships thus established affect interaction distance. Lorenz believes that territorial behavior reduces aggression by the mechanisms of both physical and social distancing.[27] Threat of invasion or violation of territory is reduced as distance increases. Security is proportional to the degree of threat reduction.

Security and autonomy are mutually dependent goals. Within the confines of a territory, a secure area, the individual senses a greater freedom and ability to control the events and objects therein. He will achieve mastery over this particular space. That feeling of potency or authority in turn augments the perception of the territory as a safe place.

Finally, territories become part of one's identity—home and temporary territories by the process of association of an individual with a space and its objects or markers, and body and self territories by development of an internalized image or concept.

Schema, Set, and Regulation of Territorial Behavior

The highly diverse but individually characteristic use of space gives credence to the hypothesis that territoriality is an acquired behavioral pattern. The overall behavioral similarity in humans points toward a genetic basis. Over time, we establish an internalized territorial schema, an outline or plan of expectations about territory against which we compare incoming data about space and an actual or anticipated interaction. The schema probably results from an experiential and learned translation of a genetically determined behavioral pattern. It provides the cognitive basis for a territorial set that is a pattern or repertoire of predictable, habitual or ritualized responses to spatial behavior by and toward others. The dynamics of this set and the development of the criterion schema arise largely out of our awareness.

Input about all of the situational variables is entered into the central nervous system together with physiologic data from the body. Operating at subconscious levels, the data are processed through the territorial schema. Congruency with the schema is evaluated.

Given a situation that is not greatly deviant from one's experience and social norms, the incoming data are interpreted as congruent with the schema. This person's territorial set will probably be fully appropriate whether that data indicate territorial invasion or expected spatial behavior. He chooses among the set behaviors for a response that fits the particular situation. Were a lack of congruence noted, that is, if the individual cannot adequately interpret the data or provide a basis for response, then the discrepancy or resultant system tension would reach the level of conscious awareness and a sympathetic response activated in accordance with the degree of threat. The reason for the discomfort may not be immediately apparent. The individual's ability to adapt is diminished. For example, if another approaches too closely, a normal unconscious response drawn from the set might be a slight turning aside or stepping back. If the other person persisted, the person whose body territory had been invaded would become uncomfortable enough to consciously tell the other to move away or to try some overt means of communicating the event of invasion. The behavior of the system is a function of interpretation of the situation as more or less congruent with the territorial schema.

Major Variables Affecting the Schema or Determining Response

Because of the limited amount of research evidence, data about the variables affecting territorial behavior are frequently conflicting or tentative. The factors discussed in this section are those that have received general empirical support.

Physiologic variables include mobility, level of consciousness, sex, and age. Territorial behavior includes defense of a territory. When an individual's mobility is limited by weakness, aging, illness, injury, or imposed therapeutic restrictions, the option of active physical defense of a territory is limited even though humans usually resort to force or violence only when the threat is intense or symbolic efforts have failed.[28] A deficit in mobility further limits acquisition, exploration, and manipulation of territory. Thus, while territorial awareness is amplified, overall control over the environment is diminished and vulnerability is heightened. Privacy may be reduced because of a need for closer contact with others to meet basic physiologic needs.

A decline in level of consciousness similarly lessens control over and defense of territory. The person is less able to stipulate who may enter his territory and/or for what purposes. In the illusion-producing haze of anesthesia, for example, closeness or touch may readily be misinterpreted as an aggressive approach in which the threat is intensified by inability to respond.

Females tend to demand less interaction space than males. Women sitting with women are likely to be found in closer proximity than males sitting with males. A male–female couple tends to maintain a closer comfortable interaction distance than like-sexed dyads.[29] Although these distances probably relate heavily to role expectations and an internalized assessment of capacity for aggression, there are also set differences in perceived body boundary vulnerability. Females seem to perceive their body boundaries as less permeable. This renders them less vulnerable and perhaps accounts for their tolerance of closeness.[30]

Spatial norms develop with the maturation process. Infants gradually learn to define body territory as they explore and differentiate the body mass from the environment. By the time a child reaches approximately twelve years of age, he will display territorial behavior normal for his particular culture.[31] Unfortunately, we have little concrete data about the precise sequence of development of the territorial schema and set.

Numerous sociocultural variables have been proposed, but few have been verified. We have long been aware of cultural differences in ideas about space, body territory usage, and the related expectations of interaction distance. Some groups have extensive and fixed home territories. Nomadic peoples seem to be content with transient use of geographic space. Northern Europeans use a far personal distance even for intimate family interaction whereas Southern Europeans tolerate greater closeness.[32] People maintain greater distances from individuals of a different race[33] and definitely increase interaction distances when confronted with a person bearing some stigma such as overweight or epilepsy.[34]

Relative social status may be partially determined by the characteristics of and amount of territory an individual holds. He may be identified with a certain body of knowledge or with a particular piece of property and enjoy the prestige and power associated with them. A landlord, the child with the largest homemade fort on the block, or the specialist in a field share the enhanced status of territory. An individual's status with respect to another determines interaction distance. People tend to maintain greater distances when in the presence of others of either higher or lower status than they do with their peers.[35]

In most cases, invasion of body territory is avoided by either defensive maneuvers or retreat by psychologic withdrawal. However, excluding other factors that vary the size or permeability of territory, especially body territory, there are occasions when intrusion is permitted even to strangers without evoking the usual stress response. By virtue of their role responsibility or occupational status, certain individuals are accorded access by "legitimate entry."[36] Doctors and nurses may move into intimate range or perform physically intrusive procedures. Lawyers may have access to confidential information. The plumber or gas man may enter the house once he is identified as a representative of a legitimate organization.

Montagu suggests that child rearing practices affecting sleep behavior may have an effect on use of space, especially as it determines acceptable interaction distance. He discusses several cultural approaches varying from family group sleeping arrangements to the Western middle class practice of separating the child from his parents for sleep, if possible putting him in his own bed and room.[37] Montagu's exploration raises several questions. Do sleeping practices per se strongly influence an adult's territorial behavior or are they just one additional force in the overall enculturation process? Does the Western child tend to grow up with a sense of separateness and thus prefer to maintain greater distances between himself and others? Does he, therefore, seek more private home territory and experience discomfort in places where communal territory is the norm?

Situations that are threatening to the self produce changes in interaction distance, usually in the direction of increased distance. Threat from an external source may, however, bring individuals closer together even to the point of invading each other's intimate body territory if by closeness they can achieve a sense of security. Occasionally, closeness may be used to reverse the threat and signal anger and aggressive intent.[38]

Spacing between individuals is determined partly by their interpretation of the meaning of touch. An individual who dislikes touch, who considers it always intrusive or always aggressive, will usually restrict others' opportunity to touch him by increasing interaction distances and using a variety of proxemic cues to indicate the dimensions of his body territory. He may also construct larger barriers to mark his territorial boundaries and increase the difficulty of invasion. For others, touch is a culturally and personally acceptable way of communicating. Their behavior indicates their tolerance for touch by closer interaction distances, fewer barriers, and more use of touch themselves. Either group's general set is modified by the specific meaning of a given interaction.

The relationship between individuals alters their use of interaction distances.[39] The closer an acquaintanceship, the less likely that proximity will produce a defensive response. Territorial boundaries are rendered more permeable. In trusting, intimate relationships, both physical and psychologic closeness is permitted.

Data about ego state effect on territoriality are mostly inconclusive, but promising as an area for exploration. Possibly, introverted people construct a larger body territory. Fisher and Cleveland suggest that persons with weakly differentiated body boundaries may create a larger body territory or even geographic territory in order to compensate for their sense of body vulnerability.[40] A person who regards himself in low esteem perceives himself as having a lower status than others and usually maintains larger distances.

Finally, the environment itself is a variable affecting use of territory. Familiarity with a territory enhances ease of functioning within it; lack of familiarity is associated with some degree of hesitancy and with a sense of vulnerability. Withdrawal is more likely than aggressive action in a confrontation with those on unfamiliar territory. In the event that interacting individuals are both in unfamiliar territory, dominance is a function of social hierarchy, or physical or cognitive power.

Density also affects territorial expression. As the availability of physical space declines, the probability of territorial invasion increases. Defensive action is likely to invite a retaliatory response and territorial expansion is more difficult if not impossible. The individual discovers that his choices are reduced to withdrawal and consolidation or fortification of territory to render it less penetrable.

Choice and Action

People respond to the field of interacting variables operating in a specific situation by a choice of territorial action that limits stress. The response is chosen from the set of territorial behaviors that have previously been succesful for that individual. His choice is manifested in action, behavior that can be assessed by observation or discussion.

There are five basic models of territorial behavior among which the individual can choose:

1. Defense of territory: This may be in expectation of or in response to intrusion; it may be concrete action or symbolic, includes vigilance, fortification of territory, and protection of information.
2. Permission for access or limited intrusion: This decreases stress response by setting conditions for entry; it includes idea of "legitimate entry" and depersonalization of invaders; is usually extended to affiliates.
3. Withdrawal: This may be a physical withdrawal into solitude or into central area of territory where security, autonomy, and privacy are maximized; it may be psychologic withdrawal into the inner self, impervious to outsiders; it may be abandonment of geographic territory; it includes anonymity.
4. Aggressive enlargement of or addition of territory: This may enhance ability to defend territory; it includes addition of physical space, ideas, areas of knowledge, social position, and aids individual growth.
5. Nonaggressive interaction: This refers to actions designed to minimize threat of invasion when on another person's territory.

Defense

Humans display a rich variety of defensive behaviors, most of which are symbolic. The most common approach uses markers, objects, or words designed to signal others that an individual has claimed the space. In home territory the markers may announce the possessor's willingness to defend his territory. Transient territory established in neutral space is less often defended. Markers include articles of clothing, signs, books, or other personal objects that will identify the space as occupied. Boundaries of fixed space are often well marked with signs, walls, and fences. On entering a new space, most people orient themselves to the space, identify what objects and space might be included in their territory, and mark it.

We arrange ourselves in space using distances and body orientations that maximize interaction distances, especially in the presence of strangers. Numerous studies of seating patterns reveal that wall seats, end seats, or seats abutting or near inanimate objects are preferred when the individual's objective is to achieve protected space and minimize interaction.[41,41a,41b] These positions decrease the possibility of being surrounded that would enhance the probability of invasion. Unless a strong motivation such as occupational achievement or desire for affiliation dominates behavior, we usually avoid establishing temporary territories located in areas of high density or movement.

Barriers clearly demarcate territorial boundaries and communicate our intent relative to use of personal territories. A fence, a locked door, a pile of books between individuals, use of a language or jargon believed unintelligible to potential invaders, physical screening, and verbal or nonverbal expressions of defense or aggression all deter territorial invasion.

Nonverbal behavior is a particularly effective and frequently used means of territorial defense.* Defensive cues include facial expressions of aggression or repudiation, direct and antagonistic eye contact, orientation of the body to exclude or directly confront potential invaders. Territorial invasion may result in scowls, frowns, or other negative expressions indicating transgression. Verbal warning is usually reserved for insensitive invaders or for those who have somehow missed the other cues.

Permission for Limited Access

With the exception of home territories whose area is concretely bounded, the dimensions of a territory vary with the characteristics of a particular interaction. At times, it is necessary to permit entry into or use of a territory by those who have no direct right to access or by those who are not affiliates of the owner. The

*Hall[42] classifies nonverbal spatial behaviors as proxemic cues. They include interaction distance, eye contact, body orientation and posture, facial display, and voice volume, and convey messages of intent in all five modes of territorial behavior. See also E. Hall, *Silent Language*,[15] J. Fast, *Body Language* Supplementary References and A. Scheflen, *Human Territories*.[32]

owner of the territory may simply fail to acknowledge the transgression, thereby rendering it a non-threat. He may depersonalize the invader. By means of the purposefully distorted vision of depersonalization, only a mechanistic nonperson with less potential for harm is considered to be invading. In a third instance, the individual recognizes the likelihood or perhaps necessity of invasion and grants the other the right of "legitimate entry." This right is extended with the expectation that the invader will observe certain nonaggressive rules of conduct for the duration of invasion.

Withdrawal

The withdrawal mode encompasses the behavior used to retreat from interaction, avoid invasion, or achieve the solitude or mind set necessary for privacy. It is a particularly effective method, accomplished by diverting energy away from the territory involved or simply removing oneself from the space in question.

Certain circumstances are conducive to use of withdrawal. Temporary territories established in public or another's private territory are marked, but often are not defended if invasion occurs,[43] especially if there is no premium on space or the space has not been occupied consistently or for very long. The characteristics of the invader (e.g., large and mean-looking, of higher status or authority) will affect the decision of whether to abandon or to attempt to retain the territory. Flight may be the most prudent choice.

From time to time, invasion is inevitable or necessitated by the need to accomplish another goal, such as health care. In crowded places like auditoriums and buses, or on busy city streets, attempts to maintain body territory are doomed to failure and will incite the ill humor of others in the area. People can minimize threat of invasion of body territory by psychologic withdrawal.[44] Investment of energy in maintenance of the territory is withdrawn with retreat into the space left, either the physical body space or the psychologic territory of the self.

The individual using psychologic withdrawal appears out of contact or remote and inattentive. There may be a delay in response to a question or statement. When possible, eye contact is avoided or quickly terminated to reduce the effect of intrusive stares of others. Staring is an especially potent form of invasion. Sleep can be a form of withdrawal, an escape from invasion by lessened awareness. Psychotic withdrawal from reality exemplifies extreme and maladaptive patterns.

Withdrawal is also an active means of establishing privacy for a task or concentrated thought, with or without the availability of physical seclusion. It may be a voluntary behavior even in the absence of others, a way of reducing outside energy expenditure by insulation within the protective confines of the territory.

Some people seek physical isolation, the degree of isolation varying from simple screening to absolute seclusion. In isolation, there is at least temporary freedom from others and their demands, from visual intrusion, disrupting noise or distracting movement, and from interruptions other than self-willed intermissions. The reduction of sensory load decreases the degree of energy output in receiving, screening, and interpreting the input, and frees the central nervous system for the task of integrating the data already in the system. The individual who has withdrawn from interaction with others has the opportunity for privacy.

Aggressive Expansion of Territory

Expansive behaviors are based in an interaction of the aggressive–protective and achievement subsystems. The manifest goal may be a larger protective zone, more status, or more control over a body of knowledge or over a set of skills. The potential result of territorial expansion is growth by enlarging the total field in which one is capable of functioning, either in physical or psychologic space.

Of the force behind territorial expansion, we can cite psychic drives for greater security, autonomy, and identity. Territorial expansion may reduce excessive tension in the system by gratifying those needs. However, growth of the individual demands a continuous effort to maintain a level of stimulation (tension) necessary for differentiation. General systems researchers note that living systems, particularly humans, are characterized by negentropy, that is, by a movement toward increasing order, heterogeneity, and complexity.[45] Repatterning of the environment or field by means of territorial expansion is tension-maintaining because the individual exposes himself to some degree of risk as well as the increased stimulation of less than familiar territory. The variables determining when territorial expansion is undertaken have not been well documented, but probably include developmental status, level of sensory input, level of intelligence, cultural values on use and perception of space, and characteristics of the environment such as density and degree of hazard present. More mundane considerations such as financial and social status and legal rights of the individuals concerned or group apply to acquisition of fixed space.

What behaviors might be observed? Physical invasion of another's territory, monetary or barter exchange, legal possession, or squatter's possession come to mind as examples of expansion of home territory. These would be followed by defensive behavior to concretize and personalize the space.

Body territory cannot be expanded beyond the range of physical awareness. Enlargement of internal or psychologic space is revealed in the behavior of knowledge and skill acquisition, or creative use of ideas to increase control over space and self.

Nonaggressive Interaction

When an individual moves through another person's or a group's space, he activates a culturally determined territorial mode that limits the threat he would otherwise create by invasion, even when he has full permission to be in or pass through that territory. He will signal his nonaggressive intent by carefully following the owner's rules, ritually asking permissions for use of objects, minimizing the amount of time spent in the territory, and generally displaying more modest if not submissive behavior than he would in his own territory. Implied or actual permission serves the purpose of limiting social aggression and lessens the threat to all parties.

In summary, we observe that people utilize a repertoire of five modes of territorial behavior in response to input they receive about use of space. Input about the space and the myriad of variables present in the field at a given moment is compared with the territorial schema. Behavioral output reflects the use of set behaviors if congruency is apparent or if there is a state of system tension in the event of discrepancy or inability to creatively develop a suitable and adaptive response. Successful territorial behavior provides a balance between privacy and community, satisfies the needs of security and autonomy, and promotes growth of the entire self-system. There will be evidence of stability in the aggressive–protective subsystems. Behavioral system stability is demonstrated by behavior that is purposeful, orderly and predictable, that is meaningful and effective for the individual over time, and that is responsive to environmental change. Energy expenditure for achievement of the goal is minimized.[43]

Preconditions

Territoriality becomes an inoperative behavioral pattern in the absence of certain preconditions. These include a social system that permits privacy, enough positive experience with territorial behavior to continue its use, an adequate mechanism for enculturation about norms for interaction and use of space, and finally, sufficient space to permit choice in spatial behavior.

In the United States, concern for privacy and indirectly for territory gave rise to legal documents insuring those rights; the individual's rights as opposed to society's were at issue. The following are examples of legal guarantees of privacy.

> Article IV, Bill of Rights of the US Constitution
>
> The right of the people to be secure in their persons, houses, papers and effects against unreasonable searches, seizures, shall not be violated. . . .
>
> Article V, Bill of Rights of the US Constitution
>
> . . .shall not be deprived . . . of life, liberty or property without due process of law; nor shall private property be taken for public use without just compensation.
>
> Privacy Act of 1974, Title 5, US Code, Section 552a
>
> . . .the right to privacy is a personal and fundamental right protected by the Constitution. . . . The purpose of this Act is to provide certain safeguards for an individual against invasion of personal privacy . . . which, by misuse of information, could endanger an individual's opportunity to secure emplyment, insurance and credt, and his right to du process and other legal protection. The law applies to agencies of the Federal Government and any organization under contract to the government.

The physical environment may facilitate or constrain expression of territoriality. It is known that overcrowding and social disorganization produce a higher incidence of social pathology such as delinquency, alcoholism, and divorce, as well as mental health problems such as despair, hoplessness, and aggressive behavior.[46] This disorder is at least partially related to territorial dysfunction. Overcrowding is associated with lack of opportunity for withdrawal from contact with others, lack of privacy, and friction over control of space. It violates the preconditions of accessibility of space and the potential ability to control invasion. It tends to produce irritability and insecurity. We do not know how much territory a single individual needs, whether opportunity for privacy supersedes a need for some amount of geographic space, or whether body territory alone is sufficient amount of territory.

Assessment of Territorial Behavior

It is far easier to isolate territorial behavior in the abstract than it is to meaningfully separate it from the intricate pattern of human behavior. Yet we recognize the influence of territoriality and find in its failure a source of stress and violation of need fulfillment. Assessment of territoriality is part of a thorough determination of the function of the aggressive–protective subsystem. The nurse will indirectly assess the structure of the schema, then determine whether her client finds his set congruent with the situation, whether the perequisite conditions are present, and whether the modes of territorial behavior he chooses are effective in need satisfaction. Does his behavior promote or diminish the functional capacity of the system as a whole?

The outline below may be used as a guide in an assessment of territorial behavior. It is not intended to be a rigorous, direct tool, but merely a guide that must be supplemented by astute observation of territorial behavior. In using it, the nurse must consider the stage of her relationship with the client and the location of the interaction. Territorial responses will vary depending on the degree of trust in a relationship and on whether the client is functioning in his own or the nurse's territory.

1. Territorial behavior as a function of the aggressive/protective subsystem:
   A. Observe the client's behavior as he moves in space. Where does he usually sit? Does he seek protected space? Does he approach or avoid social interaction? What modes of territorial behavior does he use? Are these usually adequate or does he show signs of threat? What is his response to invasion?
   B. What is his home territory like? Is it well marked—are the boundaries clear? What objects or areas of his surroundings seem to relate to his identity? Does the environment support independent behavior (e.g., adequate lighting)? How does he create safety in his environment? What is his neighborhood like? How much of it is familiar and used? Where are the central areas? Does he behave differently in home territory as contrasted with the public or nurse's territory?
   C. Estimate the dimensions of his body territory. What interaction distances does he seem to prefer? What cues does he use? How does he respond to closeness from the nurse? How does he respond to touch? How protective is he of his body? Does he violate other people's space?
   D. Does he define himself as a private person and what does he mean by privacy? Does he openly or reluctantly share information about himself? What are his areas of expertise, his range of social interaction, position in the community? Is he introspective and generally aware of the motivations underlying his behavior? Is he aware of the affect of his behavior on others? Does he anticipate his needs?
   E. Variables
      (1) Physiologic: mobility, sex, age, level of consciousness, sensory status, general state of health
      (2) Sociocultural/Psychologic: cultural dimensions of space, developmental state, social position, relationship to others in the interac-

tion, meaning of the situation, body image, ego state, presence of stigmata, perceived degree of vulnerability, perceived value of self

(3) Environmental: setting, density, familiarity, restrictions on mobility, presence of hazards, availability of resources

F. Preconditions: Adequate space, supportive social system, cultural norms, positive territorial experience

2. Status of other behavioral subsystems: Is behavior functional or dysfunctional? Are goals being met? If dysfunctional, could there be a secondary effect on the function of the aggressive/protective subsystem? Or is territorial dysfunction affecting the subsystem?

Assessment of territorial behavior is clearly not a direct question-and-answer process. The nurse must be alert to territorial cues in each interaction with the client so that she may modify her behavior or the situation as necessary. The cues from several interactions are organized gradually into an overall picture of the client's territorial pattern. The nurse seeks evidence that the client is able to function in his environment and95 . .3rs in a way that does not threaten him, that he is comfortable with the balance he has achieved between privacy and community, and that maladaptive behavior in another subsystem is not producing secondary effects in the aggressive–protective subsystem.

• *Client Situation 1*

Assessment

Mr. M. was a 72-year-old man, raised in England, who immigrated to the US at the age of 27 to work as a carpenter. His wife, dead now for six months, designed a home that he built in 1935 in a small neighborhood where a number of other immigrants lived. He had two sons and a daughter, all of whom were born in the house. One son was still living in the same town when Mr. M. first came to the clinic, but transfer to a new job several states away was imminent. His daughter lived about an hour away and travelled up to see her father about once every two weeks. The other son was a career military man, serving with the Mediterranean Fleet.

Mr. M. had been relatively active in his community although he described himself as "not an organization man." He had helped most of his neighbors with house additions. He belonged to the Masons and until five years ago had frequently helped out in small church projects, especially those that involved carpentry. He still went to meetings when he felt alright.

Mr. M. was visiting the clinic once a month to monitor his diabetes, which acquired a significantly less stable status since his wife's death. He required insulin daily in addition to some dietary modification. Visual acuity was diminishing gradually, but by his report it was not so bad that he couldn't manage for himself. He also showed early signs of congestive heart failure.

At a routine clinic visit in March, Mr. M. relayed to the nurse his distress over his family's desire to put him in a nursing home. They felt he could no longer care for himself adequately, especially after his son's transfer. At that time, his medical regimen included:

Medications: Digoxin 0.125 mg PO q.i.d., Lasix 40 mg PO q.i.d., KCL 10 mEq PO q.i.d., NPH Insulin 18 U SQ at 7 A.M. Diet: 5 Gm Na^+diet, 1800 calorie ADA diet.

He had been instructed in these measures and according to questioning and objective clinical data, he had been following the protocol well until his wife's death. He still kept his clinic appointments and reportedly was taking his medication, but stated that he found it difficult to maintain his diet. No one was there to share his meals and the exercise of shopping was becoming a burden. Driving a car was restricted by his deteriorating eyesight and his neighborhood had no public transportation to the store. He relied on his daughter-in-law to take him to the store when she did her own weekly shopping, an arrangement that would cease when his son moved. When the nurse called Mr. M.'s son for further details, the son expressed the family's concern for his father's safety as well as their recognition of his desire to remain in his own home. He stated that he could think of no alternatives. An appointment was made to visit Mr. M. and his family in Mr. M.'s home.

In his home, Mr. M. was relaxed, moved around confidently, and used expansive gestures to emphasize his points. He had a favorite chair and there were numerous photos of his family throughout the house. He took obvious pride in the house, showing the nurse all the handworked cabinetry and other projects he had made. The upper story appeared little used. The yard was bounded by a hedge. He got along well with his neighbors, but had special attachments to only a few of them who had been in the area as long as he had. The neighborhood had changed little since the house was built.

Mr. M. objected to a nursing home because it would mean loss of his own home, loss of privacy, and loss of independence. He declared himself to be a private man, confirming the earlier cues evident in the yard and in his preference for nonorganizational activity and interaction with only a few special people. The nurse had noticed that in the clinic he generally kept to himself, always sat at the end of a chair row, and turned his body away from others. In conversation with her, he volunteered little and sat further from her than most of her clients did. His family reported that he always puzzled through a problem by himself and insisted on at least one "quiet hour" a day to "let him think."

Analysis

The proposed move to a nursing home would probably decrease Mr. M.'s capacity to reach his goals of privacy and autonomy by altering his home territory and by decreasing his control over both home and body territory. The environment of the nursing home in his community would not permit the kind of physical privacy he desired, but would ensure his safety and prevent further nutritional imbalance. On the other hand, with help in the areas of resources and measures to counter an isolationist tendency, Mr. M. could probably maintain his home. Although he would require supervision to monitor his safety and physical health, his territorial behavior was functional at present. It was a vital force in maintaining his overall integrity and personal dignity, autonomy, and individuality even while age was slowly diminishing his power.

Plan

The goal set for Mr. M. was preservation of his capacity to function in his home territory for as long as possible. This required an environment that was safe, where resources could be secured, and where social isolation did not become excessive. The following plans were implemented:

1. Mr. M. understood the need for other people to be close by who could check in with him periodically. Rather than hire a visiting housekeeper, despite his reluctance to let strangers use his house, he decided to lease the upper story of his house. He supervised the renovation needed to convert it into an apartment. A middle-aged couple, both university professors, were found to lease the apartment and agreed to look in on Mr. M. daily as well as help with house and yard maintenance.
2. Arrangements were made with the Meals-on-Wheels program to deliver a hot meal each day. His daughter agreed to make monthly shopping trips for him. The dietician reviewed his plan and Mr. M. agreed to keep a log of his daily food intake so that the physician could be certain of insulin requirements and the nurse could monitor his nutritional status.
3. Certain changes were made in Mr. M.'s remaining portion of the house. Brighter lights were installed and furniture arranged to permit easy movement. Mr. M. directed the rearrangement, setting chair groupings and distances in accordance with his preference. Small area rugs were removed or tacked down to increase safety.
4. Mr. M. contracted with the Senior Citizen's transportation service to take him to clinic appointments and to Masonic meetings. Guided by his obvious pride and continued interest in carpentry, the nurse also arranged for him to join the high school shop teacher once a week to help students with their woodworking projects.
5. The tenants were given the nurse's clinic number to call if a problem developed with Mr. M.'s health or if they noticed any changes in behavior, especially toward increasing physical seclusion. Mr. M.'s daughter planned to call the nurse about her father's health status at least once a month.
6. Mr. M., his family and the nurse discussed the criteria they would use to evaluate the success of the plan.

A. Nutritional adequacy
B. Maintenance of present health status (fluid and electrolyte balance within normal limits, absence of signs of congestive heart failure, urine negative for sugar and no insulin reactions)
C. Ability to maintain the home with only occasional help from his daughter
D. Continued social interaction with the Lodge members or others of his choice
E. Continued mobility in his environment
F. Subjective report from Mr. M. indicating ability to function well within his environment and with others

Evaluation

Mr. M. remained in his home for three more years, comfortable with his independence and privacy. He achieved a reasonable balance in function between the affiliative and protective subsystems. The familiarity of his environment permitted greater security and greater control than he could have achieved in the nursing home, especially as his vision further deteriorated. Further, his involvement with the high school allowed him to continue work in his area of expertise, carpentry, even though his active participation was limited. His overall health remained stable and he showed no evidence of nutritional inadequacy. Mr. M. finally had to give up his hôme territory for a nursing home when he suffered a left-sided cerebral vascular accident that extensively limited his self-care capacity.

One of the most common situations involving territoriality is hospitalization of a client for a medical problem. The potential for invasion of body and psychologic territory is high in the individual who is at a further disadvantage because he is removed from his home territory. The variable of illness further alters the amount of energy available for territorial defense and limits the choice of behavior.

Shortly after his arrival in the hospital (or a clinic), the hospital staff request information from the client, much of it related to body function, lifestyle and finances, and other equally personal areas. A request for such information implies a commitment to use that data in caring for the client because the nurse is using her right of legitimate entry to gain access to psychologic territory. She should explain why the information has been requested and with whom it will be shared. The nurse must remain sensitive of her position, seeking only information needed for therapeutic purposes and consciously limiting unnecessary probing.

Occasionally, an anxious or hurt individual shares far more personal information than is necessary or than he would choose to share were he fully in control.

The nurse should structure the discussion to limit unnecessary exposure, validate which information is confidential, and record only pertinent data on the chart.[47] Embarrassment, shame, guilt, discomfort, and a sense of vulnerability may follow excessive disclosure, especially if the client is not assured of confidentiality.

Body territory is frequently invaded in the interest of health care even in the absence of illness. As strangers, health professionals would usually interact at personal or social distances, but in the capacity of nurse, we routinely enter into intimate space for the purpose of checking some bodily function. At this distance, we frequently engage in actual touch or manipulation of the client's body. But not all intrusions of body territory are inevitably stressful. Allekian's studies of hospitalized patients, although descriptive rather than experimental, showed that body territory invasions did not provoke anxiety except when personal parts of the body were involved.[48] She suggested that anticipation of physical contact reduces the threat of invasion. The individual has granted health professionals the right of legitimate entry. Roberts[49] suggests that the nurse deliberately organize herself to enter into body territory as few times as possible to accomplish her goals rather than making repeated unnecessary intrusions. This allows the client time to recover from an invasion instead of producing a situation in which the anxiety induced by a series of invasions accumulates and possibly reaches intolerable levels. When approaching the client, the nurse will temper the threat by clearly signaling her nonaggressive intent with open body position, orientation of her body to the client, verbal expression of purpose, gentle touch, and competent performance. Professional right of entry does not preclude the need to request a client's permission to invade. Control of territory thus remains with the client and his sense of vulnerability is not heightened.

Interactions in the general area of body territory are conducted at intimate and personal distances. Although variables such as level of anxiety, nature of the situation, and cultural background will affect the distance chosen, most initial interaction with clients should be conducted at social or far personal distances to avoid intrusion into body territory. Clients with sensory disturbances such as decreased visual or auditory acuity will need closer interaction distances to permit effective communication. With explanation of what she wishes to do and with permission of the client, the nurse may enter into closer range for the duration of her task, then move out again. However, for purposes of private communication with her client, personal distances are usually most appropriate because their use indicates that the client has the nurse's attention and interest.[50]

On admission, clients are assigned a room that becomes their temporary territory. The size of the physical territory claimed and the privacy available will of course vary with the number of people sharing the space and with the physical characteristics of the structure. An individual's territory may be as large as a room or as small as his bed and the space immediately surrounding it—in fact little larger than his body territory. The space is personalized with objects brought from home, with clothing or even with a name tag, and henceforth treated as the individual's own territory. The nurse should encourage such marking, especially if the intended duration of stay is likely to be greater than a few days. With regard to physical territory, the nurse's objectives are to structure the physical environment to preclude or limit invasion and to aid the client in creating a secure, identifiable temporary territory in which he has some privacy and autonomy.

Although the client may consciously accept the territory as only temporary and actually controlled by the staff of the institution, unpermitted entry by another is viewed as a territorial invasion. Rearranging objects in that territory, especially bedside or closet items, bumping the bed, entering without knocking, and failure to use screens or curtains may all be interpreted as territorial violations that indicate failure to respect the territory of that client. Allekian found a positive correlation between intrusion into a client's temporary territory and anxiety levels.[51] Clients described loss of personal control and a sense of depersonalization accompanying invasion. In effect, the client is rendered more vulnerable and is subjected to an additional stressor to which his response is likely limited by illness.

Equipment, although inanimate, may also constitute territorial invasions because its placement, use, and removal are not self-controlled. Further, it limits the space available to the client and may decrease his mobility in the space. The feeling of crowding as well as the noise intrusion accompanying operation of much of the equipment creates a problem distinct from the problem of fear and dependence on equipment. The nurse must advise her client of the purposes of the equipment, keep it as unobtrusive as possible, and remove it as soon as the need for it has ceased.

Finally, the nurse has the responsibility of orienting the client and his family to the space that will be his and to the public territories of the institution. Familiarity with the environment will augment the client's control over it, thus increasing his sense of security.*

Evaluation

In evaluating an individual's territorial behavior the nurse determines how effective the behavior is in maintaining need satisfaction even in the presence of inva-

*Several authors have described ways of arranging furniture and public space to permit or facilitate interaction and increased use of space. See Sommer, R., *The Behavioral Basis of Design*. Englewood Cliffs, N.J.: Prentice-Hall, 1966; Newcommer, R., and Caggiano, M., "Environment and the Aged Person," (see Supplementary References); and Scheflen, A., *Human Territories*.[32]

sion. Ideally, congruency of situation, schema, and set persists, or a discrepancy is resolved by evolution of new behaviors or adjustment of the schema. If her efforts to support the client's territorial behavior have succeeded, the nurse will find evidence of behavioral system stability.

Manifestations of failure to adequately respond to invasion or compensate for loss of territory require that the nurse reassess the situation and plan strategies to counter the dysfunction. Most of us experience invasion quite frequently. The symptoms are transient and resolved quickly with a suitable territorial response. The sustained presence of symptoms of invasion coupled with general evidence of a stress response indicate that the client's usual territorial behavior is either inappropriate or overwhelmed by the situation demands. Invasion may be signalled by a tense body posture, crossed arms, and inward curling of the shoulders, or an appearance of anxiety. He simply looks vulnerable. Occasionally, a client will very clearly state his wish that the nurse stay away or not touch him. The nurse may observe or even become the target of a hostile defensive maneuver, such as a thrown glass or other object. The client may appear irritated and uncomfortable in the presence of others, or with a slightly strained tone of voice request again that the curtains be pulled or the noise level lowered. He may physically back or turn away, erect a physical barrier when the nurse approaches, or choose the route of withdrawal.

Repeated invasion produces anxiety, defensiveness, anger, fatigue, a sense of depersonalization and indignity, and a general disquietude.[51a] These are obvious signs of instability in the aggressive/protective subsystem and reflect loss of privacy, autonomy, and security. Loss of territory may produce a grief response similar to the response to any loss.

Response to unrelenting threat may appear excessive or inappropriate to an observer, but reflect an increasingly desperate attempt to reduce the threat through more vigorous effort even if the modes used are indiscriminate and have little chance of success. Hostility and excessive withdrawal are two examples of behavior that can be dysfunctional and fail to resolve territorial needs.

In the context of territoriality, hostile behavior is a more forceful expression of the defense mode. Although the reason for the hostility may be legitimate, such as staff insensitivity to territorial requirements, the response is hazardous because of the threat of physical harm to self or to others and because of the intensity of sympathetic nervous activity. The sympathetic response draws energy that otherwise would be expended in repair or constructive activity elsewhere in the self-system.

Because our own culture generally proscribes open expression of hostility, the more extreme forms of anger and rage are less commonly witnessed than verbal attacks, sarcasm, argumentative or demanding behavior, or even overpoliteness and silence.[52] Internalized anger may appear as depression. A defensive response from the nurse only aggravates the client's anxiety and gives further impetus to the cycle of hostility. Responsibility for breaking the pattern lies with the nurse, who consciously controls her own defensive response and intervenes with a rational and supportive plan to discover the source of threat and modify the situation. For example, if analysis uncovers a problem of territorial invasion, the nurse must seek further data concerning frequency and intensity of invasion and variables affecting the client's response or increasing his vulnerability. Once she has discerned the dimensions of the problem, she has available a repertoire of methods for minimizing invasion and increasing a client's control over the environment and interactions within it. Uncontrolled or possibly harmful behavior must be reduced, with reasonable limits set as necessary. Other nursing strategies for handling hostile behavior are described in a number of resources.*

Individuals under severe territorial threat may overuse the mode of withdrawal to the point where the behavior interferes with meeting basic physiologic needs, may induce sensory deprivation, and impedes learning. In its most intense degree. withdrawal disrupts reality testing. Extreme withdrawal is unlikely in response to territorial dysfunction alone and would justify use of mental health consultants. However, significant declines in social interaction and functional capacity often follows loss of territory,[53] and invasive situations in which the individual's autonomy and security have been threatened. The nurse working with a client whose withdrawal seems related to territorial loss or invasion also must explore the situation further before deciding on a plan for intervention.

The plan will draw from a set of strategies that are designed to minimize territorial invasion and increase the client's control. Specific measures such as orientation to the environment, use of a non-threatening interaction distance[54] and continued close observation of spatial behavior may be supplemented by general strategies used in caring for withdrawn clients.

When the nurse's evaluation reveals territorial dysfunction, she proceeds to a second level assessment in which she gathers data about the source and intensity of the dysfunction, and any effects on the function of other behavioral subsystems.

Territorial Dysfunction

Territorial dysfunction may originate in the workings of the aggressive/protective subsystem or in one of the other subsystems. In the course of this section, client

*See Kiening, Sr. M., "Hostility;"[52] Lange, S., "The Violent Patient."

studies will be presented to highlight the major sources of intrasystem dysfunction.

Within the aggressive/protective subsystem, sources of territorial dysfunction include:

Constraints imposed by the physical or social environment or territorial expression
Discrepancy between the schema and the perceived situational variables
Discrepancy between the goal (privacy, autonomy, security) and set or choice of mode because of situation variables
Loss or constriction of territory

Just as a stone thrown into the water at one end of a pond produces a widening circle of ripples, a problem in one subsystem is eventually manifested in behavior of the others. Both physical and psychic energy that otherwise would be invested in the aggressive/protective subsystem is diverted to the dysfunctional system. This produces a secondary territorial dysfunction. To illustrate, suppose a person failed to sleep well for several nights. He would not achieve his restorative goal. As the problem continued, his thoughts and energy would increasingly revolve around ending his fatigue. Were his territory to be challenged by an invader at this time, his defense capacity would be attenuated by his mental and physical fatigue.

A client with a territorial dysfunction will present one of three problems: a lack of privacy, a lack of security, or a decline in autonomy. The nursing diagnosis will state which of the three needs have been violated and state the probable source of the problem, being as specific as possible. If all three needs have been breached, the diagnosis may simply read "territorial dysfunction due to . . . " Because the nurse derives her strategies from the diagnosis, the depth and precision of her analysis will directly affect the adequacy of her plan.

• *Client Situation 2: Constraints Imposed by Environment*

At 32 years of age, Mrs. W. was the mother of three preschoolers. She had been married eight years to Mr. W., a textile worker who frequently worked overtime in a mill outside of Greensboro, N.C. Mr. W.'s widowed father lived with the family because of the increasing incapacity of chronic obstructive pulmonary disease that doctors blamed on years of exposure to textile fibers. The family's relatively large trailer was located on the side of a country highway about half a mile from the nearest neighbor and beyond walking distance to the grocery store. Lacking a fence, Mrs. W. had to maintain constant surveillance over the children.

Public health service was requested for chest physiotherapy for Mr. W., whose activity was limited to the trailer. On her first visit, the nurse had to remain in her car until Mrs. W. could restrain the family's brown mutt. The dog, it was explained, was necessary to keep strangers off the property. Mrs. W. maintained a distance from the nurse of about 10 to 12 feet during this and subsequent visits to Mr. W., Sr.

Over a period of several months, Mrs. W. gradually moved in to a distance of 3 to 4 feet from the nurse and at the same time, began to share small fragments of information about herself. One day, she revealed that she found herself growing more impatient with her family, sometimes to the point of outright anger. She had smacked one child harder than she had meant to and said that she felt out of control and was very upset when it happened. Of late, she'd left the children alone in the yard to walk down the road by herself.

Assessment

Home territory The client lived in crowded trailer with physical barriers to separate personal space, but that were not useful; the trailer was personalized with many belongings, homemade items; a dog was used to defend property; there was isolation from others, no real neighborhood; noise from family members permeated entire space, interfering with sleep; the surrounding countryside was not restricted from her use except by responsibility to children; and there were no grossly unsafe features in home territory.

Body territory The client maintained fairly large body territory; she preferred the nurse to stay in front of her and kept interaction distances long; said she disliked children's clinging, constant touch; and the children were basically insensitive to nonverbal cues from their mother regarding her space.

Psychologic territory The client had little outside social interaction, had quit job when first child born; she had no time for involvement with activities she enjoyed; she did not share information about herself easily; stated she needed time to be alone, never had any privacy; she is fairly introspective person; and was concerned about her lessened control.

Territorial modes The client used a defensive mode, including force at times; there was physical withdrawal; she permitted limited entry to nurse. She experienced frequent invasion with symptoms of increasing fatigue, irritability, discomfort, decreasing control, and hostile response to children.

Variables The client is a generally healthy adult in a restricted environmental setting with several children.

Preconditions There was adequate space present in total environment but variables restricted its use.

Other subsystems The goals of affiliative, restorative, and achievement subsystems were not fully met.

Nursing diagnosis There was lack of privacy and decreased control due to close, crowded physical environment and frequent invasion of body territory. Mrs. W. experienced difficulty in all three of her territories—home, body, and psychologic. In home territory, there was no space identifiable as hers into which she could restrict entry. Privacy by means of physical seclusion was unobtainable. She could still use psychologic withdrawal, although limited by the demand to constantly monitor her children's activities. Otherwise, home territory was secure and degree of autonomy within it acceptable to her.

Invasion of body territory occurred frequently because her children stayed close, and in the environment of the trailer proximity was unavoidable. When her defenses were no longer adequate, she displayed a dysfunctional hostile response that could possibly escalate to abuse of children. The constant invasion also produced a secondary dysfunction in the restorative subsystem. Because her fatigue contributed to her inability to cope with invasion, the problem spiraled.

Psychologic territory at this point may be viewed as constricted. She had reduced the number of social connections and an area for knowledge expansion or stimulation when she quit her job. She found no time for personal, self-oriented activities. She was generally isolated from neighbors because of distance. This restriction arising in the affiliative subsystem contributed to territorial dysfunction because it isolated her in the confines of her own territories where privacy was difficult to achieve. Territorial constriction could eventually lead to diminished opportunity to reach achievement goals later resulting in decreased self-esteem.

Related diagnoses stemming from territorial dysfunction were (1) potential abuse of children due to inability to adapt to lack of privacy and frequent invasion and (2) fatigue due to impaired restorative capacity and demand to respond to territorial invasion. (Responsibilities growing out of child-rearing function may also have been a major source of fatigue).

Planning

The nurse's planning was begun with recognition of the unchangeable factor of the trailer as a residence and the children's age-related dependency that made proximity largely unavoidable. Her strategies were directed at the symptom of fatigue and increasing lack of control with the children as well as toward modification of the situation with the goals of decreasing invasion, increasing privacy, and supporting broadening of psychologic territory. The nurse developed several general objectives for herself.

1. Rule out physiologic abnormality as basis for fatigue.
2. Obtain further information on the configuration of situations impeding territorial goals or contributing to loss of control.
3. Minimize invasive activity by nurse.
4. Observe children for symptoms of abuse.
5. Support client in efforts to gain privacy and control.

Client-based objectives were:

1. Use knowledge of expected developmental behavior of children to in-

crease their involvement with self-directed activities appropriate for their age.

2. Recognize when she was particularly susceptible to loss of control. Develop means of reestablishing control.
3. Avoid abuse of children.
4. Develop plan for obtaining occasional time to be alone and engage in projects and interests of her own.
5. Obtain adequate rest to reduce fatigue.

Implementation

Working together and after much discussion with the client the following strategies were employed:

1. Physical exam and diet history. A complete blood count was drawn at the next clinic visit.
2. The client and nurse analyzed situations in which the client felt "out of control" or particularly irritable, looking for patterns preceding the symptoms. Utilized the client's introspective capacity.
3. The nurse kept personal distance or beyond, called before visiting, and explained all necessary physical invasions during clinic visits.
4. Brief physical examination of children during clinic or home visits.
5. Encouraged client's problem-solving efforts. Reassured her that control could be established and that some privacy was necessary.
6. Taught developmental sequences during Child Health Clinic visits. Helped plan activities for children and placed her in contact with Child Health worker.
7. Taught relaxation techniques as a means of rest and reducing tension.
8. Gave client Hotline number to call when she felt herself losing control with children. Frequent home visits to care for Mr. W., Sr. enabled the nurse and client to block several developing situations.
9. Client planned with neighbor for babysitting each other's children once a week. Left each woman free for a morning or afternoon. (The neighbor had a car to transport the children.)

Evaluation

There were no physiologic abnormalities to account for fatigue except a slightly low hematocrit, corrected with iron tablets and moderate dietary changes. Mrs. W. gradually began to recognize a pattern of personal fatigue, loneliness, bad weather, premenstrual tension, or a child's illness as preceding periods when it was more difficult to control her response to their invasion. She had called the Hotline number twice, and was afterwards successful in reducing tension and repatterning the situation to increase her control. There was never evidence of physical abuse of the children. She was unable to use the relaxation techniques effectively to control her tension when she "needed more space," but stated that she fell asleep more easily when she incorporated them into her bedtime ritual. She used games and projects that kept the older children's attention when they became "too clingy." She discovered that the children usually had a quiet period about 2:30 to 3:00 P.M. At that time, she could leave the children with her father-in-law for work in the yard or to go for a short walk alone. Of course, as they grew and became more independent, their invasiveness declined proportionately.

Mrs. W. and her neighbor continued the babysitting arrangement. Although Mrs. W. used her free time for housework and rarely for seeing friends or for personal projects, she said that she felt more relaxed after her private time. She reported generally less fatigue and irritability.

The nurse observed no symptoms of invasion during her interaction with the client.

• *Client Situation 3: Discrepancy Between Situational Variables and Schema*

Ms. K. was a junior nursing student on student visa to the United States from a Near Eastern country. She readily mastered the technical procedures required of her, showed reasonable clinical judgment, and could describe the framework of interpersonal relations. She was handicapped only slightly by her level of English mastery. Yet, she repeatedly experienced difficulty in communicating with clients and occasionally with her peers. Her interviewing technique, although not polished, clearly incorporated the basic principles of communication. Her clients stated that they felt uncomfortable with her, but that she was gentle and competent. Ms. K. also expressed discomfort as well as dismay because she had not experienced such difficulty when she worked as an aide in her own country.

The discussion of her experiences at home began to reveal what process recordings and tapes had not, that incongruous nonverbal behavior might be the problem rather than faulty verbal interaction. The instructor arranged to be present during several sessions when Ms. K. planned to teach clients about some aspects of their health problem. In each session, she focused her attention on nonverbal behavior. Her observation revealed the following:

With respect to the client's geographic territory, Ms. K. always knocked before entering and remembered to pull the curtains; but before leaving she would straighten the room, including rearranging the client's personal items on the overbed table or bedside stand.

Ms. K. frequently invaded the client's body territory. She habitually stood or sat within two feet of the client even when the rooms were uncrowded. She failed to inform the client when touch was needed to carry out a procedure. Touch was a constant feature of her interactions and she did not recognize clients' cues of territorial invasion.

She used her right of legitimate entry appropriately. Clients were told why certain information was needed and who would share knowledge of it. She did not probe indiscriminately and effectively used her knowledge of the client's occupation, interests, and skill in her teaching approach.

Assessment

Variables Ms. K. was of Near Eastern culture.

Analysis of Problem Clients experiencing invasion of body territory due to a cultural discrepancy between the student's and client's schema and set. The student and the clients did not share the same territorial expectations and conventions. The consequence was threat to the clients' security and autonomy overlaying the hospital and illness induced loss of autonomy. Ms. K.'s interpersonal difficulties were the result of the clients' attempts to limit invasion by either defense or withdrawal responses.

Planning The instructor's general goal was to increase Ms. K.'s understanding of territoriality. If successful, the student would:

1. Explain the concept of territoriality.
2. Describe variables affecting territorial behavior.
3. Detect manifestations of territoriality in her interactions and describe the variable operative in each.
4. Detect nonverbal cues of invasion and utilize techniques to minimize invasion.

Implementation The instructor guided Ms. K. in her study of territoriality by using the following strategies:

1. Ms. K. and her classmates were given several clinical situations to simulate. The instructor videotaped the interactions and then used the tapes to explore the students' use of space. She had deliberately avoided telling the students that she would be focusing on territorial behavior.
2. After their discussion, the students experimented with various interaction distances and explored the dimensions of each other's body territory.
3. The students were given a bibliography on territoriality.
4. Ms. K. was asked to role play interviews with clients using space as a variable.
5. After several weeks of clinical experience during which Ms. K. had observed client's territorial behavior and used her knowledge in interaction, she was asked to write a brief essay comparing territorial behavior as she saw it expressed in the United States and in her own country.

Evaluation During the semester, Ms. K. and the clients reported more comfortable and satisfactory interactions. The instructor observed fewer incidences of violation of either temporary or body territory. Most of the mistakes occurred when Ms. K. was unsure of a new task or when the situation was more ambiguous. Ms. K. could usually identify situational variables and was alert to territorial cues. She seemed to have internalized territoriality as one aspect of nursing care.

• *Client Situation 4: Discrepancy Between Goal and Choice*

Mr. Q., 29 years of age, was admitted to a neuro/orthopedic unit for a laminectomy required probably because of degenerative disk changes at the L_5–S_1 level, the result of a severe automobile accident nine years earlier. The physician elected to try a conservative approach of traction and physical therapy before resorting to surgery.

Mr. Q. was cautioned to avoid releasing traction, but had been found doing so in order to use the commode. He also had a roommate, supposedly in neck traction, who often got up and went over to talk to Mr. Q., speaking frequently of his anger at the staff and at his friends and what he planned to do "to get back at them."

Mr. Q. was uncomfortable in the presence of the staff, especially those who had to come close to him for some technical activity. Even when no technical activity was planned, he often became slightly diaphoretic, kept his arms or bedside table in front of him (between himself and staff), narrowed his eyes very slightly, and almost imperceptibly moved to the far side of the bed. His muscles were always more tense when staff approached. He jokingly chastized several of the staff for suddenly appearing in his room, clearly referring to their failure to knock. He was very pleasant to the staff and did not share his discomfort with anyone but his wife. He revealed little about himself to the staff to the point where they complained to each other that they didn't know him enough to care for him.

When he finally did undergo surgery, he described the experience of recovering from anesthesia as most frightening. As he recovered consciousness, he was aware of people around him; he was especially aware of their hands touching him and he described an intense feeling of threat. He felt that he was unable to determine their purpose, that they were violating his territory, and possibly meant him harm. He described himself as needing security and privacy, which he endeavored to guarantee by maintaining strict control over the space around him.

Assessment

Mr. Q. sent the staff many nonverbal messages about his territory which unfortunately they failed to receive.

Temporary territory The staff did not acknowledge its existence by their behavior; territory was frequently invaded; the client shared geographic space of his room with another patient; he personalized territory with books and papers; he wanted to keep curtain marking his boundary drawn, but his roommate persistently opened it; and he was in unfamiliar environment.

Body territory He was quite large; he adjusted position if a nurse moved closer to him than three feet; he kept people in line of vision as much as possible; increased muscle tension, arm position, etc., indicated attempt to block invasion; he was threatened by touch, and more defensive when in pain.

Psychologic territory He had a broad range of knowledge; he was well-educated; he shared little about himself; he described himself as private person, and was introspective.

Territorial modes The client used defense, limited entry, withdrawal, expansion (frequently requested information about physiology and medical care of the disk; physical expansion and psychologic expansion were limited by injury).

Variables The client was male; he had decreased mobility because of pain and traction; he was on medication and in hospital setting.

Preconditions No alteration.

Nursing diagnosis

Territorial dysfunction (decreased autonomy, privacy, security) due to discrepancy between protective goal and choice (limited by variable of illness) of response to invasion and reduced territory. Mr. Q. placed much importance on protection of territory. His injury, hospitalization, and therapy conspired to necessitate territorial invasion while simultaneously subverting his ability to use territorial modes that protected him. The nursing staff in this case simply were not aware of or did not apply their knowledge of territorial behavior.

Territoriality and Illness

Earlier in this chapter, the variable of illness was purposefully excluded in order to isolate the operation of territorial behavior in admission to an institution. It will now be presented and its effects analyzed.

In the presence of illness, the body's total physical energy supply is depleted and much of the remaining supply is diverted into healing and regulatory processes. The behavioral subsystem affected by illness becomes dominant with respect to the other subsystems. The physical energy available for maintenance of territory is thus diminished. Withdrawal and permission for access are the most common modes of territorial behavior during illness, both of which indicate decreased energy investment in territory.

With little empirical data about the relationship between territory and physical energy, the psychic energy investment in territory will be discussed. Illness produces obvious diversions of psychic energy away from territorial acquisition and fortification—in fact usually away from concern about all but the physical self which is the center of body territory. Territory outside of the self loses its importance temporarily. However, the individual with a chronic health problem or one that seriously affects his functional capacity could face loss or restriction of home territory and constriction of psychologic territory. Their loss will affect that individual's capacity to use territory as a means of access to security, autonomy, and privacy. When there has been an acute problem and recovery occurs, energy is once again invested in territory and more defensive responses can be expected.

The specific effects of illness depend on the type or degree of illness. Because of decreased mobility, as with pain, injury, or required bed rest, or because of communicable disease, an individual may be confined to his home territory or find hospitalization necessary. As he recognizes the limitations of illness or treatment and discovers the vulnerability of his body, that threat becomes more real. If weak or immobilized, he has difficulty in orienting himself to his territory, establishing its boundaries, or modifying it to meet his needs.[55] His defense capacity is also decreased. Verbal and nonverbal action, although the most common means of defense, suddenly seems far less potent when the potential for physical defense or flight is withdrawn. The client is both vulnerable and dependent.

As illness increases in severity, there is a concommittent loss of privacy and autonomy as the number, frequency, and duration of invasion increases, and as health professionals exert more and more external control in an effort to stem the illness. Clearly, conscious individuals in this state usually place priority on survival and trustingly grant territorial entry rights to health professionals. The Alekian study cited earlier supports this. Nevertheless, at this degree of illness, intrusions into body territory usually involve private areas and invasive procedures and such invasions are anxiety provoking. The client's protective goal conflicts with the need for dependency. The nurse's awareness of territoriality will cause her to limit invasion by herself and others, support the client's protective behavior by creating a milieu that offers safety and some autonomy, and thus will reduce a source of unnecessary energy expenditure.

Mr. Q. would have suffered less distress had the staff recognized his territorial needs. Simple courtesies such as knocking before entering would have changed a threatening invasion to a permitted entry, a far less stressful situation. Use of social or personal interaction distances for most occasions, organization of tasks to decrease the number of invasions, respect for his privacy, and at least verbal orientation to the larger space outside his room would help to alleviate his vulnerability.

• *Client Situation 5: Loss of Territory*

Eighty-six-year old Mr. H. was forced to enter a home for the elderly because he could no longer afford upkeep and property payments on the home he had lived in for 40 years. The house was small, but he no longer had the energy to maintain it. His health was good, with only occasional bouts with gout and a significant decrease in hearing not fully compensated by his hearing aid.

He had never married and no relatives lived nearby. When he decided to move, he had called several apartment houses that were advertised for the elderly and found one that was inexpensive enough, but that still had good security services. The management also offered a transportation service that he could use for clinic and shopping trips or visits to the senior citizen center he frequented. He was unfamiliar with the section of town in which the building was located, but understood it to be a nice neighborhood.

Mr. H. had been fairly active while still in his own home. He gardened, read, and often walked around the neighborhood or to the stores. At the senior citizen center, he found good talk on politics and sports (despite his hearing difficulty), and an occasional game of bocci ball.

After moving, he found it hard to meet new people. Many of the other residents stayed in their apartments and the building's lobby had only a few chairs arranged along the walls. The neighborhood was more different and seemed less secure than he had expected. He made fewer trips to the senior citizen center, where his friends found him somewhat tense and unhappy. He made less effort to hear them and eventually participated very little in conversations. He ate less and complained of more minor physical problems. He became far less active.

The nurse he regularly saw at the clinic noticed the change. Mr. H. told her that he just couldn't get used to the new apartment; it was like a hotel rather than a home. He was lonely and missed his old familiar neighborhood.

Assessment

Home territory It was an unfamiliar, less secure (in his perception) neighborhood; the apartment was also unfamiliar; protective service was available; there was poor physical arrangement for interaction with others (fostered anonymity of residents); he did not share the apartment so had access to physical privacy; he told the clinic nurse the apartment had come furnished so he had sold most of his furniture; he called his residence "the apartment."

Body territory There was no sign of discomfort until the nurse or another person was closer than about one foot (probably to facilitate hearing); he used touch occasionally to emphasize a point but generally did not violate other's territory; he kept large distance from strangers; he disliked approach from side (again probably related to decreased auditory acuity).

Psychologic territory There was a decrease in social contacts and general interest in people and environment; he complained of loneliness.

Territorial modes There were limited defense activities; withdrawal was beginning to be excessive, resulting in decreased nutrition and affiliation, possible depression, loneliness, tension, and constriction of psychologic territory.

Variables Age, slightly decreased mobility secondary to gout and age, arrangement of apartment environment, and poor auditory acuity.

Preconditions No alteration.

Other subsystems Ingestive and affiliative goals not met.

Nursing diagnosis

Decreased security and autonomy due to loss of territory. Related diagnoses were (1) excessive withdrawal due to diminished capacity to develop a new territory; (2) loneliness due to altered affiliation patterns (withdrawal, environment and removal from known neighborhood); and (3) decreased nutrition due to excessive withdrawal.

Mr. H.'s familiarity with his old territory afforded him some protection, an advantage over those who did not know the area so well. His neighbors had been friends, ready to help if necessary. Despite his age, he had moved with relative impunity in that well-known and predictable territory. Once he had moved, he felt the loss of his home and with it some of his identity and was forced to established a new territory. He was overwhelmed by the task, was not successful, and tried to compensate for his vulnerability by withdrawing. His options were limited and the withdrawal became dysfunctional.

Planning

Age was an unchangeable factor; nor could the client return to his former home. The nurse's activity would have to be directed toward alleviation of the symptoms by supporting Mr. H.'s attempt to establish a new home territory. Further evaluation of his home situation was needed. The following behaviors would indicate progress in resolution of territorial dysfunction. He would:

1. Begin to refer to the apartment as home and would increasingly personalize it.
2. Resume former activities commensurate with level of health (e.g., walk around neighborhood, visit senior center and engage in conversation as formerly) and decrease complaints of loneliness.
3. Manifest no further nutritional deficit.
4. Evidence continued desire to care for self and maintain capacity for independent living.

Strategies

The nurse implemented several strategies, using a social worker as a resource person.

1. She referred the client to social worker for evaluation of the building and the apartment as well as for advising Mr. H. of community programs for senior citizens. From the environmental evaluation, the nurse learned that the apartment was well lighted and adequately furnished, but almost totally lacking in any personal effects. They had been left in a large box in a storage room of the building. The public spaces of the building provided few environmental arrangements that would facilitate interaction among the residents.
2. The social worker and the public health nurse who served that district agreed to organized a group in Mr. H.'s building, which Mr. H. agreed to

attend. Their focus was self-care and included discussion of the environment. A secondary effect was the opportunity to meet other residents.

3. With the nurse's suggestion, Mr. H. decided to put up his pictures after all. His chair and a few lamps that had been stored were brought up and exchanged with the building's furniture.
4. A diet history was taken and Mr. H. was counselled by a dietician about low cost, easily prepared meals. He also decided to eat at the senior citizens center a few times each week.
5. The nurse spent a few minutes with him during clinic visits talking about his new home and neighborhood.

Evaluation

Mr. H. was beginning to work through the loss of his former home. He did put up his pictures and mementos and reported that "the place felt better." Because of his membership in the group, he began to know people in his building and through them the neighborhood became more familiar and less threatening. As his apartment gradually developed into home territory, Mr. H. began to increase his level of activity. His use of withdrawal gradually decreased but he never reached his previous level. His demeanor revealed a man of less assurance and less outgoing personality.

His nutritional status did not deteriorate further. He occasionally shared meals with new acquaintances. With the help of some city programs for the elderly, Mr. H. was able to maintain his independent status.

Addendum

Stimulated by Mr. H.'s situation, the nurse and the social worker suggested a few simple environmental changes to the building manager, explaining the need for social interaction. Chairs in the lobby were rearranged in small groupings instead of being lined along the wall. Larger apartment-identifying plaques were installed gradually and more lighting was used in the halls. The changes resulted in increased use of the common areas, decreased isolation of residents, and reports of better security.

Summary

Research is needed to clarify the range of behavior subsumed by or related to territoriality. What motivations truly underlie it; what are the cognitive processes involved? Is the basic pattern a genetically ordered one and/or a learned one? How does spatial behavior proceed developmentally? How may territoriality as a concept be more meaningfully applied to the cognitive domain of ideas, values, and opinions?[56] What is the extent of influence of territoriality on social organization? How much does autonomy and security depend on it? How strong a force is territoriality? Is there a relationship to electrodynamic fields and if so, what variables affect it? What tools can be used to validly and systematically measure territoriality? How much territory does a person need?

Nurses cannot afford to ignore the territorial force and treat space as a static enclosure. We cannot divorce ourselves from it nor understand behavior without considering the field of variables that includes space. It molds us while we change it. Each of us patterns space into territories in the process of trying to meet the needs of privacy, security, and autonomy. Yet, we have not operationalized the concept in daily nursing practice. We frequently work with clients who have lost territory or whose illness alters their territorial expression. The elderly and people who live in crowded or restricted settings are particularly vulnerable to territorial disorder. We make home visits, interact with clients in clinics, hospitals, or other institutions and often come away with less than success, but fail to consider whether a territorial invasion might underlie the poor result. Territoriality is clearly a behavioral pattern for nurses to explore and use as they give nursing care.

References

1. Edney JJ: Human Territoriality. Psychol Bull 81: 960, 1974
2. Ardrey R: The Territorial Imperative. New York, Dell, 1966, p 3
3. Sundstrom E, Altman I: Relationships between dominance and territorial behavior: A field study in a youth rehabilitation setting. From Edney, op cit, p 961
4. Pastalan LA: Privacy as an expression of human territoriality. In Pastalan LA, Carson DH (eds), Spatial Behavior of Older People. Ann Arbor, University of Michigan Press, 1970, p 4
5. Sarwer-Foner GJ: On human territoriality. A contribution to instinct theory. Can Psychiatr Assoc J 17: (Suppl) 2:55, 175, 1972
6. Altman I: Territorial behavior in humans: An analysis of the concept. In Pastalan LA, Carson DA (eds), Spatial Behavior of Older People. Ann Arbor University of Michigan Press, 1970, p 8
7. Auger JR: Behavioral Systems and Nursing. Englewood Cliffs, N.J., Prentice-Hall, 1976, pp 33–86
8. Maslow AH: Motivation and Personality, 2nd ed. New York, Harper & Row, 1970, p 39
9. Ardrey R.: op cit, p 48
10. Sarwer-Foner GJ: op cit, p 169
11. Colman AD: Territoriality in man: A comparison of behavior in home and hospital. Am J Orthopsychiatr 38: 464–68, 1968
12. Horowitz M: Body buffer zones: Exploration of personal space. Arch Gen Psychiatr 11:651–655, 1964

12a. Shaw M: Group Dynamics: The Psychology of Small Group Behavior. New York, McGraw-Hill, 1971, p 126
13. Heald F: Treatment of obesity in adolescence. Postgrad Med 51:110, May, 1972
14. Horowitz M: op cit, p 655
15. Hall E: The Silent Language. Garden City, N.Y., Doubleday, 1959, p 97
16. Hall E: The Hidden Dimension. Garden City, N.Y., Doubleday, 1966, pp 113–125
17. Horowitz M: Human spatial behavior. Am J Psychother 19:27, 1965
18. Pederson D, Shears L: A review of personal space research in the framework of general system theory. Psychol Bull 80: 370, 1973
19. Sommer R, Becker F: Territorial defense and the good neighbor. J Pers Soc Psychol 11: 88–89, 1969
20. Fried M, DeFazio V: Territoriality and boundary conflicts in the subway. Psychiatry 37: 53, February, 1974
21. Edney J: op cit, pp 964–965
22. Hein EC: Communication in Nursing Practice. Boston, Little, Brown, 1973, p 109
23. Ibid, p 112
24. Proshansky HM, Ittleson WH, Rivlin LG: Freedom of choice and behavior in a physical setting. In Proshansky HM, Ittleson WH, Rivlin LG (eds), Environmental Psychology. New York, Holt, 1970, p 180
25. Westin AF: Privacy and Freedom. New York, Atheneum, 1967, p 35
26. Fischer C: Privacy as a profile of authentic consciousness. Humanitas 11: 27–43, February, 1975
27. Lorenz K: On Aggression. New York, Bantam, 1969, pp 23–48
28. Sommer R: Man's proximate environment. J Soc Issues 22:61, 1966
29. Evans G, Howard R: Personal space. Psychol Bull: 80:335, 1973
30. Fisher S: Sex differences in body perception. Psychol Monogr 78:21, 1964
31. Evans G, Howard R: op cit, p 337
32. Scheflen A: Human Territories. How We Behave in Space–Time. Englewood Cliffs, N.J, Prentice Hall, 1976, pp 90–91
33. Duke M, Nowicki S: A new measurement and social learning model for interpersonal distance. J Exper Res Personal 6:126
34. Sommer R: op cit, p 69
35. Shaw M: op cit, p 129
36. Schuster EA: Privacy, the patient and hospitalization. Soc Sci Med 10:248, May, 1976
37. Montagu A: Touching: The Human Significance of the Skin. New York, Columbia University Press, 1971, p 248–250
38. Meisels M, Dosey M: Personal space, anger, arousal, and psychological defense. J Personal 39:340, September, 1971
39. Little K: Personal space. J Exper Soc Psychol 1:241, 1965
40. Fisher S, Cleveland S: Body Image and Personality, 2nd ed. New York, Dover, 1968, p 355
41. Fried M, DeFazio V: op cit, pp 52–54
41a. Sommer R, Becker F: Territorial defense and the good neighbor. J Personal Soc Psych. 111:88–89, 1969
41b. Becker F: Study of spatial markers. J Personal Soc Psychol 26:440–45, June, 1973
42. Hall E.[16]: op cit, p 97
43. Becker F: op cit, p 442

44. Lyman S, Scott M: Territoriality: A neglected social dimension. Soc Prob 15:246, 1967
45. Rogers ME: An Introduction to the Theoretical Basis of Nursing. Philadelphia, Davis, 1970, p 51
46. Graham H, Gurr T: Violence in America: Historical and Comparative Perspectives. New York, Bantam, 1969, p 758
47. Smith D.: Patienthood and its threat to privacy. Am J Nurs 69:509-13, March, 1969
48. Allekian C: Intrusions of territory and personal space: An exploratory study of anxiety-inducing factors in hospitalized patients. Intern J Psychiatr Med 5: 37–38, 1974
49. Roberts SL: Behavioral Concepts and the Critically Ill Patient. Englewood Cliffs, N.J., Prentice-Hall, 1976, p 269
50. Ibid, p 271
51. Allekian C: Intrusion of territorial and personal space. Nurs Res 22:240–241 May/June, 1973
51a. Felipe, NJ, Sommer, R: Invasion of personal space. Soc Prob 14: 213, 1966
52. Kiening M Sr: Hostility. In Carlson C (ed), Behavioral Concepts and Nursing Intervention. Philadelphia, Lippincott, 1970, p 194
53. Lieberman M: Psychological effects of institutionalization. J Gerontol 23: 343–353, July, 1968
54. Engebretson D: Human territorial behavior: The role of interactional distances in therapeutic interventions. Am J Orthopsychiatr 43: 111, January, 1973
55. Roberts SL: op cit, p 263
56. Edney JJ: op cit, p 973

Supplementary References

Block D: Privacy. In Carlson C (ed), Behavior Concepts and Nursing Intervention. Philadelphia, Lippincott, 1970, pp 251–268

Fast J: Body Language. New York, Evans, 1970

Minckley B: Space and place in nursing care. Am J Nurs 68: 510–516, March, 1968

Newcomer RJ, Caggiano MA: Environment and the Aged Person. In Burnside IM (ed), New York, McGraw–Hill, 1976, chap 39

———: Understanding hostility. AJN Programmed Instruction. 67: 2131-2150, October, 1967

Lange S: The Violent Patient. ANA Clinical Sessions, 1966. New York, Appleton-Century-Crofts, 1967, pp 54–60

Chapter Four •

The Need for Air

Sister Loretta Spotila

Air is an element essential for well-being: yet it is often taken for granted by the healthy person. For the person who is ill, obtaining air can become a matter of basic survival. In this chapter, the client will be discussed in terms of both healthy* and illness states, with a demonstration of how the nursing process is used to meet his need for air.

The Healthy Person

Assessing the Need for Air

Assessment is the first step of the nursing process and involves a review of the client situation to obtain data that will enable the nurse to identify health-related problems.[1] Using observation, perception, and communication skills, the nurse

*The term *healthy* is used in reference to the need for air and could apply to the client in any setting; e.g., the client hospitalized with a nonrespiratory ailment, as well as the client outside the hospital setting.

secures information by interviewing the client and/or significant others, by conducting a physical examination and by reviewing data already recorded. To establish a data base, the nurse reviews the client's past health history, his present physical, psychologic, and emotional status, his pattern of daily living, and his family and home situation.

A basic framework within which the interview is to be conducted is necessary for the systematic collection of data. Often, the experienced nurse had compiled her own list of factors to be included in assessment. Today, however, there are increasing demands on the nurse and a growing recognition of the importance of quality care for all clients. As a result, many health care facilities have developed nursing history forms to facilitate data collection and assessment. The nursing history should be obtained on the client's admission or as soon as possible thereafter. The nurse sets a specific time and place for an admission interview with the client to obtain the necessary information. She uses her professional skills to make the client feel at ease during the interview process. Because of the differences in every individual client's degree of illness and immediate needs, the nurse needs to be flexible in the assessment process and adapt the interview to each client's situation.

To relate the process of assessment to the healthy client's need for air, the factors that produce the best air input for survival will be considered. In order to define what is expected, required, and necessary to meet one's need for air, the discussion will concentrate on knowledge that the nurse needs in four major areas. First is the air itself—its functions and its components: second, the physical structures necessary for breathing; and third, the physiologic mechanisms involved in breathing. The fourth major area concerns the client himself—his individual characteristics, background, and personal concerns.

The Air Itself

Few of us could dispute the fact that air is a basic human need. It is valuable and taken for granted; it is one of the most used and perhaps one of the most abused of our natural resources. Air is the breath of life; this essential is usually maintained by automatic body processes.

From the perspective of health care givers, air is usually defined as somcthing necessary for breathing—for respirations. It is this need that will be emphasized throughout the chapter. Air is needed for the gas exchange process that is vital to life. In respiration oxygen is taken in and carbon dioxide given off; air acts as a reservoir for both. Yet, if the need for air is truly to be filled, a consideration of the many other functions that air has in our life and in our environment is necessary.

In addition to permitting respiration, air distributes moisture, transmits odors, insulates the earth, filters various sun rays, and effects the weather. Because of these functions, air provides the temperature and humidity necessary for human life; it serves as protection, especially for the skin, from dangerous sun rays, transmits pleasant and unpleasant odors, and enables us to communicate sounds to one another. The communication of sound highlights some of the more specific functions of air and breathing. The air we breathe enables us to talk, sing, whistle, laugh, cry, and play a musical instrument. In this way, it helps us not only to communicate but also to both give and receive pleasure, to develop talents, and strengthen self-esteem. Therefore, the need for air extends beyond the physiologic to needs that are psychologic and social in nature.

Air, or the atmosphere surrounding the earth, has two major components. Air is most often and simply classified either as a gas, such as oxygen, carbon dioxide, and even carbon monoxide, or a non-gas. The non-gases, or particulates—a word now frequently heard in the daily weather reports, are the solid particles and liquid droplets found in the air. For example, dust, soot, pollen, lead, and other minerals, water vapor, and aerosol products are particulates. However, for the purpose of specifically relating it to health, air can be divided into its natural components and its manmade components. The natural components of air are the mixture of gases (oxygen, nitrogen, carbon dioxide, argon), water vapor, and contaminants from sources in nature such as pollen and forest fires. The manmade components, those considered contaminants and pollutants, can be either gaseous or particulate in nature.

Gaseous pollutants include carbon oxides, sulfur compounds, nitrogen oxides, hydrocarbons, and ozone. The major source of these pollutants is the burning of gas, coal, and oil for heat and power. This includes the use of transportation vehicles, power plants, industrial processes necessary for manufacturing, and solid waste disposal. Particulates that pollute the air include smoke, fumes, dust and soot, mist and aerosols, infectious organisms, elements such as lead, beryllium, and asbestos, and the poisons of pesticides, herbicides, and insecticides. The sources of most of these pollutants are fuel combustion and industrial processes, agricultural processes, and spraying and use of aerosols.

The Physical Structures for Respirations

Respiration is a complex process accomplished by the coordination of a number of body functions and body parts. Air is inhaled as a result of excursions of the rib cage and the diaphragm, as well as changes in the size of the airway passages. As the thoracic cavity volume increases and decreases, the lungs expand and contract, with air flow determined by the degree of chest expansion. This movement can also be influenced by body position, abdominal distention, limited diaphragmatic movement, and poor muscle coordination and power.

The movement of air through the respiratory tract to and from the lungs is known as ventilation. When air is breathed in, it travels through the nose, pharynx, and larynx, which filter, humidify, and warm it. From here, the air continues through the trachea, right and left main bronchi, lobar and segmental bronchi, bronchioles, and eventually to the gas exchanging units in the lungs. These units consist of the alveolar ducts, alveolar sacs, and millions of alveoli.

The patency and flexibility of all these structures are essential for air intake and are maintained by tissue function. With the exception of the partially bony structure of the nose, the tissues of the respiratory structures are cartilaginous and muscular in nature. Alveolar patency is maintained by surfactant, a lipoprotein substance produced by the alveolar cells. Pulmonary surfactant reduces alveolar surface tension and equalizes alveolar pressure during inspiration and expiration, thereby preventing alveolar collapse. Other factors that help to maintain airway patency, as well as serve as the defense mechanisms of the lungs, are the cilia, mucus secreting cells, and rich blood supply that line much of the respiratory tract. The mucus lining moistens and filters out from the air particulates such as dust and bacteria. The cilia constantly sweep the mucus to the oropharynx to be expectorated or swallowed. In the alveoli, phagocytic mechanisms ingest materials and microorganisms to keep the lower airway sterile. The cough reflex, stimulated anywhere in the respiratory tract, enables removal of mucus secretions and particles.

Physiology of Respirations

Regulation of breathing is normally automatic and controlled by neurologic and chemical processes. The respiratory center in the midbrain, together with peripheral chemoreceptors, is responsible for the transmission of neural activity, response to chemical changes in the blood (e.g., arterial oxygen tension and arterial blood pressure), and the rhythmicity of respiration. Although voluntary control of breathing occurs in the cerebral cortex, one's spontaneous respiratory activity will eventually adjust the rate and depth of respirations to meet oxygen needs.

Effective respiration involves not only ventilation but also adequate alveolar perfusion and diffusion. Perfusion is the pulmonary blood flow through the alveolar capillaries. Pulmonary circulation is traced from the right ventricle of the heart, to the pulmonary artery, through the pulmonary arterioles, capillaries and venules, and back through the pulmonary veins to the left atrium. The effectiveness of this circulation depends on cardiac output, the integrity of the pulmonary blood vessels, and the pressures and resistances within the pulmonary system.

Diffusion, or the actual gas exchange process, occurs in the pulmonary unit. The exchange of oxygen and carbon dioxide takes place across the alveolar–capillary membranes and the rate of exchange is influenced by the integrity of the diffusion pathway. For example, oxygen molecules cross the alveolar linings of surfactant and fluid, the alveolar membrane itself, through the interstitial space, across the capillary membrane, and into the red blood cell to combine with hemoglobin. If any component of this pathway is defective, then the diffusion process as a whole is impeded. In addition to the diffusion pathway, the amount of surface area available for diffusion, the pressure gradients of the gases, and the degree of blood flow and air intake also influence the rate of the diffusion process.

Individual Factors

A number of individual factors are important in data collection. The client's age, especially in regard to the phase of growth and development, is significant. The aging process affects lung structure and breathing processes and must especially be considered in the elderly person. The type and length of occupational experiences should be taken into account, especially if the person works in an environment with a high concentration of air and chemical pollutants.

The client's psychosocial and economic background must be considered. Current and past places of residence and travel experience should be reviewed because problems stemming from environmental pollution may be present. Also, one's financial ability to provide a nutritional diet and a clean, well-ventilated, temperature-controlled environment may influence data interpretation. The client's outlook on life and his personal goals, independence in living and self-care ability, degree of motivation and self-esteem, his role within the family, and his interest in socializing and in leisure activities should also be considered in order to effectively assess his needs. The client's own personal concerns and his emotional state will greatly influence his needs and response to treatments and must be included in the assessment process.

Summary

To assess the need for air in the healthy client, the nurse considers three physiologic areas: the air itself, the status of the client's respiratory structures, and the status of his respiratory mechanisms. In addition, the client's age, occupation, socioeconomic background, home environment, and personal goals and concerns are considered.

Understanding the data collected in these areas and viewing the client as an individual, the nurse can identify whether or not there are problems requiring nursing intervention. After reviewing and organizing the data, the nurse analyzes it and determines the client's strengths and his needs or problem areas, as well as any potential problems.

With specific reference to the healthy client and his need for air, the following factors have been selected as examples for discussion throughout the remainder of this chapter. The fulfillment of the healthy client's need for air requires the presence of:

The air itself

1. Clean air in the immediate environment
2. An environment conducive to well-being
3. A method of verbal communication with others

The respiratory structures

4. Maintenance of protective mechanism of lungs
5. Intact structures
6. Patent airway

Respiratory physiology

7. Optimum breathing movement
8. Optimum energy level
9. Systemic and pulmonary tissue perfusion
10. Optimum exchange of oxygen and carbon dioxide

Individual needs

11. Independence in self-care
12. Optimum self-esteem and positive outlook on life
13. Financial stability to provide optimum living situation
14. Maintenance of role in family/social structure

Clean air with a minimal amount of pollutants is obviously first on this list; the remaining factors are related to physiologic, psychologic and socioeconomic aspects of the client's status. Assessment of the client according to this list will indicate either that no problems exist or that there are deficits requiring nursing intervention. If all required factors are present and no problem is identified, the nurse supports and reinforces the client's health behaviors by various strategies. These strategies, or methods of maintaining the client's healthy status, will be discussed in the following section on planning.

Planning for Need Fulfillment

Planning is the second phase of the nursing process. It begins after the nurse has identified those factors necessary for the client to maintain his healthy status. During this phase, the nurse assigns priorities to the client's identified needs and determines which ones can be met by nursing actions, by the client and/or significant others, and which can best be resolved by other health team members.[2] In addition, the nurse, together with the client, identifies long- and short-range goals and determines nursing strategies or actions necessary to support and fulfill the client's needs. These goals, at present frequently referred to as the expected outcomes of the client, are the basis for nursing care planning.[3] They take into consideration not only the client's desired physical state but also his emotional state and personal concerns. The goals, or client outcomes, should be stated in behavioral terms so they may be more easily evaluated. For example, goals should indicate what change is expected in the client's physiologic symptoms, what activities the client should perform, and what elements of his care he is knowledgeable of and should be able to verbalize.

The actions identified should be clear and concise, purposeful, and relevant to the client situation. It is also helpful for optimum client outcomes if the nurse who has collected the data and identified the problems or needs initiates the nursing care plan. It is most likely that this nurse best knows the client and has rapport with him and his family. This nurse–client relationship fosters communication throughout the hospital stay and can result in more effective nursing care planning. It is important to note here that the nurse plans nursing care measures to either maintain the client's current health status or to correct deficits. She also anticipates future needs and plans preventive nursing care measures designed to avoid potential problems or health deficits.

After the client goals and nursing actions are identified, it is essential that they be recorded on the nursing care plan in a concise, clearly stated manner. The care plan should be readily available to all the staff and used as a guide on a day-to-day basis to assure continuity of care.

Utilizing the data base established during assessment, the nurse employs certain actions to assure fulfillment of the healthy client's need for air. For the purposes of discussion, the actions identified are designed specifically for the client in the hospital setting. They are intended as examples of nursing strategies and are not considered a complete care plan for the client's needs.

Table 4.1 lists the factors necessary for the fulfillment of the client's need for air and the nursing strategies planned to meet this need. As illustrated in this table, many of the nursing strategies that have been identified are applied to several different factors. In writing a nursing care plan, it is helpful for the nurse to determine if there are common elements in the problems identified and then to design general, or standard, nursing actions applicable to similar problems.

To promote an environment conducive to the client's health, comfort, and safety, the nurse can employ simple measures that are very often forgotten in the midst of highly sophisticated and technical hospital care. These basic measures may prevent the occurrence of serious health problems in the client already hospitalized with other health deficits.

Table 4.1 *Nursing Care Plan for the Healthy Client*

Factors for Need Fulfillment	Nursing Strategies
1. Clean air in immediate environment	1. A. Discourage smoking (emotional support for ex-smokers) B. Discourage use of aerosols, sprays C. Eliminate dust D. Provide good ventilation E. Control airborne, infectious organisms (instruct to cover mouth and nose for cough and sneeze; restrict visitors with upper respiratory infections)
2. Environment conducive to well-being	2. A. Control temperature and humidity at comfortable, health-promoting level (prevent drafts, extreme hot/cold temperature, dry air) B. Minimize offensive odors C. Control noise to avoid over-/under-sensory stimulation
3. Verbal communication with others	3. A. Signal cord/system within reach B. Encourage socialization with visitors and by phone C. Encourage expression of feelings and questions
4. Maintenance of protective lung mechanisms	4. A. Provide good hydration and nutrition B. Avoid irritants and smoking C. Encourage deep breathing and effective coughing techniques D. Provide sufficient rest and avoidance of stress
5. Intact structures	5. Nursing strategies as in No. 4.
6. Patent airway	6. A. Maintain good posture B. Correct head-neck-chest alignment/position according to degree of health (e.g., lying, sitting) C. Use effective coughing and deep breathing techniques
7. Optimum breathing movement	7. A. Provide good nutrition for body strength, muscle tone and coordination, neural activity B. Maintain weight control C. Support automatic breathing rate and techniques (via instructions and alleviation of anxiety) D. Maintain good body position to support adequate chest cage movement
8. Optimum energy level	8. A. Maintain good nutritional intake B. Provide sufficient rest and sleep periods C. Plan paced activities

Table 4.1 *Nursing Care Plan for the Healthy Client (Continued)*

Factors for Need Fulfillment	Nursing Strategies
9. Systemic and pulmonary tissue perfusion	9. A. Reduce client's energy demands B. Avoid over-fatigue and stress C. Provide good nutrition and hydration D. Limit fluid and salt intake as needed E. Use support hose and antiembolic exercises
10. Optimum oxygen and carbon dioxide exchange	10. A. Maintain patent airway and oxygen intake as necessary B. Use effective coughing, deep breathing techniques and provide for body position changes C. Avoid respiratory irritants D. Provide humidified air E. Maintain good nutrition and fluid intake
11. Independence in self-care	11. A. Monitor client's self-care ability B. Monitor personal habits and routines, especially if elderly C. Encourage self-care and decision making D. Pace activities with rest periods
12. Optimum self-esteem and positive outlook on life	12. A. Provide for client's interests, hobbies, other diversional activities B. Encourage questions and decision making C. Monitor emotional stability, personal goals and expectations
13. Financial stability to provide optimum living situation	13. A. Inform client of available community resources B. Provide contact with Social Service/ Business Office representative regarding financial concerns C. Promote preventive care to offset unnecessary health care expenses
14. Maintenance of role in family/ social structure	14. A. Encourage interaction with family and friends B. Modify visiting hours if necessary

To maintain integrity of the respiratory tract and to support normal physiologic respiratory processes, the nurse concentrates on strategies to promote good health practices. Sufficient rest and avoidance of stressors, adequate hydration and nutrition, good skin care, and conservation of energy are some measures that will maintain the client's health status. Other measures, such as avoidance of respiratory irritants, promotion of automatic breathing rates and techniques, and humidification of air as needed are specifically designed to assist with the breathing processes.

To maintain the client's integrity as a person and to support his role in society, the nurse encourages self-care and independence within the client's limitations, provides for the client's interests, and promotes interactions with others.

Having identified the client's needs and designating nursing strategies appropriate to his situation, the nurse records this information on the care plan format provided. After the care plan is written, the planning phase of the nursing process concludes and the implementation phase begins.

In addition to identifying strategies for maintaining clean air in the hospital environment, the nurse should extend her role beyond the health care setting. As a citizen and as a professional, she should be actively concerned and accept responsibility for providing clean air in the community.[4]

As a citizen, the nurse can learn more about environmental problems in the local area and support antipollution legislation at local, state, and federal levels. When possible, the nurse can actively participate in citizen groups that work to achieve a clean environment. On a more personal level, the nurse can take measures to conserve energy resources that ultimately will decrease air pollution. She can avoid use of aerosols, cigarettes, pesticides, disposable products, and unnecessary use of private transportation vehicles.

As a health care professional, the nurse should promote good health practices that include mantaining a well-balanced, nutritional diet, avoiding smoking, and immunizing children. She should encourage health screening and casefinding programs, especially for children with allergies and adults with poor health habits. Efforts directed toward educating the public about the health hazards of pollution can also be effective. The nurse might also become actively involved in professional organizations to inform the membership of and promote group action for effective environmental control legislation.

Implementing the Nursing Care Plan

Implementation is the third phase of the nursing process and involves application of the nursing care plan to achieve the defined goals.[5] During this phase, the professional nurse uses technical, intellectual, and interpersonal skills to implement the plan of care. Using these skills in the interactions with the client, the nursing staff and other health team members, the nurse determines how the nursing care strategies can best be carried out. She uses her knowledge of the self-care abilities of the client, the abilities and availability of the family and/or significant others, the number and level of preparation of the nursing staff members, and the roles of other health team members. This enables her to direct and coordinate the actions that have been planned to assist the client. Specific actions may require direct intervention by the professional nurse, some may be delegated to other levels of nursing personnel, and still others need only to be coordinated. For example, instructing the client in good health practices, encouraging him to express his feelings and then listening attentively to what he says and encouraging him to make decisions and to ask questions are responsibilities of the professional nurse. Controlling the temperature of the client's room and preventing drafts, minimizing noise, encouraging good body posture in ambulatory clients and good body position in those who are bedridden, and monitoring vital signs may be delegated to other nursing team members. Maintaining a nutritional food intake and providing humidified air and diversional activities require coordination of the services offered by dietary, central supply, and occupational therapy department personnel.

The professional nurse is also responsible for involving the client in implementing the actions planned for his care. Depending on the client's health status and the degree of need violation, if any is present, the client may be independent of nursing assistance or very dependent on the nurse to meet his needs. For example, the healthy client should be able to pace his own activities with rest periods throughout the day, cough and deep breathe as directed by previous instructions of the nurse, drink sufficient fluids to remain hydrated, and record his intake and output of fluids.

The delegation of nursing actions to various persons may change from time to time. This change in nursing care assignments will depend on the client's response, the availability of nursing staff members, and the coping abilities of the client and significant others. In some client situations, it may be desirable that simple physical care measures be performed by the nurse in order to give the client an opportunity to discuss his feelings and fears in a more relaxed environment. Much of the success in filling the client's need for air is closely interwoven with the nurse–client relationship and the positive outlook and motivation of the client. For example, the depressed or apathetic client will have energy expenditure and muscle activity that are insufficient for adequate ventilation and as a result may become hypoxic.

The nurse continues to assess the client's status and adapts the plan to the current situation. Thus, the steps of the nursing process are used both recurrently and concurrently. The action involved in the implementation phase can be effective only if assessment, planning, and evaluation continue. By being flexible in approach and adaptable in intervention, the nurse promotes the optimum level of the client's physical, psychologic, and social health status. In the healthy client, the factors necessary for need fulfillment can be maintained by skillful implementation of the nursing care plan.

After the nursing actions have been completed, they should be documented together with the client's response to them. Today, greater emphasis is being placed on the need for accurate documentation by the nurse. With the increased demands for quality care and the subsequent emphasis on patient care evaluation, the documentation of nursing actions and the client's response to them is an essential part of the nurse's responsibility. Having worked closely with the client during assessment of his needs and strengths, planning for his care, and communicating with others during these activities, the nurse assigns high priority to recording the results of these activities on the client's permanent health record.

Many health care facilities have developed special forms for taking a health history and for formulating a nursing care plan; they are similarly developing other forms that facilitate documentation of nursing actions and client response. Nurses' Notes are general forms that usually record information about the client's symptoms, treatments given, procedures done, and the client's response. Nurses' Progress Notes are forms that record client information related to the outcomes or goals identified on the nursing care plan.

Two forms which have been recently developed are Client Education Records and a Nursing Discharge Summary form. The Education Records are used for specific topics. Each contains a checklist of the knowledge and skills the client needs to have. This not only provides a record of what the client has been taught but also serves as a guideline for instructions given to the client. Sufficient space is provided to record his learning progress, response to instructions, and need for further review and reinforcement. The Nursing Discharge Summary form was developed to facilitate the discharge of the client from the hospital and to improve the quality of nursing documentation. This is accomplished principally because the form reminds the nurse of her responsibilities to the client during that time. In addition, as a result of this form, the nurses have become more aware of discharge planning and the need for review of homegoing instructions previously given to the client. The use of this form is also of assistance in the data retrieval process necessary for patient care evaluation studies. Thus sufficient and appropriate documentation of nursing action and client response not only records what has already occurred, but also in some instances directly effects nursing care yet to be given.

Once the nursing documentation is completed, the implementation phase ends and the evaluation phase begins.

Evaluating the Outcomes of Nursing Actions

Evaluation is the fourth phase of the nursing process; it involves reviewing the client's status in order to determine the effectiveness of the nursing actions.[6] Evaluation is accomplished when both nurse and client appraise the degree of the client's progress according to the preestablished outcomes and goals of therapy. Thus, the evaluation phase is purposeful and goal-directed.

Evaluation of the client in view of short and long range goals is done frequently. As goals are met, the nurse modifies the nursing care plan and establishes additional goals appropriate to the client's program. This surveillance continues throughout the client's hospitalization and, like the other steps of the nursing process, evaluation continues on a concurrent and recurrent basis. Evaluation naturally follows nursing assessment and planning. By evaluating nursing actions and their outcome, the nurse accepts responsibility for her actions, shows interest in a person-centered approach to the client, and demonstrates a willingness to alter the plan of care as necessary.

With specific reference to the healthy client's need for air, methods the nurse may use to evaluate the outcomes of the nursing strategies identified earlier will be examined.

By means of client interview and observation, the nurse can determine if the client's environment remains conducive to his well-being and communication with others. Did control of pollutants, room temperature, and noise promote client comfort or cause symptoms of infection or breathing difficulties? Was the client able to reach the signal cord or did he have problems communicating his needs because of difficulty in speaking? Was the client able to maintain his body defenses and normal respiratory processes or did deficits occur that resulted in various symptoms such as cough, elevated temperature, or dyspnea? Did the client remain as independent as possible and cope with his family and financial concerns? Did he maintain a positive outlook and interest in his progress?

If the client's needs have not been met, that is, if healthy status has not been achieved, then the nurse needs to determine the causes. Did the nursing staff implement the plan consistently? Were the plans appropriate or did they need revision? Did the client and/or significant others cooperate in the care as planned?

In addition to observation of client outcomes, the nurse uses her communication skills to obtain feedback from the client and his family, members of the nursing staff, and other health team members. Feedback is an aid to her evaluation of the client situation because it permits accurate interpretation and validation of the data that have been collected. Based on the inferences made about the situation, the nurse determines if actions can be redirected or repeated to enable the client to attain or maintain the outcomes established earlier.

In evaluating the client, the nurse must determine whether the data collected at this time resemble that collected during the original assessment. If the client's outcomes were maintained as expected, no variations in nursing actions are needed. If the client remains hospitalized, the supportive nursing actions should continue, with periodic evaluation of their effectiveness. If the data collected on evaluation of the client vary from the original assessment and indicate undesirable changes in the client's healthy respiratory status, for example, the presence of breathing difficulties, then the client's ability to meet his need for air has been violated to some degree. At this point in the client's care, the nurse must begin reassessment of his health status in order to identify the extent of the violation of need fulfillment.

The cycle of the nursing process activities continues in the following discussion of the person experiencing an alteration or a violation of his basic human need for air.

The Person With a Human Need Alteration or Violation

In this section of the chapter, the discussion will focus on the clinical use of the nursing process as it applies to the care of the client with certain health deficits. The emphasis continues not on the care of the client with pulmonary problems but rather on how the nursing process is used to assist the client in meeting his need for air.

Beginning with reassessment, the nurse collects data that give evidence of the unmet need for air. Having collected new data, she plans actions for resolving the client's newly identified deficits and coordinates these actions with the previously used plan of care. After implementing these new strategies designed to offset the deficits, the nurse will again evaluate their effectiveness. Each of these steps of the nursing process will be discussed in detail as it relates to the client whose basic need for air has not been met.

Reassessing the Need for Air

Reassessment of the client begins when the client's expected outcome is not attained. At this time, the nurse reviews the client situation in the manner described earlier in the chapter. Using interview, observation, communication, and intellectual skills, she collects additional information on which to establish the nursing diagnoses—those client problems that can be resolved by nursing intervention. Because the nurse in this situation is focusing on the client's need for air, certain areas are of particular concern.

When obtaining a general health history, the nurse usually addresses the following: general appearance, physical and emotional condition, physical disabilities, use of medications or prosthetic aids, patterns of daily living (mobility, sleep, nutrition, and elimination), home, family, and occupational situations, and the client's own description of the symptoms of his present illness and his perceptions and expectations of his current illness and hospitalization.

However, because the nurse's primary concern here is with the ill client's need for air, she can use as a basis for respiratory assessment the fourteen factors listed earlier that are necessary for need fulfillment. With this list as a framework and using various methods of data collection and analysis, she can determine the extent of the client's unmet need for air.

When assessing the client's physical status, the nurse uses observational skills, diagnostic instruments, and the results of diagnostic testing. Via observation and client interview, the nurse collects specific data about the client's respiratory status. Information obtained about breathing functions includes the rate and quality of respirations, muscles used (abdominal, diaphragm, accessory), type of breathing sounds present (wheezing, congestion), symptoms and characteristics of distress (e.g., cyanosis or dyspnea: degree, frequency, and associated activities), symptoms of neurologic distress (restlessness, irritability), and mental state (forgetful, confused). Also, data are needed about presence of impairments such as cough (type, frequency, and if productive), secretions (color, amount, and consistency of mucus), allergies (types and usual symptoms), and use of cigarettes (amount per day). Also of importance to data collection is the client's use of any respiratory aids such as certain posture or body positions, general strengthening or breathing exercises or purselip breathing, use of oxygen or mechanical devices such as atomizers or positive pressure breathing machines, and use of medications (name, dose, and frequency).

Inspection and observation of the client for body weight and configuration, chest shape and symmetry, skin color and turgor, skeletal development, and muscle strength and use will help identify the client's physical status. Palpation of the chest cage for movement and symmetry, percussion of the thoracic cavity for lesions or fluid accumulation, and auscultation of breath sounds for presence and quality are additional tools for physical assessment.

Review of diagnostic test results should include the two groups of pulmonary function studies: those evaluating the lung's mechanical functions (lung volume, air flow, and compliance–resistance properties) and those measuring the gas exchange process (oxygen and carbon dioxide tensions, pH, and oxyhemoglobin). Other diagnostic test results to be reviewed include basic hematology and blood chemistry studies, skin tests for tuberculosis and allergies, analysis of sputum, nose and throat cultures, and any diagnostic bronchoscopy or biopsies performed. An understanding of the purpose and procedures required for these studies can enable the nurse to more fully assess the client on a day-to-day basis. She may use the knowledge gained from the testing to prevent further problems by adopting anticipatory nursing care measures. In addition to the data collected for physical assessment, the nurse also considers data previously collected about the client's socioeconomic background, home situation, personal concerns, and goals.

Table 4.2 *Factors and Corresponding Nursing Diagnoses*

Factors for Need Fulfillment	Possible Nursing Diagnoses
1. Clean air in immediate environment	1. A. Wheezing and symptoms of respiratory distress (due to allergic reactions to dust, smoke, pollen) B. Breathing difficulty (due to poor ventilation) C. Cough and elevated temperature (due to airborne infectious organisms)
2. Environment conducive to well-being	2. A. Bronchial irritation (due to dampness, air drafts) B. Irritated mucous membranes with potential for infection (due to dry air) C. Fatigue (due to increased breathing efforts from overheated room) D. Mental confusion (due to over-/under-sensory stimulation)
3. Verbal communication with others	3. A. Speaking difficulty (due to inadequate air flow B. Withdrawal (due to difficulty speaking) C. Increasing anxiety (due to difficulty speaking)
4. Maintenance of protective lung	4. A. Cough, elevated temperature (due to decreased ciliary activity and presence of infectious organisms) B. Excessive amount, thick tenacious sputum (due to mucous membrane irritation) C. Chronic cough (due to excessive sputum)
5. Intact structures	5. A. Dyspnea and orthopnea (due to swollen, inflammed mucous membranes, alveolar collapse, loss of lung tissue elasticity, tumor growth)
6. Patent airway	6. A. Partial airway obstruction (due to swelling, mucous collection, bronchial spasms, poor body posture)
7. Optimum breathing movement	7. A. Decreased breathing movements (due to poor body posture/position/alignment, poor muscle tone and coordination, abdominal distension) B. Hyperventilation (due to anxiety)
8. Optimum energy level	8. A. Excessive, chronic fatigue (due to increased breathing efforts and cough) B. Anorexia and dehydration (due to fatigue)
9. Systemic and pulmonary perfusion	9. A. Cardiovascular collapse, symptoms of shock B. Lung congestion

Table 4.2 *Factors and Corresponding Nursing Diagnoses (Continued)*

Factors for Need Fulfillment	Possible Nursing Diagnoses
10. Optimum oxygen and carbon dioxide exchange	10. A. Fatigue (due to hypoxia) B. Mental confusion, somnolence (due to hypoxia) C. Dyspnea and air hunger
11. Independence in self-care	11. Frustration (due to physical dependence on others)
12. Optimum self-esteem and positive outlook on life	12. A. Inability to cope with necessary life-style changes B. Views rehab activities as useless C. Fears own ability for care at home
13. Financial stability to provide adequate living situation	13. Concern regarding posthospital expenses for equipment, transportation, home modifications
14. Maintenance of role in family/social structure	14. A. Feels alienated from family B. Lack of interest in others

With an analysis of all these aspects of data collection, the nurse can again determine the ill client's problems, deficits, or unmet needs as well as his potential problems and personal strengths. For the purposes of discussion, refer again to the fourteen factors listed earlier for the healthy client and to Table 4.2 for some corresponding nursing diagnoses that may occur in the ill client. The nursing diagnoses and the nursing strategies necessary to offset them will be discussed in the following section.

Planning to Offset Nursing Diagnoses

Having identified the client's deficits and determined the nursing diagnoses, the nurse begins the care planning process to revise previous or develop additional nursing actions. The first step is to establish priorities based on the client's condition. If life-threatening deficits are present, they take priority and require immediate response. For example, the problem of airway obstruction due to accumulated secretions requires immediate suctioning. Following this immediate treatment, the nurse revises the plan to provide closer observation and suctioning of the client at frequent intervals to prevent recurrence of obstruction.

The nurse and the client are involved in establishing the long and short range goals of nursing intervention. These expected behavioral outcomes of the client can be established in several ways. In addition to her knowledge of the client's condition and the factors identified as necessary for fulfillment of air needs, the nurse should assess the client's expectations of his outcomes, especially in relation to his understanding of current pathologic processes. For goals to be realistic and attainable and to avoid conflicts in establishing them, nurse and client need to have the same understanding of the client's status. Both nurse and client need to understand the influencing factors present during goal setting. Not only the disease process itself (e.g., emphysema) but also the resultant physiologic and psychologic changes in the client can alter his activities. Limited physical activities, for example, can result in role and lifestyle changes that in turn can cause alterations in the client's perception of himself, his occupational ability, and his intrafamily and social relationships.

General overall goals of therapy that can be considered include:

1. Restoration and maintenance of respiratory function at an optimal level.
2. Prevention of functional disabilities.
3. Assistance for the client in accepting and coping with the known (or unknown) medical diagnosis.

Examples of general client outcomes that can be developed and made more specific for clients with respiratory problems are listed here:

1. Verbalizes knowledge of disease condition and reasons for therapy.
2. Demonstrates ability for performing self-care measures and therapeutic treatments.
3. Verbalizes understanding of limitations and adapts to activities permitted.
4. Follows maintenance aspects of health and recognizes symptoms of recurrence.
5. Follows dietary and fluid intake prescribed.
6. Demonstrates knowledge and skills for use of medications and equipment.
7. Verbalizes importance and willingness to continue follow-up care.
8. Demonstrates ability to cope with lifestyle changes necessitated by respiratory limitations.

Within this broad delineation of overall therapy goals and client outcomes, the nurse and the client can establish short-range goals appropriate for his physical as well as emotional and personal well-being.

Examples of nursing strategies and short-range goals that can be developed are identified in the care plan in Table 4.3. These goals and nursing strategies are directed to assisting the client in regaining, as much as possible, the fourteen factors identified earlier as necessary for fulfilling one's need for air.

Table 4.3 *Nursing Care Plan for the Client with Air Deficits*

Deficits and/or Nursing Diagnoses	Desired Goals	Nursing Strategies
1. A. Wheezing and symptoms of respiratory distress due to allergic reactions to dust, smoke, pollen	1. A. Absence of wheezing and symptoms of respiratory distress	1. A. Maintain clean room and free of flowers and smoke
B. Breathing difficulty	B. Breathing easier without discomfort	B. Provide adequate ventilation via open window/door and air conditioner
C. Cough and elevated temperature	C. Afebrile; decreased cough	C. Aseptic use of equipment; restrict contact with personnel and visitors with infection
2. A. Bronchial irritation	2. A. Breathing without complaint of dry, irritated throat or cough, afedbrile	2. A. Provide comfortable temperature and humidity level (e.g., humidifier) and adequate air ventilation
B. Irritated mucous membranes with potential for infection	B. Desired goals as in No. 2. A.	B. Nursing Strategies as in No. 2. A.
C. Fatigue	C. Giving own care with assistance and eating all meals	C. Control room temperature; pace activity according to available energy
D. Mental confusion	D. Appropriate mentation	D. Provide restful, quiet environment; provide clock, calendar, and personal articles
3. A. Speaking difficulty	3. A. Calls for and receives assistance as needed	3. A. Signal cord/system within reach; provide materials for writing if unable to speak
B. Withdrawal	B. Verbalizes need and feelings; interacts with staff and family	B. Assign same staff member for daily care; encourage client in listening and letting others speak

(Continued)

Table 4.3 *Nursing Care Plan for the Client with Air Deficits (Continued)*

Deficits and/or Nursing Diagnoses	Desired Goals	Nursing Strategies
C. Increasing anxiety	C. Relaxed, calm manner, uses written communication	C. Reassure with touch and calming manner; provide for written communication
4. A. Cough and elevated temperature	4. A. Afebrile; decreased cough	4. A. Restrict visitors and personnel with symptoms of infection; cover mouth/-nose for sneeze and cough; proper disposal of tissues
B. Excessive amounts of thick, tenacious sputum	B. Clear lungs; less tenacious sputum	B. Auscultation of breath sounds; avoid smoking and aerosols; fluid intake to 2400 cc/day unless contraindicated
C. Chronic cough	C. Less frequent cough; decreased amount sputum	C. Postural drainage; effective coughing and deep breathing techniques
5. Dyspnea and orthopnea	5. Verbalizes easier breathing; less rapid respirations and pulse rates	5. Semi-high fowlers position (lean over bedside table as necessary); avoid inhaled irritants; effective breathing techniques (especially purse-lipped breathing); plan activity and rest periods
6. Partial airway obstruction	6. Improved airflow; clear lung sounds and absence of wheezing; relaxed facial expression	6. Maintain airway patency (artificial as necessary; position as necessary); maintain good body alignment and change position every hour; calm, unhurried approach to client
7. A. Decreased breathing movements	7. A. Chest movement adequate for respirations	7. A. Maintain body position which enables thoracic movement; gradually incréase exercise and activity to increase muscle tone
B. Hyperventilation	B. Controlled, relaxed breathing	B. Instruct in controlled, relaxed breathing techniques; alleviate anxiety with supportive measures

8. A. Excessive, chronic fatigue	8. A. Energy for activities of daily living	8. A. Plan pace of activities; conserve body energy
B. Anorexia and dehydration	B. Eating all meals; moist mucous membranes and good skin turgor	B. Measure intake and output; small, frequent, attractive feedings
9. A. Cardiovascular collapse	9. A. Vital signs normal for client; skin warm and dry; oriented to surroundings; relaxed facial expression	9. A. Monitor cardiac status: vital signs and EKG/monitor pattern; maintain ventilation and oxygen intake; conserve body energy and avoid unnecessary care; support circulation with body position, elastic hose to lower extremities; assess fluid and electrolytes status and maintain via accurate measurement; provide reassurance and emotional support
B. Lung congestion	B. Clear lung sounds	B. Auscultate breath sounds; maintain best position for ventilation; assess and monitor fluid intake and output
10. A. Fatigue	10. A. Energy for activities of daily living	10. A. Planned activity and rest periods; emotional support; alleviate anxiety with explanation of causes of fatigue
B. Mental confusion, somnolence	B. Alert and oriented	B. Assess level of consciousness at appropriate time intervals; maintain appropriate oxygen level; avoid oversedation
C. Dyspnea and air hunger	C. Easier breathing without distress	C. Monitor respiratory rate; position for optimum ventilation

(Continued)

Table 4.3 *Nursing Care Plan for the Client with Air Deficits (Continued)*

Deficits and/or Nursing Diagnoses	Desired Goals	Nursing Strategies
11. Frustration	11. Coping with current limitations; self-care according to maximum ability	11. Encourage to verbalize feelings; explain pattern of progression to greater independence (emphasize strengths and abilities); encourage questions regarding treatment rationale; allow self-care as able; allow decision making regarding own care
12. A. Inability to cope with necessary lifestyle changes	12. A. Verbalizes feelings regarding lifestyle changes	12. A. Assess understanding of disease implications and relation to self and own goals; evaluate motivation and emotional stability; support client in coping efforts
B. Views rehab activities as useless	B. Participates in own care	B. Assist client to plan realistic goals; assist family to accept client's limitations
C. Fears own ability for care at home	C. Asks questions regarding progress and goals of treatment	C. Client and family instruction; arrange visiting nurse referral as necessary
13. Concern regarding post-hospital expenses for equipment, transportation, home modification	13. Participates in discharge planning; financial concerns met	13. Involve client and family in all discharge planning; arrange for home evaluation as necessary; arrange for post-hospital follow-up by visiting nurse; consult with Social Service representative; explain financial resources available
14. A. Feels alienated from family	14. A. Participates in family decisions	14. A. Allow and encourage ventilation of feelings; assist family to include client in family matters
B. Lack of interest in others	B. Looks forward to visitors; interacts with hospital staff and other clients	B. Encourage socialization with other hospitalized clients; encourage participation in group activities (diversional and educational)

In developing a nursing care plan such as this, the nurse relies on her knowledge of the air and its components and of respiratory anatomy and physiology, on her professional skills and past clinical experiences, on her knowledge of a particular client and his individual needs, and on the medical plan for care. The nurse can also benefit from nursing department committee work that is directed toward establishing standards of nursing care for clients in that institution, developing standard nursing care plans and identifying expected outcomes for specific types of clients during each phase of their hospitalization. In addition, the nurse now has access to a variety of recently published texts, standard nursing care plans, and similar references that can be of assistance in nursing care planning for hospitalized clients.[7,8]

Having identified the client's needs and appropriate nursing care strategies, the nurse concludes the planning phase of the nursing process by writing the care plan and making it available for nursing and other health team members.

Implementing Actions to Offset Nursing Diagnoses

Once the nursing care plan has been formulated, the implementation phase can begin. The nurse relies on a broad base of knowledge, highly developed skills, and an understanding of people to determine how best to carry out the various strategies that have been planned. Delegation of nursing care to someone other than the professional nurse must now take into consideration the client's degree of illness and severity of his condition as well as his self-care abilities, family interest and abilities, and nursing and hospital staff availability.

It is important also to consider the cause of the client's deficits and his prognosis for wellness in order to effectively implement his care. For example, if the client's unmet needs for air are due to a chronic disease process such as emphysema, then the focus of the initial care will probably be an alleviation of acute distress but then it will progress to the rehabilitative aspects of care. Keeping in mind that the concept of rehabilitation involves a holistic approach to care and the client's reintegration into society, the nurse must elicit the client and family's participation in his care as much as possible. Once the client regains some independence in his self-care, he can be encouraged to participate more fully. His participation will be determined by his awareness of the disease condition and an understanding of how various treatments assist him. Also, it depends on whether he is given an opportunity to express his feelings and fears about his health and whether he is given directions to assist him in understanding his own behavior. As the client begins to accept his condition and cope with it as best he can, he will participate more fully.

The nurse must create an environment conducive not only for the client's physical healing progress but also for his continued development as an individual with dignity and self-worth. Implementation of care involves direct intervention by the professional nurse, delegation of some care to others, and coordination of care not only between hospital departments but also between the hospital, home, and community settings. Throughout this intervention, the nurse provides emotional support, encouragement, and learning opportunities for the client and his family so that the client may successfully reach the expected outcomes that both he and the nurse have established.

The professional nurse should also be aware of the fact that both the client and members of his family usually require assistance in understanding the client's problems, their causes and, more importantly, their implications. The client needs direction and encouragement in giving his own care and the family needs help in understanding their role in relation to the client and his illness. The family, as a major support system, helps the client to maintain his self-esteem and identity.

When providing learning opportunities for the client, the nurse should include both client and family in the plan and its implementation. Having assessed what the client already knows, needs to know, and wants to know, the nurse plans the content of the learning program. It is helpful if she also uses the expected client outcomes as a basis for client instructions. Use of effective teaching and learning principles will aid in the client education process. Giving clear and simple directions, relying on previous client experiences, encouraging participation and repetition, and obtaining feedback via verbalized knowledge and demonstrated skills are only some examples of these principles. An approach that is individually designed for each client, that has specific objectives planned for each learning session, and that is supported by good nurse–client rapport and open communication will greatly contribute to the client's learning progress.

After implementing the various strategies, the nurse must give evidence of this nursing activity and of the client's responses to it. Complete and accurate documentation of this information on the client's permanent health record is an important responsibility of the nurse. Nurses are encouraged to develop more specific forms to guide nursing care and also to facilitate nursing documentation. When these forms become available, more accurate descriptions of nursing care and client responses will be recorded. Until that time, nurses are challenged to set priorities in their clerical as well as clinical activities and accept accountability for both.

When nursing documentation is completed, the implementation phase ends and evaluation begins.

Evaluating Outcomes of Revised Nursing Actions

In the evaluation phase of the nursing process, the nurse and the client review the client's progress toward the goals identified earlier. This is a process that continues from day to day during hospitalization. Both the nurse and the client reflect on the nursing actions taken and determine the client's response to that care.

Is the client breathing easier without symptoms of discomfort or distress? Is he afebrile and free of symptoms of infection? Are lung sounds clear and air flow improved? Does he have sufficient energy for self-care, eating meals, and walking in his room or corridor? Are his breathing movements controlled and relaxed? Is he alert and oriented? Is he interested in his own care, participating in discharge planning, verbalizing his feelings and concerns, and coping with his current limitations? In other words, has he reached the short-range goals that were established earlier? Has nursing intervention eliminated the deficits or do the goals need revision?

If this evaluation is being done shortly before discharge, to what degree has the client met the expected outcomes previously determined for him? Can he explain in simple terms what his disease condition is and the reasons for his therapy? Can he demonstrate self-care measures and use of necessary equipment to maintain a healthy respiratory status? Does he pace his activities and adapt to his limitations? Has he expressed a willingness to continue follow-up care and verbalized the symptoms requiring immediate medical attention? Does he know the names, actions, doses, and side effects of any medications he will be taking at home? If the client's physical status has stabilized and yet he has not achieved these outcomes, he needs an extended hospital stay for additional learning opportunities and development of necessary self-care skills. If the client's physical condition has improved and his discharge from the hospital is deemed necessary, then the nurse can make provision for posthospital follow-up care. Visiting nurse or other home health services are often available, thus permitting the remaining outcomes to be met on an ambulatory basis in the home setting.

In the light of the fourteen factors described as essential for need fulfillment, in review of the client's outcomes, and in consideration of the overall goals of therapy, the nurse determines if the client's need for air has been fully or only partially met. If desirable outcomes have been achieved, then the client has regained his healthy state and needs only supportive action. If the client still experiences health deficits, the nurse and the client continue to work together to assess his current respiratory status, implement new nursing strategies, and continue their evaluation until the most optimal level of health can be attained and it can be assured that the client's requirement for air is filled.

The Clinical Specialist and the Nursing Process

Greater emphasis is being placed on the need for high quality nursing care services. Faced with the demands of governmental regulations, voluntary accreditation agencies, consumer pressures, cost control, and demands for professional growth and worth, quality assurance has become one of the key phrases in the current nursing vocabulary.

To assure the delivery of quality care, nurses must continue to develop a high degree of sophistication and level of competence among the administrative, educational, and clinical personnel. Development of the clinical nurse specialist role is one means of providing clinical leadership. The clinical nurse specialist, an expert clinical practitioner, is prepared on a Masters level in nursing, demonstrates a high level of knowledge and skills, and is responsible for favorably influencing the quality of nursing care for a specific group of clients.

It is from the perspective of a clinical specialist that I will present my experiences in using the nursing process with both nursing staff members and clients. I will share the approaches I have utilized in assisting nurses to become more conscious of the nursing process itself.

Having completed graduate studies, I accepted the position of clinical specialist for medical nursing in a 517-bed, acute care, teaching hospital. Having a staff position and working closely with the nursing care coordinator for medical nursing, I was involved primarily on five general medical divisions and occasionally in the medical intensive and coronary care units. As the first clinical specialist in the hospital, I was continually orienting the staff personnel to my role and stressing the need for high quality nursing care. In my first position as clinical specialist, I faced the challenge of integrating graduate studies with my expectations of the reality of the everyday nursing world. One of the key responsibilities of my first job was to provide leadership in the use of the nursing process. In addition, I was to work cooperatively with the staff in implementing goals and standards of nursing care.

During the first several months, I became acquainted with the hospital and nursing staffs, further developed my technical and communication skills, and demonstrated my expertise in clinical care. My clinical activities included establishing and maintaining a limited client caseload. As time progressed, I received an increasing number of referrals from house and private physicians, and social workers assigned to the medical divisions. These referrals requested an assessment of their client's learning needs and abilities and an assessment of the home and family situations influencing their client's current health status. In addition, they requested an evaluation of the client's self-care activities that may have caused the health deficit(s) that resulted in the current hospitalization.

When working with my client caseload, I utilized my expertise in assessing and planning for the client's self-care abilities and learning needs, the general nursing care required, and his discharge planning needs. I implemented and evaluated these plans both independently and with the nursing staff. It was via a client caseload that I initially demonstrated to the staff the use of the nursing process. Each level of nursing care giver, including the clinical specialist, has a different degree of expertise in using the nursing process. Two questions that kept recurring to me as clinical specialist were: "What was it that I could contribute to its use besides demonstrating it in direct patient care?" and "What other means could I employ to provide leadership to the staff in the use of the nursing process?"

As I continued to work with the nursing staff, I found that the term nursing process was little known. When I did see evidence of the nursing process, it was used neither consistently nor continually around the clock, and not for every client throughout his hospitalization. Realizing the staff's need for use of the process with a greater awareness and frequency, I planned future approaches that included not only demonstrating the phases of the nursing process but also using the terms to assist the staff with integrating theory into everyday nursing practice.

I found, as time progressed and the needs of the nursing staff became more apparent, that several things could be done to facilitate the use of the nursing process. To accomplish this, I directed my energies into what may be called special projects. Actually, these projects served as the various modes by which I demonstrated and explained the values of the nursing process to various nurses.

Planning

Having recognized the need for a workable nursing care plan format and being interested in its use as a vital avenue of communication, I led a subcommittee of staff nurses to revise the current format to a more desirable and comprehensive one. By indicating spaces for long- and short-range objectives, nursing approaches, and client's progress, we provided nurses with a tool to record their plan for nursing actions based on the client assessment.

Assessment

Although the phase of planning usually follows assessment, in this instance the need and readiness for a workable planning format preceded that for a usable assessment form. As the staff became more adept in using the new care plan card they realized the need for a more detailed nursing admission assessment. After months of trial and error and several revisions, a nursing admission history form was developed and is being implemented this year. In addition to these two forms, others have been developed to facilitate nursing documentation of not only the care given but also the client's responses to that care. For example, we have in use new client education records for diabetes and for postpartum and infant care.

As emphasis continued to be placed on the client's learning needs and discharge planning, the nursing department realized the need for formalized client education programs. Having developed teaching guidelines for use with diabetics, I initiated, with a multidisciplinary team approach, a Diabetes Group Teaching Program for hospitalized clients. Since the initiation of this program in April 1974, the nursing personnel have become more aware of their responsibility in planning for and reinforcing necessary client education and began to give this area of client need greater priority. One outcome of the program was the development of the role of Diabetic Class Instructor in mid-1975. The responsibility for the in-hospital diabetic classes was delegated, on a rotation basis, to staff nurses throughout the hospital who serve in this role under the direction of the clinical specialist for medical nursing. The major functions of this nurse are to conduct the diabetic classes, coordinate the diabetic learning of clients attending the classes, and assist other members of the nursing staff with the implementation of nursing standards of clients with diabetes. In their practice, these nurses now demonstrate improved skills in assessing the client's learning needs and greater creativity in individualized teaching methods. They have broadened their perspective of client education, continuity of care, and the nurse's responsibility. These nurses have also become knowledgeable and responsible resource persons regarding diabetes for peers on their own nursing divisions.

Intervention

Another method I utilized to increase the staff's awareness of the nursing process was more formalized. Working closely with the staff development and quality assurance coordinators facilitated many of my teaching activities as well as gave me the opportunity to share professional ideas, approaches, resources, and trends in nursing care. As a lecturer in the hospital-conducted coronary and critical care course for nurses, a pulmonary nursing workshop, the quality assurance program inservices, and the orientation classes for registered nurses and licensed practical nurses, I discuss the nursing process in theory and direct the staff in its application to client situations. These formal presentations supplement my one-to-one and group sessions held with nurses in the clinical setting.

Evaluation

In addition to my involvement on the medical divisions, I accepted the additional challenge of chairing the Nursing Standards and Professional Review Committee. This committee was formed by the director of nursing to establish and implement nursing care standards, to audit the effectiveness of nursing actions on client's outcomes, and to provide more effective documentation methods for nursing personnel. The committee has been one major focus of my efforts to significantly influence the level of nursing care throughout the hospital. Under the direction and leadership of this committee, nursing care criteria have been established, nursing peer review is in progress, and the need for application of the nursing process as the core of nursing activity has been highlighted. The committee has since proven to be an important force within nursing for improving clinical care via the nursing process.

By means of contact in the clinical setting, informal conferences, and committee work, I developed close working relationships with the nursing care coordinators and assistant directors for nursing. These working relationships also provided opportunities for us to generate and share ideas about nursing today. With the continued support and direction of the director of nursing, this leadership group of the department worked at length in revising the statement of nursing philosophy by which we would practice. A key point of that philosophy was including use of the nursing process as an expected part of professional nursing activity.

All of these collaborative efforts encouraged and fostered our own growth as well as aided us as leaders of the nursing staff in applying the nursing process in the care of all clients.

As the above account indicates, I have found answers to my earlier questions regarding my use of the nursing process and use of leadership methods with the staff to increase their use of the process. As is often the case, time provides us with answers; or rather, perhaps it is that time give us opportunities for growth and, through our own efforts, we find the answers.

Since my employment nearly four years ago, I have acquired a better understanding of the scope of my responsibilities. Through the roles of teacher, consultant, and practitioner, I have worked to meet both client and staff needs. I recognize, even more, that the effectiveness of the clinical nurse specialist as a clinical leader is the result of an ongoing process. And, much of the success of this position depends on strong administrative support, a climate for change, and flexibility for development.

References

1. Yura H, Walsh M: Nursing Process, 2nd ed. New York, Appleton-Century-Crofts, 1973, pp 25–26
2. Ibid, p 28
3. Mayers M: Systematic Approach to the Nursing Care Plan. New York, Appleton-Century-Crofts, 1972, pp 56–57
4. Murray R, Zentner J: Nursing Concepts for Health Promotion. Englewood Cliffs, New Jersey, Prentice-Hall, 1975, pp 264–265
5. Yura H, Walsh M[1]: p 29
6. Ibid, p 31
7. Tucker SM, Breeding MA, Canobbio MM, et al: Patient Care Standards. St. Louis, Mosby, 1975
8. Mayers M: Standard Nursing Care Plans. Palo Alto, California, KP Medical Systems, 1974

Additional References

American Lung Association. Air Pollution Primer. New York, American Lung Association, 1974

Brecher E, Brecher R: Breathing . . . What You Need to Know. New York, American Lung Association, 1973

Early M: Gaseous exchange process: nursing implications. In Kinsel K (ed). Advanced Concepts of Clinical Nursing. Philadelphia, Lippincott, 1971, pp 207–235

Maxwell KE: Environment of Life. Encino, California, Dickenson, 1973

Orem, DE: Nursing Concepts of Practice. New York, McGraw–Hill, 1974

Shapiro BA, Harrison RA, Trout CA: Clinical Application of Respiratory Care. Chicago, Year Book Medical Publishers, 1975

Sitzman J: Respiratory Problems and the Nurse's Changing Responsibilities. Cardio-Vascular Nursing 6:41–45, May–June, 1970.

Turk A, Turk J, Wittes J, Wittes R: Environmental Science. Philadelphia, Saunders, 1974

Wade JF: Respiratory Nursing Care: Physiology and Techniques. St. Louis, Mosby, 1973

Chapter Five •

The Need to Love and to Be Loved

Kitty S. Smith

The recorded history of man gives evidence that love in its many forms has been present in all cultures from the beginning. Art, dance, rituals, sculpture, and the written word reflect the need to love and to be loved. Expressions of love are found in Ferruzzi's painting of the mother tenderly pressing the infant to her breast, the Swan Lake ballet, the wedding ceremony, Shakespeare's sonnets on love, and the love story of Evangeline and Gabriel.

Every person, regardless of race, sex, culture, or age, has a need to love and to be loved. Because it is the professional goal of nurses to assist clients to fill their self-care deficits to achieve optimum health, it would follow that nurses should possess the knowledge, skills, and attitudes required to aid their clients in achieving the maximum health potential. Because love has been identified as a basic human need,[1] its fulfillment becomes a primary concern for the nurse as clients' abilities and capabilities are assessed. The relationship between two people that is conducive to the optimum development of both is foundational to fulfilling the love need.

Although nurses verbalize a concern for caring for their clients and loving their fellow man, little has been written about love by nurses that is helpful to the practitioner. Where normal healthy relationships, including love, are acknow-

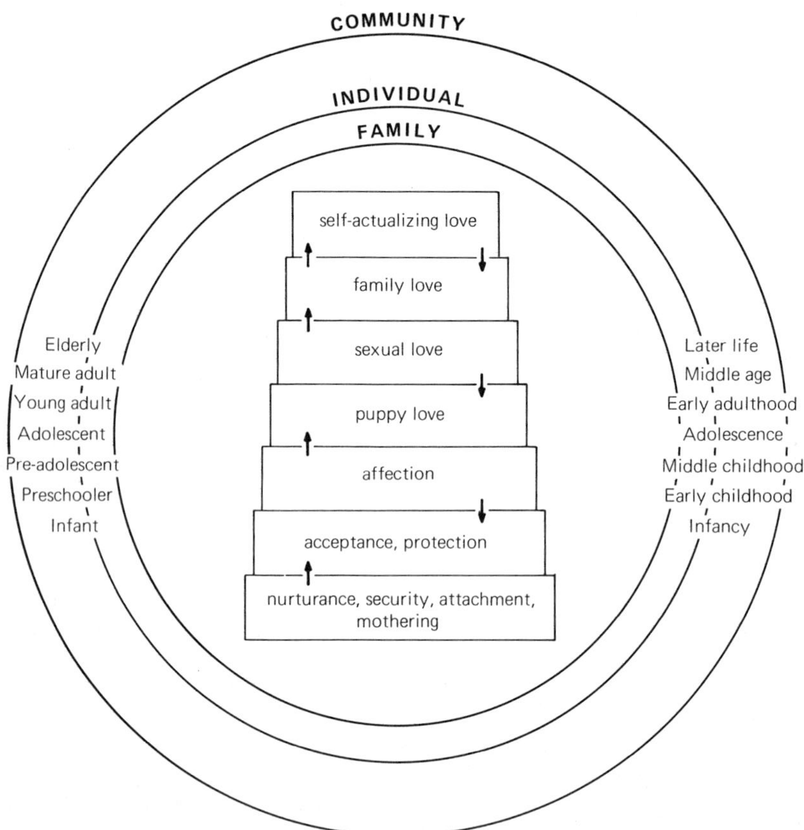

Figure 5.1: *Developmental model of love*

ledged, the presentation is usually stated in general terms. The normal healthy state of clients in the various age groups receives much less consideration in the nursing literature than do the deviations from normal. Research into human needs and behavior has been carried out primarily by psychologists. The age groups that have received the greatest attention are infancy, early childhood, preadolescence, adolescence, and old age.

There is a dearth of literature relative to the role of the nurse assisting a client to meet his need to love and to be loved. In this presentation, an attempt is made to explore in some depth the concept of love, the means leading to its fulfillment, and the roles played by the client and the nurse. Love is viewed as being developmental. In the developmental approach one views the individual as passing through the stage of infancy, when he is totally dependent on another for nurturance, security, protection, and mothering, to the giving of affection in early childhood and preadolescence, first to the caretaker, then to others, to puppy love

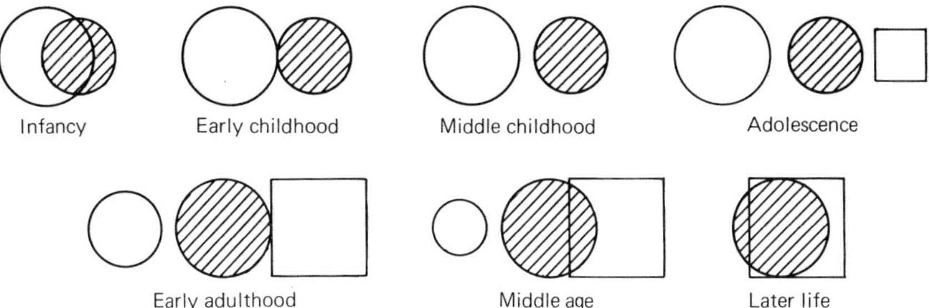

Figure 5.2: *Love relationships. The shaded circle represents the individual, the unshaded circle, the mother, and the square the significant other.*

in adolescence, sexual love in adulthood, and finally to self actualization in later years. The diagram in Figure 5.1 represents the developmental idea of love. The concept of love as developmental is also viewed in terms of the relationship between individual, mother, and significant others. At first the infant is completely dependent on his mother. As he grows and develops he gradually leaves his mother for another person; in that relationship he achieves self-actualization. The relationship between the individual and others as his love object changes is shown in Figure 5.2.

The components of the love need are presented for each age group—infancy, early childhood, middle childhood, adolescence, young adulthood, middle adulthood, and old age. The variables of sex and the ethnic, cultural, educational, and socioeconomic factors are explored as they affect the individual of a specific age group and his membership in a family, group, and community. For each age group the presentation includes the assessment of the healthy love relationship, the violation of the need and the strategies needed by the client and nurse to meet the need. Because of space limitations, a plan cannot be implemented for each age group; a plan is developed for the stage of infancy only. Using a nursing system model based on self-care competencies, we will analyze a situation and design a nursing plan for action. The model is one method the nurse can use to carry out the nursing process in an organized fashion to assist clients in meeting love needs. Evaluation as a part of process is considered in relation to the plan developed and to the presentation as a whole.

What Is Love?

Love as a concept is complex, universal and both comprehensive and vague. Love is everywhere in the universe, in all things of God's creation. Love between man and woman is unique, but no more than other kinds of love: the parental, filial and fraternal ties, the friendship and love of one person for another regardless of gender, and the love man has for himself, his fellowman, his country and his God. Man's love of self, if true, can lead to love of neighbor, but its extreme form becomes narcissism. Love is of both the spirit and the body and from this flows love of charity, friendship, doing service and sexual love.[2]

Great literary works of confession, history, meditation, poetry, revelation and biography reveal several major facts about love. First, there is a plurality of loves, which means there are different kinds of love, depending on the object of the love. Socrates teaches that one arrives at absolute beauty through the true order of love.[3] In his analysis of different types of friendships, Aritstotle classifies different kinds of love.[4] Aquinas makes a distinction between love as the realm of passion and love as an act of will.[5] According to Freud the origin of love is found in sexual instincts.[6] St. John wrote "God is love; and he that dwelleth in love dwelleth in God, and God in him."[7] In the Divine Comedy, Dante sees heaven as the realm of love and hell as the place of absence of God's love.[8] The second fact about love is that quite often it turns to hate. One can both love and hate the same object, since love when threatened by jealousy, fear, or anger can become its opposite, hate. Third, there seems to be no happiness more perfect than love. Lastly, love has privileged status, in that it retains some of its honor when it defies morality.[9] Some form of love or its antithesis abounds in all of literature.

Man needs to love and be loved. Love is a basic human need; but what is love? According to Webster's dictionary the word *love* is derived from the Old English *lufu,* which is akin to the Old High German word *lupa,* love; the Old English word *lèof*, dear; and the Latin words *lubere*, *libere*, to please. Love as a noun is defined as (1) "strong affection for another arising out of kinship or personal ties" as a mother for her child; (2) "attraction based on sexual desire," that is "affection and tenderness felt by lovers;" (3) "affection based on admiration, benevolence or common interest," as for schoolmates; (4) "warm attachment, enthusiasm or devotion," as of the sea; or (5) "object of attachment, devotion or admiration," as football. Love as a verb means (1) "to hold dear, cherish," (2) to feel a lover's passion, devotion or tenderness," a caress; (3) "to fondle amorously;" (4) "to take pleasure in;" and (5) "to feel affection."[10]

Exploration of the synonyms and antonyms of *love* gives further clarification to the meaning of the term. Synonyms for the object of love are *beloved, lover, dear, dearest;* those related to feeling love are *passion, charity, goodwill, devotion, adoration, fondness, tenderness, affection, warm feeling, compatibility* and *affinity;* and those concerned with having love are *strong liking, fondness, devotion,* and *attachment*. Antonyms of the word *love* are *hate, dislike, distaste, aversion, loathing, contempt, resentment, hostility,* and *ill will.*[11]

In his writings on the hierarchy of human needs, Maslow has identified belonging and love as the level of need man strives to fulfill after meeting his basic physiologic, safety, and security needs. Although love and belonging are common topics in the literature, there is a lack of empirical study on love, which prompted Maslow to pursue research in the area of love and self actualization.[12] Maslow sees love as being subjective rather than objective; concerned with affection and tenderness, happiness, and satisfaction; desiring physical and psychologic closeness; sharing; perception of the loved one in a unique way; sexual arousal of lover; and the purest love is the love of grandparents for each other. He asserts that a healthy love is a self actualizing love, one in which self is given freely and honestly, a love in which the person does not have to be guarded in any way.[13]

In *The Art of Loving,* Fromm delineates five somewhat different love relationships.[14] Brotherly love is the most basic kind of love. It is the orientation to all human relationships and finds expression in the Biblical command "love thy neighbor as thyself." Motherly love involves the parent taking the responsibility for a life entrusted to his care and finding happiness in seeing that life fulfilled. True motherly love is nonpossessive. Erotic love is the craving for union with another person. It is in erotic love that we usually see the greatest investment of self in the happiness of the other person. Self-love is a necessity for emotional competence. Each person has a need for self-acceptance and self-esteem; therefore, the person who is able to love productively loves himself and others. Finally, the love of God emphasizes the individual's need for union with God, the highest reality he can perceive.

Teilhard de Chardin in his scholarly treatise on human energy argues that love is a higher form of human energy that can be verified both psychologically and historically. He states, first, that the totalizing principle of human energy is love. This includes totalization by love of individual actions, totalization of the individual as related to himself, and totalization of the individual in regard to others. Secondly, love must be viewed in a specific frame of reference, which is love as an historical product of human evolution. He examines this from the viewpoint of the phenomena of Christianity and Christian monism.[15]

Love is not synonymous with sex; however, there is confusion in much of the present day writing. Sex can be viewed solely as a physiologic need, although it is usually associated with human needs such as love and affection. In the love need the person both gives and receives love.[16]

Love Needs

Accepting the premise that love is a developmental process, it is appropriate to consider the components of the love need and the deprivations that may occur for each age group—infancy, early childhood, middle childhood, adolescence, young adulthood, middle adulthood, and old age. Because the nurse is concerned with assisting her clients to meet their basic human needs with love as one of these needs, it is also appropriate to identify the nursing strategies that can be used with each age group to guide the client to fulfill his love need.

Infancy

What each human being becomes depends in great measure on his early relationships among humans. Deprivations in these human exchanges can culminate in varying degrees of illness.

Assessment of Love Needs

The unborn infant is well protected in his mother's womb as he is supported in an aquatic environment with a consistency of temperature and pressure. His existence is abruptly changed by birth. Following birth both mother and infant need each other. The mother needs the sight of her baby, his closeness to her body, his cry. She needs to fondle, touch, caress, make loving sounds, and to nurse the baby at her breast.[17]

The physiologic and safety/security needs of the infant take priority immediately after birth. He needs to be warm to feel protected, nursed at intervals to feel nurtured, held firmly to feel accepted, and stroked, talked to, and cuddled to feel attached. Tender loving care by the mother or maternal figure such as grandmother, father, or caretaker is highly significant in fulfilling the newborn's need for support through acceptance by human contact. It is necessary that this interaction with the infant be consistent and provide stimulation because psychologic care is as important as physical care. For the infant tactile stimulation is basic to the development of healthy emotional and affectional relationships.[18] Montagu uses this premise to explore the many ways in which a mother can provide for this need.

Breastfeeding not only benefits the mother physiologically, but also makes the infant feel secure and loved.[19] He responds not so much to what he is fed but to how he is fed. He is warm as he lies against his mother's body; he can hear the rhythm of her heart, feel the security of her arms, and learn how to root and nuzzle. The warmth, nourishment, and security of mother is his. The mother who formula feeds her baby needs to hold and cuddle him during feedings so that he gains the sensations of security and support in association with satisfying the hunger need.

Skin is the primary sense organ in the infant. It is through this sense that the baby first receives the imprints of the quality of care and affection being given to him. Babies respond quickly to temperature and air and are soothed by warmth. Hey and O'Connell, in examining the neutral thermal zone of babies, learned that an environment of 75 F is necessary to provide a neutral thermal environment for breast fed babies.[20] According to Cooke, the caloric intake of infants decreases as environmental temperature increases from 81 F to 90 F and vice versa.[21] This raises the question about how heavily an infant should be wrapped when being nursed.

In his contact with humans, the infant needs to be held firmly, to feel body contact, and to feel secure. To put one's arms around another is to communicate love. In a study on the handling of the infant by the mother, Rubin finds a definite progression and sequence in the nature and amount of contact made by the mother. At first the fingertips, rather than the hand, are used in exploring the infant. The fingertip traces the profile and the contours of the infant's face, and determines the texture of the hair. The index and forefingers are used to support the infant's head when bathing. The mother uses her arms in a rather rigid manner and tends to carry the baby away from her body.[22] With experience she relaxes and uses the whole of her hand and arm to hold the infant close to her body. Rubin notes that the mother, who has an experience of meaningful touch during the intrapartal or postpartal period, uses her hands better in handling the infant.[23]

Patting, stroking, caressing, and fondling are stimulating, soothing, assuring, and comforting. The physical holding of an infant is a form of loving. The differences in the quality, frequency, and timing of tactile experiences from one culture to another are found in all possible variations.[24] The Balinese infant[25] is always in someone's arms and the Ganda tribe infant of East Africa[26] is carried on his mother's back. In the United States, the infant is bathed, fed, clothed, and placed in a bed by himself, a straight nonmovable crib, and the bed clothes are neatly tucked around him. Where is the cradle? Where is the rocking chair? Montagu believes that tactile contact for the American infant expresses caretaking and nurturance rather than love and affection.[27] The taboos on interpersonal touching in our society may be related to the Christian tradition of the fear of bodily pleasures.[28]

The infant learns to trust his mother through being kept warm, fed, and made comfortable. He trusts that when in need he will be cared for. Erikson in *Childhood and Society* stresses that the primary personality development task of the infant is to develop a sense of trust.[29]

During the first year of life the infant progresses from a state of complete dependency at birth, to responding to social stimulation by three months of age. At this time he can make small throaty noises in response to faces, voices, and the sight of food. By six months of age he is forming ego boundaries; at nine months he is becoming an active person in his social environment and is seeking control over his physical environment. At this age, the quality of the time the mother spends with the infant is more important than the amount of time. By one year, the child can give affection and show jealousy and anger. He loves rhythm, is egocentric, and is usually involved in solitary play.

It is in the system involving parental contact, interaction, and reaction that the infant first learns that he is being loved. This conclusion was drawn by Brazelton from research in child development being conducted at Boston Children's Hospital Medical Center.[30] All experiences of the first year of life are believed to leave an imprint at the unconscious level and thus contribute to the formation of all future associations. Emotional development is dependent on the quality and consistency of the early relationships. If the first building block for satisfying the love need of the person is inadequate, then all subsequent blocks will be lacking in some degree of adequacy. The end result will be an adult who is insecure and unable to give and instill trust and love. If the foundation for meeting the love need is well developed in infancy, then it is assumed that all future steps in the development of the person will lead to a healthy love, to the ability to give and receive affection, to establish satisfying relationships, and to love and to be loved.

Love-Need Deprivation

Maternal deprivation—the lack of consistent, appropriate, and satisfying mothering by the caretaker during infancy—may lead to many emotional and physical problems for the individual during his life cycle. The infant who is separated from his parents for a long period of time or who is exposed to a multiplicity of caretakers with varying techniques for scheduling and handling relative to bathing, clothing, feeding, and playing has his need for love fulfillment violated. He may respond by failure to thrive. If deprived of the accustomed maternal body contact, he may develop depression with lack of appetite and even marasmus.[31] In a study on the development of six-month-old infants in an orphanage, Bakwin concludes that the symptoms of relative immobility, poor sleep habits, unresponsiveness to stimuli such as a smile, and proneness to febrile episodes are due to a lack of stimulation by caretakers.[31] Province and Lipton, in comparing institutionalized infants with infants reared by their families, found that institutionalized infants are unusually quiet, sleep excessively, and react strangely to being held. They do not adapt to the warmth and arms of the adult.[32]

Lack of love is manifested in the guise of a multitude of physical and emotional problems. Crying that does not cease with appropriate care may be a distress signal. Feeding problems may develop. There may be scratching and itching of the skin, even eczema. If inappropriately held and fondled, the infant may suffer from affect hunger as an adolescent and adult.[33] Hollender, in studying prostitution, reported that one call girl used sex so that she could be held.[34] Adequate mothering is necessary for the development of healthy sexual behavior. The way the mother holds and cuddles the infant and handles his genitalia affects subsequent sexual development and behavior. It may affect the manner in which all aspects of the sex act are approached and handled. As the unloved child grows he may be awkward in his demonstration of love and relationships toward others.

Nursing Strategies

Any nurse who has professional contact with the pregnant woman and the mother and infant has the responsibility to support and use those helping and assisting actions that facilitate the fulfillment of the love need. The following are suggestions for nursing assistance:

1. The nurse can foster prenatal courses, natural childbirth, breast feeding, rooming in, well child clinics, classes in parenting.
2. The nurse with the newborn can (a) place the newborn in the mother's arms as soon as possible after birth, (b) let the infant remain at her side as long as desired, (c) put the newborn to nurse, preferably breast, as soon as possible, (d) involve significant others (mate, other children, family, close friends) with newborn as soon as possible in the hospital or home, (e) avoid disruption of fondling and touching, and (f) restore the cradle or its substitute.
3. The nurse can teach the mother and/or substitute caretaker (a) to express love to infant by cradling, cuddling, caressing, (b) ways and means of providing appropriate stimulation for the infant, (c) how to touch and handle infant in feeding, bathing, clothing, diapering, playing, (d) steps of growth and development, and (e) basic appraisal skills for determining deviations from normal growth and development.
4. The nurse can identify the strengths of the mother and significant others and give support, reassurance, and reinforcement.
5. The nurse should explore any problem with the mother and together they should plan for its solution.
6. The nurse should act as a role model to demonstrate the use of techniques that will enhance love need fulfillment.

Early Childhood

Assessment of Love Needs

To become loving and caring the human being must be tenderly loved and cared for in his early years from the moment of his birth. Thus it is necessary that consistent loving care of the child by his mother or caretaker be continued as he enters the early childhood years of one to six. These are years when he explores and enjoys the world around him and sets the stage for his behavior with others. Even as he moves toward independence he needs to have the feeling of belonging and being wanted, of being wanted and appreciated for himself and not for what he can do.[35]

During the early childhood years he acquires a sense of trust in self and in others; he develops a healthy concept of self; he learns to give and to receive affection, to be a member of a family group, to understand and use language, and give personal care; he achieves motor coordination skills; and he begins to learn physical and social realities, distinguishes between right and wrong, and respects rules and authority. The child then enters the developmental stage in which initiative is the primary task.[36]

These behaviors for the preschool child are delineated further as tasks for specific stages of development are identified. During the second year of life, the child makes increasing personal contacts and gets involved in the environment around him. Loving care is the best safeguard against fear and anxiety as the child is led and guided in his explorations. He tries to please his caretaker, which in turn leads to toilet training and language development.[37] By his second birthday he has learned that he can exercise choice over what he does, notes responses to his choices, and gains a feeling of independence. He would like to make friends but does not know how.

In his third year the child develops his self-concept from reflected appraisal from significant others and begins to know self as a separate person. The child who is loved by others has little difficulty accepting himself. He develops some social awareness outside of family. An example is the nursery school child who likes to share candy or carry packages. Love begets love. He senses his parents' cultural expectations and identifies differences in race and sex. As he discovers and identifies his sexual identity, male or female, he acquires a romantic interest in his parents.

The child at four is generally independent in most activities of daily living. He has a desire to emulate his parents; this leads to the emergence of conscience and the incorporation of the values of the parents. The need for intense and frequent contact decreases.

At five years, there is a strong interest in family, especially extended family, and enjoyment of group activities with playmates. At six the child is ready to enter the world of competition in the form of school, and to be separated from his mother or caretaker for periods of time.

The child must be nurtured and enculturated. His development into an integrated person is the responsibility of the family, who perform a number of functions in this regard. Parental nurturance fulfills the child's physical, security, and affection needs. The mother is usually accepted as the primary nurturant figure and the nature and caliber of her care will affect the quality of trust developed by the child. Family structure forms boundaries for the integration of the child's personality. The child is dependent on parental figures and the parent's sex linked roles are models for his behavior. The family as a social system provides for teaching of female and male roles and inculcation of language and social values; the various socio–cultural phenomena of the system influence the child.[38]

Different child-rearing practices exist in and reflect the various cultures around the world. In the United States the child lives in a time-oriented society where schedules are dictated by clocks. There are certain toys for specific age groups, and a time to do and a time not to do certain things. This provides the climate for implementing specific activities for the child at specific times and if it is not the appropriate time, the child is left alone. The child also becomes the possessor of certain things that are his to own and his to use. In contrast, the Hopi Indian child lives in a timeless world where there is a belief that everything already exists although some things may not be evident. He is not in a hurry. The Fijian child has no concept of acquiring possessions or gaining wealth, as there is no concern for private possessions. There is a cultural taboo on ambition and personal advancement; thus the child becomes an integral part of the family and its society, sharing everything with all others. Even within American culture there are social class differences in customs, as well as ethnic differences among groups who preserve separate identities such as the Mennonites, the Greek Orthodox, and the Hasidic Jews.[39]

Home and the bosom of a caring family is the environment conducive to the development of affection. Warmth, understanding, and mutual support are the elements needed. For healthy development a certain amount of protection, control, and nurturance are necessary. Parents must give the child enough contact, help, recognition, attention, and closeness without discouraging independence.[40]

The young child is very busy with his own affairs, and therefore may need only interest, an accepting voice and kind treatment, whereas another child of his same age may need more demonstrative care.[41] The child who is loved can be busy with his own activities, but he knows that when he is in difficulty he can reach out for adult assistance. This child accepts physical routine, is happy and relatively calm, and has a real excitement for life. What the caretaker does for the child is to lead him to a sense of trust, and autonomy.[42]

Throughout his precious but vulnerable early childhood years the child needs guidance and support in self-direction and thinking, acceptance of rules and regulations, and the beginning development of values and beliefs. The permanent building block for all future behavior of that person is established during these years. Hopefully the child will become a person who will have self-actualizing love in his later years.

Love-Need Deprivation

If smothered by love and overindulged during the preschool years, the child may become egocentric and inconsiderate of others. Too much love may hamper his emotional growth and development and protect him from life's hardships.[43]

Children who are loved thrive better than those who are not so fortunate. If there is a loss of maternal love or that given by the primary caretaker, there is an interference with the child's desire to improve and advance. When rejected by a parent one child may become aggressive and destructive and another may become anxious and withdrawn. If there is coldness on the part of the mother, the child may react by developing eating problems or bedwetting. The punishment given by the parent for such activities tends to reinforce the child's behavior. An unloved child is apt to take feelings of insecurity into adulthood and may never learn to give and receive affection or establish satisfying relationships.

Nursing Strategies

Nurses in many health settings have the opportunity to assist the mother and preschooler in developing those behaviors which are viewed as being important to meeting the love need. The following strategies may be used. The nurse can:

1. Foster mothers' discussion groups, well-child clinics.
2. Assist the mother in developing techniques for control of behavior and allowance of freedom for the child relative to feeding himself, toilet training, playmates, exploration of environment, demonstration of affection, and sibling rivalry.
3. Guide the mother in making decisions relative to setting sensible limits so that the child cannot harm himself and yet can participate in things interesting to him; separating out tasks that the child can do independently; and selecting activities, toys and books to provide stimulation for furthering communication, interpersonal relationships, and acquiring knowledge and skills.
4. Teach the stages of growth and development in the area of motor, cognitive, and social skills.

Middle Childhood

Assessment of Love Needs

As he enters the world of a structural school system and meets many strangers of his own age and older, the schoolage child has the ability to trust others and has a sense of respect for his own world. He is leaving the ever present security of the home and the caretaker and entering an environment where he must fend for himself. His teacher becomes a significant other together with his peer group as he gains self-control and independence, and develops and achieves.

This is a period of accomplishment or industry according to Erikson.[44] The child will gain wider knowledge and understanding of his physical and social world. He will build wholesome attitudes toward self and learn the appropriate masculine or feminine social role. He will also be developing intellectual skills—reading, writing and calculating—and physical skills. These will be tempered with development of conscience, morality, and a scale of values. He will be learning to win and hold his place among peers, to give and take, and to share responsibility.

More specifically, as he strives to achieve the seven-year-old is subjected to increasing challenge and competition and wants and needs support and praise. He needs assurance that what he is doing is being carried out correctly. As he adapts to school life he misses his freedom and home, but he gradually develops endurance. In striving to develop an ethical sense, he wants to be good, but worries his parents with his contradictory ethical behavior, which ranges from prudishness to callousness and impropriety. He wants to be like his own peers and to be liked by them. He assesses himself in comparison to them. His choice of friends is uninfluenced by social and economic factors. There is manifestation of the developing awareness of self as an independent individual and as a boy or a girl. Play behavior reflects gender identity and he illustrates his growing confidence in himself by his careless disregard of parental requirement. He may insist that he has washed his hands when they are actually covered with grime. The reality of the universe is explored; thus he may be increasingly concerned with God, the universe, death; his belief in Santa Claus is waivering; and his imaginings may lead him to fear the natural environment.[45]

The eight-year-old is no longer a child but not yet a youth. This is the maturity level where the two sexes begin drawing somewhat apart. Boys and girls participate as equals in school and recreational activities but are becoming aware of differences. The interest in babies, their origin, procreation, and marriage begins at this age. The child is speedy, expansive, and can appraise what happens to him and what he causes to happen. He is building up an ethical sense and has a lively property sense as demonstrated by his collections. He challenges himself by spreading out into new territory with backyard shows and lemonade stands. The eight-year-old is cosmopolitan with a deep interest in life. During this period of development, the child demands maternal attention, but it is a psychologic rather than a physical interchange. He is no longer as dependent on his teacher. He and his group are making their own decisions and developing a group consciousness.[46]

The nine-year-old is no longer a child but not yet a youth. He is more self-organized, self-motivated, and persistent. He becomes very absorbed in activities, and is an individualist with positive likes and dislikes. He has considerable ability in social as well as self criticism and is more refined and discriminating. He is anxious to please, wants to be liked and can be trusted. Girl–boy associations have an impersonal matter-of-fact quality. The mother no longer needs to be home when the child returns from school. He likes to discuss things with his father; he gets along well with siblings and cares well for younger brothers and sisters for short time periods. He likes solitary activities, enjoys school but wants to be independent of the teacher. He thinks in terms of right and wrong, and lacks interest in God and religion.[47]

An adult in formation is the ten-year-old. Sex differences are pronounced, and companionship between the sexes is strained. The child works with speed, is receptive, easily responsive to appeals to reason, and demonstrates with fair indication what type of man or woman he/she will be. He has greater self possession and is aware of individuality in himself as well as others. At this age he may esteem his peer group more than family.[48]

Gesell's basic premise about humans is that the foundation and most of the framework for man's behavioral system is formed during the first ten years of his life and that these ten years cannot be ignored, as they form the building block for the maturing youth.[49]

There is probably no such person as a typical preadolescent, who is the eleven- to twelve-year-old. These years represent the period of growth spurt. The dormant reproductive organs begin to activate and secondary sexual changes take place. Probably the most frustrating aspect of this age is that the youth wants the rights of being grown up but cannot assume the responsibilities. Group membership and belonging increases in importance and every individual needs one close intimate friend of the same sex. There is a need to gain independence from adults, especially from parental control, and clarify the emerging adult world. The preadolescent still loves his parents but cannot face being ostracized by his peers; thus he is torn between pleasing both groups. Acceptance by others is important. There is a need to be listened to, to explore, to test truths and limits, and to make decisions. The twelve-year-old can handle a great deal of responsibility.[50]

The schoolchild develops a wholesome concept of self as he gains independence, self-control, self-development, and achievement. The family must meet the child's needs to allow him to have experiences and to provide him with the feeling of love and security. He needs assistance in handling all of the changes being experienced within and around him. The significant others in the school setting should be cognizant of their roles in promoting the developmental tasks of learning and assisting in gratifying needs of the individual.

As the youth moves into the preadolescent years, he begins to look at the adult world in contrast to the child's world. Somc conflict with parental authority arises in this process. Parents must know and appreciate the importance of the customs outside of the home and family. Achieving freedom from adults is in the realm of both psychologic and physical freedom. Family should avoid overstructuring the child's life and imposing a too-restrictive disciplinary program.[51] Whether or not the child learns to give and receive affection is determined by the family relationships and his experiences with his peer group. It is important for him to be able to identify with his peer group and to have intimate friends. While providing guidance and security the parents and teacher should allow him freedom to explore, give him time to find the answers, provide for varied peer contacts and be near and ready to guide whenever needed. The passage into teen years is a struggle with sexual tensions and need for increased self-esteem, autonomy, and independence.

Love-Need Deprivation

Behavioral problems arise from lack of fulfillment and the inability to accept and cope with the situations encountered. The lack of nurturance, support, security, and acceptance from mother, caretaker, family or peers, the discord displayed in the home between and among family members, and the stress in the school environment may be evidenced by such behaviors as (a) poor eating and sleeping habits, (b) peer maladjustments, (c) psychophysical disorders such as nailbiting, thumbsucking, headaches, bedwetting, (d) speech disorders, (e) school problems such as learning difficulties, attention seeking, negativism, (f) sexual problems such as masturbation, inspection, and premature heterosexual activity, (g) withdrawal reactions, and (h) aggressive reactions.

The overprotected and overdependent child has difficulty adjusting to the new experience of attending school. His fear of separation from his family is stressful and may be manifested in crying, nailbiting, and vomiting. An older child in a family may believe that his younger siblings will usurp his parents affection while he is away from home.[52]

As members of an industrialized society, Americans are very mobile. Frequent moves sever people from their roots, their family, friends, and neighbors. The frequent mover is a newcomer or a transient, and therefore never belongs to any permanent group. In this kind of an existence, if moving occurs too frequently the child can become frustrated and disoriented.

The child's having to take on increasing responsibility in family roles when parents do not or cannot assume and handle the situation may result in immediate behavioral problems or lay the foundation for future deviant behavior. If the demands on the child are carried out within a loving, sharing family environment, no significant deviant behavior is apt to occur.

If there is no parent sex role figure present in the home with whom the child can identify, he/she may become more confused than the average preadolescent seeking role identity.

Nursing Strategies

Nurses in the school, office, clinics, and private practice are especially concerned with the schoolage child and his healthy growth and development toward fulfillment of his basic needs including love. At this stage in the life of the child, the nurse needs to work with not only the mother, but with the child and his teacher. Some of the nursing activities that can be employed are:

1. Foster mothers' discussion groups, mothers' clubs, multidisciplinary conferences, PTA sessions or school health and rap sessions to aid parent(s) in understanding growth and development patterns, and methods for handling these normal developmental behaviors and their deviations.
2. Support the mother by allowing her to express her feelings, and assisting her to understand and deal with separation anxieties relative to child going to school.
3. Work with the parent(s), teacher and preadolescent to enhance their knowledge and abilities to cope with a healthy approach to sexual changes which will be occurring in the child's body and the overt behaviors anticipated with these changes.
4. Assist the teacher in working with children with diverse backgrounds and growth/behavior patterns.
5. Use the classroom setting to teach the children about their stage of growth and development, what to anticipate, and how to handle it.
6. Provide one-to-one assistance in helping children understand and deal with overt behaviors such as nail biting, scratching, thumb sucking.
7. Refer parent(s), child and/or teacher to other resources for assistance if deemed necessary and appropriate.

Adolescence

Assessment of Love Needs

The adolescent, the youth of twelve to eighteen years of age, is not someone different, but a continuation, an extension of his infancy, preschool years, and the years from six to twelve. The development during these teen years is a period of transition between childhood and adulthood, a phase of development toward maturity. The adolescent is embarking on a phase in his life where he is concentrating on two tasks: (1) the formation of a clear sense of identity as to who he is and what kind of person he is; and (2) a formation of a sense of intimacy or the ability to form close heterosexual relationships.[54] He is adjusting to body changes, developing new and more mature relationships with peers, achieving emotional independence from parents, selecting and preparing for an occupation, achieving mature values and social responsibility, preparing for married life, and developing concern beyond self. The adolescent is moving from dependency on the family into the greater community of life where he will become and be responsible for his own person. Adolescence ends when the individual reaches a new plateau of relative stability.

This gradual progression toward adulthood can be divided into three phases, which may overlapping: early adolescence, midadolescence, and late adolescence.[55]

Early adolescence encompasses the spurt in growth during the prepubertal phase in which developmental changes and onset of puberty take place. The onset of puberty does not upset the monosexual peer groupings to any noticeable extent, but there is a shift of interest to the opposite sex. The acceptance of the sex role and the stability of gender identity depend on the definitive gender designation during the first several years of life.[56] Hollander states that adequate mothering is necessary for the development of healthy sexual behavior.[57] The way the mother holds, cuddles, touches, and plays with the young child affects subsequent sexual development.[58] Girls become aware of the significance of the reproductive processes and often are embarrassed about menses. They have romantic cravings, maternal cravings, and some sensual feelings; boys seem to experience an urgency concerning sex and must deal with these feelings. Masturbation is almost a universal practice among boys, but it is not as common among adolescent girls. Sexual impulses are drained off in pursuit of many activities, especially in the arena of sports. In moving from self-love to love of another person, the adolescent forms intense crushes on older persons—a teacher, a club counselor, an older sibling of a friend. For this early teenager home remains the center of his life as he strives toward independence. In this process he is neither ready to assume responsibility nor capable of handling his feelings. He may feel unloved and unwanted unless the parents provide safeguards to assist in the adjustment.[59]

In the wake of the onset of midadolescence, one to two years after pubescence, the increase of the sexual drive moves the adolescent toward the opposite sex, thus breaking up peer groups and intimate friendships. In this movement, parents are put at a distance, their values and standards are questioned, and the youth surges ahead to try things his way. This sets the stage for conflict and lack of communication within the family circle. The peer group gains importance and its mores dictate what is accepted as appropriate behavior. Establishment and maintainance of affectional and sexual relationships with persons outside the family proceed slowly. With necking and petting the young couple explore and enter into the riddles of sexuality; however, this has little to do with being in love. In forming a bond with another, they yearn for their infatuation to mature into true love. Falling in love four or five times a year does not render the love less strong nor the ache any less painful when the relationship is ended.[60] Going through this phase prepares the adolescent for later fulfillment of heterosexual love.

By late adolescence the young person should have freed himself from his family to the point where he is comfortable with sexual expressions and is ready to be concerned with his future, the acquisition of identity through career decisions, and capabilities of intimacy through marital choices. Identity formation has much to do with the individual's past identification with parents, idols, and both friends and enemies as individuals and in groups.[61] Achievement of identity is the recognition by another. Identity and the capacity for intimacy are interrelated. Even though the adolescent may have been involved in many sexual experiences it is usually not until late adolescence that he is interested in and ready for intimate relationships. Due to the changes in the sexual mores in Western culture, sexual intercourse and cohabitation have become an integral part of experimentation with intimacy. Intimacy and identity have merged in an adolescent when he has gained the feeling of being needed and wanted by another person. When he has achieved this level of development he sees his parents as individuals with lives of their own, involved in each other and their occupations, rather than as just parents.[62] At this time in his life, he has overcome the dependency on family and is ready to redirect his energies away from those persons who have for a number of years been the primary objects of his affectual attachments.

Today's American teenagers are forced into a long period of dependence—intellectually, economically, and socially.[63] Education, as a valued acquisition, is extensive and is becoming more prolonged. This process hinders an earlier achievement of independence and autonomy. Jobs are scarce for the unskilled and labor laws make it difficult for the young to be employed, so economic independence is hard to attain. In Western culture, women, especially the mother and female teacher, have been most influential in shaping the lives of children. This has not been intentional, but has resulted from urbanization and industrialization, as the father is absent from the home a large part of the time. In studying personality adjustment, Heilbrum learned that boys and girls who have more male influence during childhood and adolescence reveal better personality adjustments in later life.[64] Becker found that when fathers are active in child rearing, their sons reveal more masculine behavior and a higher development of conscience than do sons of fathers demonstrating less affection, parental responsibility, and activity in child rearing.[65]

As the adolescent encounters the many conflicts and demonstrates a variety of behaviors along the way to achieving independence he needs support and guidance from all adults who know that these are passing phases of his development. Parents must be tolerant and be satisfied that their past guidance was carried out well enough to permit their child to seek and gain autonomy. Parents need to recognize that their child's acceptance of his gender role is conditioned by their love and trust of him and that his self-concept is influenced by the roles they gave him as models.[66] Although this may be a frustrating period for both the parents and the adolescent, the parents must be willing to utilize all of their knowledge and intellectual skills to provide an acceptable climate in which the adolescent can meet the many crises to be encountered in his search for self-identity and intimacy. Parental guidance must be subtle to be appreciated by the teenager. This includes knowledge of the task to be achieved, providing open communication for exploration of task implications, contributing in many ways to achieve the task, and making him feel worthwhile by helping to find acceptable employment.[67]

Love-Need Deprivation

For the adolescent failure to attain the sex role or a diffusion of the sex role, may have an enduring influence on the remainder of his life's experiences. Girls who are sex delinquents often have not polarized their sex role. A cruel father can make his son resent his male role, and a daughter her female role because she does not want to be under male domination.

The young teenager who feels unwanted, unloved, or neglected may turn to animals as love objects. He can love and care for them, and in turn feel needed. The older teenage girl may seek sexual relations so she can feel loved, or she may become pregnant so she can have a baby to love. By way of rebelling, striking back at parents or proving to be grown up, pregnancy may be used as a weapon.

Youth rebellion grows out of the need for love and hunger for group membership. Cases of maladjustment are found when belongingness is thwarted.[68] Peer pressure and rebellion against parental authority may lead to use of drugs, intimate sexual relations, and cohabitation. When unable to cope due to lack of support and affection, the adolescent may carry out extreme behaviors such as molestation, rape, or suicide. He may turn to the use of drugs or alcohol as a crutch for his ego.

Nursing Strategies

The nurse, whether in the school, office or clinic, has the opportunity and responsibility to serve as a confidant, advisor, and teacher to the teenager and his parents as he struggles with the changes brought about by adolescence. In order to give assistance, the nurse can:

1. Be a good listener, and support and educate parents as to expectations relative to teenage behavior and suggest methods for coping.
2. Work with teachers in the school setting to provide instruction on changes and differing growth rates, physiologic adjustment, reproductive anatomy and sexual responses, sexuality, coping with homosexual fears and masturbation, venereal disease, drugs, and family planning.
3. Support physical education classes and rap sessions for the handicapped, convalescents, obese, and late maturers.
4. Be available to the adolescent for one-to-one counseling in privacy.
5. Work with teenage groups at youth centers, churches, social agencies, or wherever appropriate to offer guidance and counseling in the areas of sex, venereal disease, sexuality, family planning, and drugs.
6. Be available to work with other disciplines in relation to youth and the inherent adjustment problems.
7. Know the community resources and be ready to refer the adolescent and/or his parents to appropriate resources for assistance.

Early Adulthood

Assessment of Love Needs

The developmental process draws to a close as the individual attains an identity and an ability to share life with a member of the opposite sex. The developmental building blocks, from infancy to eighteen years of age, have been formed and placed in his life's structure by his parents or their substitutes with his assistance. Now he is at the stage where he is responsible for the continuation of building his life, and he experiences that his adult life is only as firm and healthy as its foundational underpinnings. As he proceeds with the process he in all probability seeks another person with whom to share his tasks. Building satisfying love relationships with others is one of the means of establishing connections with the world.

The time that adult life starts is not always set chronologically, as the individual may have launched his life's career and chosen a spouse some time during adolescence. If he has not committed himself, then as he begins to see meaning in his life he becomes involved in an occupation, selects and learns to live with a mate, starts a family and supplies his children with their material and psychologic needs, manages a home, finds a congenial social group, and assumes civic responsibilities. Erikson proposes that development of the capacity of intimacy is the central task linked to early adulthood and that couples in this stage are moving toward autonomy, the next stage of development.[69]

There are important differences between the development of men and women during this period. For the man this is a period of relative vigor and activity during which he establishes himself in a variety of roles and different relationships. If not attending school, he is generally involved in some type of career or professional training and is developing his role as a working member of society. His success depends on achievement and ability to work through new types of relationships with peers and superiors. He has a more permanent goal for intimate relationships—that of love, courtship, marriage, and family rather than sexual experience only. He seeks out other types of social experiences with men, such as membership in clubs and lodges. Psychologically, he has moved away from his parents; however, they may begin to develop a somewhat dependent relationship on him, rather than the reverse, as before.

The woman matures earlier than the man both biologically and socially. Women do not require as long a preparation for the role of wife and mother as the man does to establish his career. Women seem to possess a drive toward conception and motherhood. They are more accepting of a relatively dependent role both in relation to husband and to society in general. Although the acquisition of career training and working have been goals secondary in importance to raising a family, the former are gradually assuming a major role in American society. During early adulthood, the woman maintains closer links with her own family, especially her mother.

For the adult love is viewed in the total developmental setting and not as an isolated phenomenon. The person no longer fits in the home of his parents; therefore, he must seek an attachment that will provide for the direction of his life outside of his home. He finds that he needs to satisfy his peers and his superiors in the work situation. He needs to satisfy his inner urgings by selecting a mate to complete himself. Adult love can be conjugal or illicit, normal or perverse, sexual or idyllic, infantile or adult, romantic or procreative. D'Arcy speaks of two kinds of love, active or passive and self-centered or self-effacing. In healthy people, however, the dichotomies are resolved.[70] Before the person can give or accept real intimacy, he must acquire a reasonable sense of personal identity.

Romantic love is a phenomenon of Western culture. In seeking his mate the young man may invent a romanticized version of the loved one—a seductress, a soother of his anxieties, a mother of his children, or an image of his mother. The woman usually sees the man as the one person in her life who understands.[71] In the United States there is a trend toward living together to test a relationship before making a legal committment of marriage. In the relationship both without and within the bonds of matrimony there can be a freedom of sexual expression, the use of contraceptive measures, and the act of abortion to terminate an unwanted pregnancy. Relationships between the sexes are pursued for mutual satisfaction as well as for ego fulfillment. As human awareness of the other heightens and there is a committment to a long-term bond, an engagement and marriage generally follow. Courting may culminate in marriage for many reasons other than the true union of two individuals.

Although love is not synonomous with sex, the two are at times equated in the minds of many, particularly as the young couple learns to gain fulfillment from the sexual act. The sexual act should imply involvement, concern, responsibility, tenderness, and the awareness of the needs and the weaknesses of the other. The female is more responsive to and more dependent on touch for erotic arousal, whereas the male depends more on visual stimuli. Although differences may be partly genetic, cultural differences are significant.[72] In American culture mothers are closer to their daughters than to their sons and demonstrate more affection with girls than with boys. The mother stimulates girl babies, but soothes and rocks boy babies. Touching the girl child is not as restrictive as the mother touching the son. This early experience of the individual affects relationships throughout life.[73]

The basic love needs of man are met in the intimate relations of marriage and family. Love is present when the needs of the other person are the needs of the lover, and this involves care, respect, responsibility, and knowledge. Love and sex are enjoyed by healthy people.[74] Sheehy claims that the young adult is ignorant of his inner life and his mate and deals primarily with external forces, as the growth patterns of the partners are uneven. Stabilization occurs during the twenties.[75] The young adult, ages 22 to 28 years, becomes involved in the adult world, and life becomes less provisional and more rational and orderly. With the passage into the thirties, the person has a sense of wanting to be something more and this requires a willingness to change and to settle down in earnest pursuit of goals.[76] If the union of the couple has materialized into a solid relationship, they will weather the change together; otherwise, they may become one of the many divorce statistics for the late twenties age group.

Love-Need Deprivation

Many families have deprived their members of adequate warmth and love, thus making the foundation for development into an adequate adult a very tenuous one. The early impairments to the ability to love another person may have been early rejection, generalized attitudes of suspicion and distrust, emotional immaturity, egocentricity, or scars of trauma such as deaths, separations, severe illnesses, or accidents. These flaws in the building blocks of a healthy life are carried into adulthood.

An unloved or rejected child may become an adult who enters marriage for unsatisfactory reasons such as to get away from his parents, to prove that he can do something, or to have someone to care for and to be cared for. The deprived individuals may find it difficult to give and to receive love; they may be overly possessive of the ones they love and insatiable in their need to be assured that others love them; they may become insulated or have feelings of loneliness and isolation. The adult with love deprivation will surely transmit to his offspring the lack of love, attachment, security, and nurturance that he needs to develop into a healthy individual.

An adult who lacked tactile stimulation as a child may be awkward in his body relations to others and in his demonstrations of love. Men may be clumsy during intercourse due to limited tactile stimulation.[77] Women may become promiscuous as they search for warmth and contact with another human. For some the sexual act is regarded as a release of tension rather than a meaningful communication between two persons in a deeply involved relationship. Physical violence may be done to the body in forms of slapping, spanking, pinching, biting, scratching, gripping caresses, and tying the extremities. This type of behavior may become a part of the daily living pattern and the battered woman becomes a concern for society. Many physical complaints of the young adult are thought to be essentially displacements of sexual problems.

Nursing Strategies

Unless she is an expert in a special area of the health field, the nurse serves the adult population best by being a good listener and referring the adult or a couple to a specialist and/or community service who can assist them with their problems, such as marriage counselor, genetic counselor, religious advisor, and sex counselor.

The occupational health nurse sees more well adults than any other nurse and in the work setting can carry out a number of activities to assist the young adult in meeting his love needs. She can:

1. Counsel the person, in relation to his family, on growth and development problems, pregnancy, marital discord, care of aging parent or relative, and sexuality.
2. Support the establishment of special services and discussion groups on the job for the worker.
3. Develop and teach programs oriented toward fulfillment of love needs.
4. Refer the person to community resources for appropriate assistance.

The clinic or office nurse has opportunities to work with the pregnant woman and her family to assist them in building the first developmental block their child will have to use toward fulfilling his love need, and at the same time the couple are gaining a fuller appreciation of each other. The nurse can:

1. Foster maternity clinics, prenatal classes, parenting classes, and regular medical supervision.
2. Support the woman in making choices about type of delivery, breast feeding versus bottle feeding, caring for her other children, and working.
3. Provide classes on a formal or informal basis including all aspects of pregnancy and parenting.
4. Serve as an advisor and confidant.

Middle Adulthood

Assessment of Love Needs

The passage from young adulthood to the middle years of 35 to 60 is more a state of mind than an actual state of change. The mature adult experiences the results of full development of earlier tasks, trust, autonomy, initiative, industry, identity, and intimacy. It is the time when the adult is moving toward the pinnacle of his career, which when achieved will show a gradual decline. After the survey of where he has been and a critical look at where he wants to go, the man is put to the test for making a decision to either stay with his established career pattern or to strike out on something new; the woman makes judgments about her hopes or fears of what the future holds for her. Erikson describes this period as the crisis of generativity versus stagnation.[78]

These years find the adult relating to his spouse as a person; helping teenage children become responsible and happy adults; adjusting to physiologic changes of middle age and to aging parents; establishing adequate financial security for the remaining years; achieving full civic and social responsibility; and developing adult leisure time activities and extending interests. This person is predominantly independent and responsible.

The woman watches the dependency of her children come to an end and her nurturing functions cease. At this point, if not already involved in a career, she may enter the occupational field either by reentering a deferred vocation or choosing a new one. The care of grandchildren may give new pleasure. The man moves to the heights in his career, and, with the responsibility for children ceasing, has the freedom to focus on his own life. Having achieved his goals, the man begins to take great pleasure in teaching others and becoming involved in correcting social injustices.[79]

At some time during this period the adult experiences a rearrangement of the body's hormone system. This is followed by wrinkles, graying hair, and the shrinking of the body, which is responsible for loss of height. Self-esteem suffers as body changes take place. With menopause the woman gains a sense of freedom and increased sexual activity. The man in midlife may complain of sexual impotence. According to Masters and Johnson all but a very small percentage of the impotence cases are psychologic in origin.[80]

Although these are years of many developmental crises, the couple who gains pleasure from seeing one another grow adjust to each other and to their needs. Satisfaction with partner and marriage develops tolerance and contentment. Techniques are worked out for facing problems and change. The older person becomes more practical and knows what does and does not work. The mate can be a faithful and valuable source of companionship. There are shared interests and a healthy respect for and honesty with themselves. They do not have to pretend. The partner is certain of his spouse's affection and, even if the couple is neglected by their children, they have each other to love. Through all crises they support one another. If they have a good marriage the couple usually has the respect and affection of their children. As grandparents they feel freer to give and indulge the grandchildren as they seek to love and to be loved and needed by the grandchildren.[81]

Love and caring for the aged parent is an acknowledged and accepted responsibility of the adults who have loved and been loved from their infancy through life by their parents.

Love-Need Deprivation

The adult makes restitutive efforts during the middle years. If he has difficulty accepting the passage into middle age he may resist change or he may deny his age and experiences and try to recapture his youth. This problem may have arisen from his inability to achieve a clear self-identity during adolescence.

The couple who has stayed together for the benefit of providing a home for their children may now find it convenient to divorce and use their freedom in search of the happiness and love they have not experienced. The feeling of being unloved, whether true or not, leads to many psychologic problems. These feelings may grow out of the inability of the person to accept changes such as the end of fertility, the end of nurturance, body changes, and nearing the end of a career. In struggling with impotence and a need for change, the man seeks out female companionship, usually a younger woman, to boost his ego. The woman may isolate herself and develop self-pity or completely break her habit pattern and acquire different means of satisfying her love needs.

There may be too little or too much love in the family. If the children have presented problems that have caused great anxieties and discord, the parents may literally toss them out of the home when they come of age. As a consequence, the parents may have to cope with feelings of inadequacy and guilt. The opposite extreme is the parent who has great difficulty in permitting his children to assume the adult role and be free of parental guidance.

Nursing Strategies

The nurse serves the middle-aged population best by being a good listener, referral agent, and helper whenever needed. The greatest contact will be with the work force and those persons seeking specialized assistance. The nurse can:

1. Foster discussion groups and specialized clinics for the person who may need guidance with marital problems, sexual problems, and hormonal changes.
2. Support programs for guidance in changing occupations for both the worker and the mother entering the job market.
3. Become involved in programs for the battered woman and the alcoholic.
4. Be available to provide guidance on a one-to-one basis.
5. Work with other members of the health professions to provide comprehensive assistance.

Later Years

Assessment of Love Needs

When the adult has reached 60 years of age, is in a healthy state, and has passed through all other stages of development without deprivations of any consequence, he has achieved in all probability the attainment of the highest of all human needs, self-actualization.[82] According to Erikson, his developmental task as a mature adult is concerned with ego integrity.

These later years bring the need to adjust to retirement, reduced income, decreasing physical strength, and death of spouse and friends; to meet social and civic obligations within one's ability; to establish an explicit affiliation with one's own age group; and to maintain interests beyond oneself. Self-esteem diminishes with a marked decrease in all physical and mental activities, and there is an increased need to be perceived as someone of value. Dependency again becomes apparent and there is an increased need for tenderness and affection.

Because of the increased amount of leisure time available after retirement and the heightened emphasis on maximum personal development, the life of the adult can be further enriched. Although there is more time to do and enjoy things of interest, often the man has to prove himself capable of continuing in the world of work and in many instances the woman in this age group continues to work. If the retired couple are in the home fulltime, they have to cope with learning how to live for 24 hours each day in each other's presence.

A couple who has been closely related throughout their lives become more dependent on each other in old age. They accept the individuality of and have great respect for each other. False teeth and wrinkles do not get in the way of their relationship. Love to them is a spontaneous experience, an admiration for each other, which is more passive than active. Maslow believes that couples, especially grandparents, achieve self-actualizing love in their later years.[84] Self-actualizing love occurrs when the couple love because of the very essence of the other. This is complete fulfillment of the two as one in being.

Decreased income and waning health many times force couples to give up their homes for smaller living quarters or to move in with their children. The single adult may have to share living arrangements with an aging sibling, relative, or friend. If the home for the aged is the choice, there is a need for understanding, concern, and compassion as the elderly adjust to living with those of their age group, who demonstrate varying degrees of decreased physical and mental abilities. There is a great need to be in the midst of those who care. The person must cope with loss and bereavement of loved ones, not only of his spouse but also friends and children. Reestablishment of the personality in face of such separation is necessary and must be achieved. As these crises are worked through, the aged person begins to plan in some manner for his death.

Behavior patterns and coping mechanisms developed in early life still exist in old age and will determine whether the ability to love and to be loved are to be an integral part of the behavior of the elderly person in his declining years.

Love-Need Deprivation

At this late stage in life the adult may reexperience demonstrations of behavior in his children that were troublesome to him at an earlier age. The child who felt unloved or overprotected and was glad to get away from home is usually not very happy to have his parents back in his own home. When a parent comes into the home under these circumstances he is treated as an intruder and not as a member of a loving family. His physical and social needs may be met either by a rigidly planned life dictated by the family or by the dictates of extreme necessity.

The absence of someone to love and be loved by is devastating. Each person needs to feel that someone is interested in and cares for him. Loneliness becomes more of a reality as the individual becomes decreasingly active. If family is far removed or nonexistent the lack of having someone to at least care for him may be associated with the inability to afford appropriate living accommodations and medical care. To become reliant on community agencies for assistance in being cared for further decreases self-esteem.

Physical debilitation causes much stress among the elderly, particularly when they can no longer actively demonstrate their love by doing. The wife with arthritis must be transported everywhere in a wheelchair. She can no longer walk arm in arm with her husband. The grandparent with palsy cannot hold his first grandson and looks distressed, with tears in his eyes for his inadequacies. The husband can no longer handle his monies in taking care of his household and feels a loss in his inability to take care of his wife.

Nursing Strategies

The nurse who is usually associated with geriatrically oriented programs becomes involved with the elderly in assisting them to meet their love needs. She can:

1. Foster clinics, programs, discussion groups, and special interest groups to meet specific needs.
2. Serve as an advisor or consultant to the homes for the aged.
3. Assist the nursing homes to develop a philosophy that includes loving care.
4. Assist the nursing home personnel in implementing techniques and skills to achieve loving care.
5. Serve and teach in health care programs for senior citizen centers and senior citizen complexes.
6. Provide assistance in planning for stimulation of the older person.
7. Be available for comforting in time of stress and crisis.
8. Assume a helping role when the adult is unable to perform.
9. Support the adult in making decisions in times of crisis.
10. Be available to support the family and the client when death is anticipated.

Planning to Fulfill Love Needs

In confronting any situation requiring nursing assistance, the nurse must assess its assets and limitations, or its strengths and weaknesses, and from this assessment determine the needs of the client(s). The nurse then looks for areas that are conducive to change and growth in the client and herself. In this process the nurse must know how he responds to the identified needs. How does he feel about the situation? What strengths and weaknesses does he have that will or will not assist in bringing about desired outcomes? Whenever feasible (hopefully most of the time), the client(s) are involved with the nurse in establishing the plan for action to meet the identified needs. By contract, either implicit or formal, both the client and nurse know what is expected to be achieved and within what parameters. The focus of nursing is to increase the ability of an individual to care for himself. The process for planning in any health situation is also applicable for planning to fulfill love needs. It must be remembered that love is a basic human need.

It is not practical in this chapter to develop a nursing plan for action to demonstrate assistance provided by the nurse in fulfilling the love needs for all developmental stages of man; therefore, for demonstration purposes, a plan is designed for the first stage of development: infancy. Due to the complexity, involvement, and length of such a plan, a selected segment of each step is developed in detail. The framework used is the Nursing System Based on Self Care Competencies (Fig. 5.3). Although the system is outlined in steps, all steps are interrelated and the system may be entered at any point. Explanation of each step of the system is offered as the assessment and plan unfold for infant Danny Dale and his family.

• *Situation: Infant Danny Dale**

At the first visit by the community health nurse, Danny Dale is one week old. He is tucked carefully in his crib, which is located in the bedroom of a one-bedroom apartment in a low-middle class suburban area. Danny's mother, Louise, a 25-year-old attractive woman is home recuperating from a normal spontaneous delivery at the local hospital and is caring for her infant son. Louise is quite anxious about the care she is giving Danny. Joe, Danny's father, 26 years of age, has returned to his job as bank teller after taking a week's vacation to help his wife after Danny's birth. They have no extended family nearby.

Danny has regained his birth weight of 7½ pounds, is 21 inches in length, is breast feeding on demand and averages four stools per day. Inspection reveals an apparently normal infant. Danny, the first child of Louise and Joe, had been planned.

Louise states that during her uneventful pregnancy, she had attended the local health department maternity clinic regularly, and that she and Joe had attended some of the classes for parents. Louise is a high school graduate and had worked as a department store cashier before Danny's birth. She and Joe agree that she will stay home to raise the family. Joe, a community college graduate, earns $10,000 annually as a bank teller and has fringe benefits including health insurance. The family is white, and Protestant in religious affiliation. The young couple appear to be in good health.

They plan to use the local health department Well-Child Clinic for routine check-ups for Danny and they have a general medical practitioner in the neighborhood, to whose office they will go for emergency care.

Assessment

Step 1: Data Collection. *Family Type and Members* The Dale family is a nuclear family composed of Joe, age 26 years, a community college graduate,

*The application of the Nursing System Based on Self Care Competencies to the Dale family situation was carried out in collaboration with Doreen Harper, MSN, Assistant Professor, George Mason University, Fairfax, Virginia.

I. **Assessment**

Step 1 – Data Collection
Family and individual members: include age, sex, education, occupation
Socioeconomic structure of family
Cultural-ethnic influences
Religious influences
Value system
Family role relationships
Developmental stages
Health state
Health care situation
Health care resource used by families
Behavioral organic disorders
Basic needs of individual family members

Step 2 – Therapeutic Self Care Demands (TSCDs)
(Actions to be taken to maintain or regain health or wellness.)

Step 3 – Determination of Client's Assets and Limitations for each TSCD

Step 4 – Self Care Deficits (SCDs)
(Nursing diagnoses relating to each TSCD and client's inability to meet that need.)

II. **Plan for Nursing Intervention**

Step 1 – Nurse/Client goals (for each SCD)

Step 2 – Methods of Nursing Assistance
(Methods to be used by nurse)

Step 3 – Nursing Plan for Action

Specific Nursing Actions	*Rationale for Actions*

Step 4 – Performance Criteria

III. **Implementation**

(Include determination of nurse assets and limitations)

IV. **Evaluation** of plan, and nurse and client competencies. Use performance criteria.

Fig. 5.3: *Nursing System Based on Self-care Competencies.*

who is presently a bank teller; Louise, age 25 years, a high school graduate, formerly a department store cashier and presently a housewife and mother; and Danny, the first child of Joe and Louise, who is one week old. The family is in the child bearing stage of the family life cycle.[85]

Socioeconomic Structure The only source of income is Joe's salary of $10,000 annually plus fringe benefits that include health insurance. They are living in a rented apartment, which will become too small in the near future.

Cultural-ethnic Influence The family is a low-middle class, white, Protestant family. They have a strong sensė of family responsibility.

Value System Joe and Louise have a committment to family life and health care and demonstrate mature moral judgment.

Roles Joe assumes the role of breadwinner and head of the household and Louise is mother, homemaker, and wife. They apparently have made decisions together, and are interested in and have accepted their parenting roles. There are no relatives nearby to assist and serve as role models.

Health Assistance The couple shows reasonable concern about health care in that Louise attended maternity clinic regularly and there are plans to take Danny to the Well-Child clinic. The community health nurse is available for home visits. They have health insurance and access to a general practitioner in the neighborhood. There are no apparent organic behavioral disorders in the family.

Physical/Psychologic Needs of Danny The infant is being breast fed on a demand schedule. His elimination is normal for a breast fed baby. He has his own crib and there seems to be adequate space. There is need for exploration of the areas related to temperature, rest, activity, solitude, and social interactions such as holding and cuddling, and hazards of the environment.

Step 2: Therapeutic Self Care Demands[86] From the assessment of the situation requiring nursing assistance, the nurse must next identify the specific sets of actions that are needed to be performed by the client in order to accomplish objectively beneficial self care. These specified sets of actions are known as therapeutic self care demands (TSCDs). The demands are stated in terms of need for action. Three TSCDs are identified relative to the Dale Family as follows:

TSCD1—Mother needs to provide an environment conducive to meet the love needs of the newborn

TSCD 2—Family needs to adjust to new role of parenting
TSCD 3—Family has need for knowledge of neonate's growth and development

Step 3: Determination of Assets and Limitations With the identification of TSCDs the nurse isolates the assets and limitations for each TSCD in the situation that will affect the ability and capability of the client to achieve positive results. The measures utilized by the client to bring about favorable results and the influence of all data need to be considered by the nurse in order for client strengths to be identified.

In the assessment of the Dale family, only one therapeutic self care demand, that is TSCD 1, will be considered for identification of assets and limitations. The enumeration of the assets and limitations follows:

Assets:

1. Highly motivated family
2. Intelligent parents
3. Adequate minimal income
4. Skilled worker—father
5. Mother—normal postpartum progressive
6. Healthy infant
7. Breast feeding
8. Parents interested in child care
9. Parental communication relative to infant
10. Oriented to family life

Limitations:

1. Crowded living space
2. No extended family in immediate area
3. Anxious mother
4. Lack of practical experience with infant
5. Inadequate knowledge of tactile and auditory stimulation
6. Cultural restriction of tactile stimulation
7. Lack of knowledge of the development of the process of love
8. Territorial isolation of infant

Step 4: Self-Care Deficits When the client, the self-care agent, or the substitute self-care agent is unable to accomplish the usual and therapeutic self-care demands (TSCD) because of conditions or disabilities, then deficits result in his self-care.[87] The conditions or disabilities the self-care agent encounters may cause him to be unable to act for himself, to refrain from acting for himself, or to act ineffectively in caring for himself. From the limitations identified with any TSCD, the nurse can determine the self-care needs or deficits for the client. These deficits are expressed in terms of inability to do or lack of adequate or appropriate means. The self-care deficits (SCDs) delineated for TSCD 1 for the Dale family are as follows:

SCD 1—Insufficient knowledge regarding the relationship of love to basic infant care
SCD 2—Lack of practical experience regarding basic infant care

SCD 3—Inability of mother to control anxiety relative to infant care
SCD 4—Lack of familial support system in immediate environment
SCD 5—Lack of knowledge concerning the relationship of touch and verbal communication to infant's need for love

Plan for Nursing Intervention

Step 1: Nurse/Client Goals The phase that logically follows assessment is one for planning action for intervention to bring about change in the situation. Specific goals or objectives for intervention by the nurse and expected behavioral outcomes for the client (self care agent) need to be stated and accepted as realistic by both parties before any methods of assistance are determined.

Although all self-care deficits for TSCD 1 in the Dale family situation are important for fulfilling the infant's developmental needs for love, SCD 5 is chosen to be developed in detail for planning nursing intervention. The nurse/client goals for SCD 5 follow.

Nurse Goals	*Client Goals*
1. To teach mother regarding relationship between sensory communication and love need of the newborn.	1. To learn about the relationship between sensory communication and the fulfillment of the love need for the newborn.
2. To support mother in utilizing touch and verbal communication in care of newborn.	2. To utilize touch and verbal communication effectively in care of newborn.

Step 2: Methods of Nursing Assistance There are many ways a nurse may assist the client, and one or all methods may be used at varying times in a single situation. (1) The helping method, to act for or to do for another, requires the nurse to use her own physical or mental abilities. For example, the nurse may need to bathe the infant if the mother is physically unable to. (2) Guiding another to make a choice or to follow a specific course of action is an acceptable method of assistance. The nurse may guide the mother in choosing breast feeding over formula feeding for her newborn. (3) The nurse may give physical and/or emotional support to the client. This means the nurse assists in sustaining client so he can endure that which he is doing, thus avoiding failure. The nurse may support the mother in breast feeding her newborn. (4) Provision of a developmental environment so that client may meet present and future demands implies that the nurse helps the client to set goals and adjust behavior to achieve them. (5) Teaching another is a method of assisting a client, who needs instruction to develop skill. An example of this kind of assistance is the nurse who teaches the mother

how to hold her newborn.[88] (6) The client may need to be referred to another health resource if the nurse is unable to assist in meeting the client's need or there is a resource more appropriate. For instance, the nurse may refer the breast feeding mother to La Leche League for assistance and support.

When the client or the substitute self-care agent is able to perform and can learn to do the required activities to provide self-care, but needs assistance through guidance, support, provision of a development environment, teaching, and referral, the nurse designs a supportive–educative system of care.[89]

Step 3: Nursing Plan for Action In developing the nursing plan for action, the nursing actions are expressed with specificity and the rationale for each action is stated. Nursing actions, when implemented, should lead to effective achievement of goals.

For the Dale family a supportive–educative system of nursing assistance is designed for SCD. This includes the following methods of assistance as appropriate: guidance, support, provision for a developmental environment, teaching, and referral. Specific nursing actions with rationale are identified in the following plan of action.

Nursing Plan for Action: Dale Family

TSCD 1—Mother needs to provide an environment conducive to meet the love needs of the newborn.

SCD 5—Lack of knowledge concerning the relationship of touch and verbal communication to infant's need for love.

Nurse Goals:

1. To teach mother regarding relationships between sensory communication and love need of the newborn.
2. To support mother in utilizing touch and verbal communication in care of newborn.

Step 4: Performance Criteria Criteria for performance by both nurse and client are built into the plan for action. Criteria should be developed for each specified nursing action. It is these criteria that will be used in the evaluation process. One type of format for developing performance criteria is a listing of questions to be answered by the nurse and the client to determine if goals are being met.

Using specific nursing action 7 from the nursing plan for action for the Dale family, a detailed listing of questions is developed for purpose of evaluating the performance of the nurse and client.

Table 5.1 *Nursing Plan for Action*

Specific Nursing Actions	Rationale for Nursing Action
1. *Teach mother with infant present* Nurse observes a. Mother's reactions to infant, b. How mother handles infant, c. Infant's reactions to mother as caretaker. Nurse instructs mother by demonstrating on infant.	Having mother and infant together for teaching purposes provides the real-life situation for mother as caretaker and the nurse as the teacher. The mother can relate teaching to her own infant more realistically than when telling or a model is used. The nurse can serve as a role model in demonstrating handling of infant.
2. *Identify specific behaviors mother performs that are conducive to relationship, such as cuddling, caressing, handling.* Nurse identifies a. How mother uses body and hands in handling infant, b. How mother holds infant – firmly, loosely, timidly, c. How mother holds infant when breastfeeding, bathing, d. When mother holds infant other than while breastfeeding, e. When mother picks up infant, f. Where mother holds infant – standing, sitting, rocking, walking, g. Presence of patting, stroking, h. Presence of talking to or cooing over infant, i. Place where talking/cooing takes place – breastfeeding, diaper changing, bathing, holding, at cribside, j. Presence and use of rocking chair and cradle, k. Mother's reaction to diaper change, l. Where diaper change takes place, m. How genitalia are handled, n. Type of daily schedule.	By identifying behavior the nurse can assist mother to acquire more appropriate actions that lead to fulfilling the infant's love need.
3. *Teach mother how to communicate to infant primarily through tactile sensation.*	Physiological and safety/security needs are priority at birth; therefore, infant needs warmth to feel protected, milk to feel nurtured, held firmly to feel secure; and stroked, talked to, and patted to feel accepted. Tactile stimulation is basic to the development of healthy emotional and affectional relationships.[90]
Nurse to teach mother to a. Use the full palm of hand and arms in holding infant,	Mothers have a tendency to use fingertips and fingers to handle infants when born, causing insecurity and fear of falling. The physical holding is a form of loving.[91]

Table 5.1 *Nursing Plan for Action (Continued)*

Specific Nursing Actions	Rationale for Nursing Action
b. Hold infant close to her body,	Offers security to infant as he can feel body rhythms and hear the mother's heart beat.
c. Handle infant's body caressingly and firmly when bathing, dressing, diaper changing,	Provides safety, security, and the feeling of acceptance by another.
d. Speak softly and pleasantly as baby is handled,	Voice and touch provide a pattern of affection and acceptance.
e. Pat and stroke infant gently,	Provides feeling of affection and acceptance.
f. Breastfeed properly,	Provides a way of holding, loving, mothering.
g. Provide a constant temperature for infant.	Skin, being the primary sense organ of infants, they respond quickly to temperature and air changes. It is recommended that a room at 75° F is best, especially for breast fed babies.[92] It has been found that as room temperatures increase from 81° F to 90° F infant's intake decreases.[93]
4. *Describe behaviors that will get at conducive relationships by using audiovisual materials and demonstrations.* Nurse a. Identifies behaviors which can be learned by use of AV materials and demonstration, b. Selects appropriate materials for showing and demonstrating, c. Presents AV materials and/or gives demonstration, d. Seeks feedback from mother by asking questions re: content or having redemonstration, e. Evaluates with mother the value of use of AV materials and demonstration.	Pictures and demonstrations are worth thousands of words. Mother can see that infant is content if held in a certain manner. Through demonstration the nurse can act as a role model. By redemonstration, the mother becomes more familiar and comfortable with techniques being learned, and can receive guidance and instruction on the spot for improvement.
5. *Adapt behaviors demonstrated by mother to more suitable methods.* Nurse plans with mother to a. Use palms of hands and arms when holding infant, b. Hold and cuddle infant at times other than feeding,	By adapting more suitable methods, mother increases skill, is more functional, and can do things better. She and the infant should be more satisfied.
c. Use rocking chair or cradle,	Rocking provides a rhythmic contact that is soothing.
d. Place infant on a schedule with constancy,	Feeling of security is achieved

Table 5.1 *Nursing Plan for Action (Continued)*

Specific Nursing Actions	Rationale for Nursing Action
e. Cuddle, coo, embrace, pat and stroke infant tenderly, f. Talk to infant at various times and places, g. Handle genitalia without fear, h. Diaper as often as needed, i. Keep infant in a regulated environment regarding temperature and ventilation.	through regularization. Warmth develops trust.
6. *Reinforce positive behavior.* Nurse rewards mother with a. Verbal approval, b. Reassurance, c. Pat on the back, d. Praise.	Identification and acknowledgement of human strengths assists the individual in coping with human limitations.[94] By rewarding the mother as she moves towards acquisition of tactile skills, the mother's self-esteem is maintained. The mother knowing she is doing some things well will more readily acquire other knowledge and skills.
7. *Act as a role model to demonstrate use of tactile and verbal communication.* Nurse shows mother as she teaches a. How to hold infant, b. How to bathe infant, c. How to talk to infant, d. How to pat and stroke, e. How to diaper infant.	By seeing an act performed correctly by one who is deemed a skilled performer, the observer is more apt to accept the performance as a model and strive to emulate it. It is anticipated that the mother will adapt as some of her mothering behavior the actions performed by the nurse as she teaches the mother.
8. *Recommend appropriate literature.* Nurse recommends literature at a. Mother's level of comprehension such as Montagu's *Touching.*[17]	Mother will have authorities other than the nurse to guide her in forming skills and attitudes and acquiring knowledge about infant care and child rearing.

Specific Nursing Action 7—Act as a role model to demonstrate use of tactile and verbal communication.

Questions to be answered by mother:

1. Did nurse act as an acceptable role model?
2. Did nurse demonstrate techniques for touching, i.e., patting, stroking, cuddling?
3. Did nurse demonstrate how to hold baby when nursing, cuddling, bathing?
4. Did nurse show how to hold baby firmly, yet tenderly?
5. Did nurse show mother how to use her hands and arms when holding baby?
6. Was nurse explicit enough in instruction?
7. Did nurse demonstrate and teach at mother's level?

8. Did nurse allow mother to ask questions?
9. Did nurse answer inquiries satisfactorily?
10. Did mother perceive infant as comfortable with nurse during demonstrations?
11. Did mother perceive demonstration as necessary?
12. Did mother feel comfortable with nurse?
13. Did mother feel comfortable with redemonstrations?
14. Did mother feel she received positive reinforcement?
15. Did mother feel she learned new skills?
16. Did mother feel she has been able to apply new knowledge and skills comfortably?
17. Does mother feel she understands the relationship between handling the infant and the fulfillment of the infant's love needs?

Questions to be answered by nurse:

1. Was the mother interested?
2. Was the mother motivated?
3. Was the mother responsive?
4. Did the mother learn from role demonstration?
5. Did the mother improve her techniques of touch? Use of hands and body? Patting, Stroking, Cuddling?
6. Did the mother talk or sing to the baby while caring for him?
7. Did the nurse feel knowledgeable?
8. Did nurse feel adequately prepared to demonstrate and give support to mother?
9. Did nurse feel comfortable in situation?
10. Did any biases or value judgments get in the way of performance?
11. Was the nurse satisfied with her job performance?

Implementation of Plan

In implementing any course of action, the nurse needs to remember that to gain the best results she must use the knowledge gained from the assessment of the situation astutely and wisely. The beginning point for any interaction is where the client is in relation to his degree of maturity, intelligence, education, emotional stability, motivation, knowledge, attitude, skills, and values. In order for the nursing plan for action to be effective it needs to be planned and/or approved by the client(s) involved. The nurse may find that some goals will need to be redetermined and some specific nursing actions and responding client behaviors reworked as to priority, degree of expected change, and/or usefulness.

In working with mothers in attempting to promote the building of the foundational block for developing love, the nurse brings to the setting her own value system, biases, skills, knowledge, and attitudes relative to the concept of love and the role of mothering. She needs to know herself as a person, her strengths and limitations, and how she can best assist the young mother and the infant to grow in love. In moving ahead to achievement of the nursing goals, the nurse must be aware that the degree of constancy and consistency in assisting the client affects outcomes, and that reciprocation may not be evident. But to make the whole process work, the nurse needs to be a caring person—caring for the client and caring for herself. In caring the nurse needs to develop faith and to be grateful. If a caring person, she should be able to give the appropriate assistance to the mother and her infant for developing the love need.

Evaluation

Evaluation includes ascertaining the effectiveness of the plan in terms of outcome behaviors demonstrated by the client and the effectiveness of the nurse. The nurse and the client are the agents in the the evaluation, although at times there may be others involved. They make the judgments about the degree of achievement anticipated in relation to the previously set goals. The plan for evaluation is an integral part of each step in the development and implementation of a nursing plan for action.

The evaluation of the nursing plan for action for the Dale family is achieved by using the performance criteria developed for each specific nursing action as the evaluation guide. If there is satisfaction on the part of the client and the nurse, then it can be assumed that the goals are met.

Conclusion

The human need for love and its deprivation at each age is a concern for all nurses. Practitioners of nursing have a responsibility to assist with the development of the love need in their day-to-day contacts with clients. To be of assistance in this mission, it is evident that further exploration into the delineation of the specifics responsible for the fulfillment of the love need is necessary for making astute nursing diagnoses and plans for nursing action. Tools must be developed for measuring outcomes of assistance. From these measurements guidelines can be established to assist parents and caretakers in providing the appropriate environment and behavior for developing love. Further inquiry into the phenomenon of love as related to other human needs and the art of nursing is anticipated.

To teach love one must understand love. To give love one must possess love. Can all nurses teach love? Do all nurses give love? Can the nurse teach love and give love if she has not been privileged with acquiring the developmental foundation in her early years? If one believes love is learned and each individual is in the continual process of becoming, perhaps love can be taught. This inquiry has implications for those in nursing education and nursing service. Are nursing students chosen according to their ability to give loving care, or do the individuals, who seek nursing as a career, possess those qualities that understand and provide love? What criteria can be used to determine the faculty or staff members who can provide the teaching of love and the giving of tender loving care? The task ahead is challenging and can be rewarding. To love and to be loved involves responsibility, dedication, and sharing.

References

1. Maslow A: Motivation and Personality, 2nd ed. New York, Harper & Row, 1970, pp 43–46
2. The Great Ideas: A Syntopicon of Great Books of the Western World. Vol I. Adler (ed) J. Chicago, Encyclopaedia Britannica, 1952, pp 1051–1053
3. Ibid, p 1053
4. Aristotle: Nicomachean Ethics. Book VIII, Ch 2, 1155^{b}; Ch 6, 1158^{a}1
5. Aquinas: Summa Theologica. Part II–III, Q 26–Q 28
6. Freud S: Instincts and Their Vicissitudes, The Major Works of Sigmund Freud. In Great Books of the Western World, Vol 54. Chicago, Encyclopaedia Britannica, 1952, pp 418–421
7. New Testament: I John 4:16
8. Dante: Hell. Canto III, ll. 1–148. Paradise. Canto XXVIII, ll 1–22
9. The Great Ideas[2]: p 1058
10. Webster's New Collegiate Dictionary. Springfield, Massachusetts, G C Merriam, 1976, pp 681–682
11. Roget's College Thesaurus. New York. New American Library, 1962, p 481
12. Maslow A[1]: p 182
13. Ibid, p 183
14. Fromm E: The Art of Loving. New York, Harper Brothers, 1956, pp 47–83
15. Teilhard de Chardin P: Human Energy. Translated by JM Cohen. New York, Harcourt, 1969, pp 145–160
16. Maslow A[1]: p 45
17. Montagu A: Touching: The Human Significance of Skin. New York, Columbia University Press, 1971, p 68
18. Ibid, p 31
19. Ibid, p 72
20. Editorial: At what temperature should you keep a baby. Lancet 2:556, September 12, 1970

21. Cooke RE: The behavioral response of infants to heat stress. Yale Biol Med 24:334–340, February, 1952
22. Rubin R: Maternal touch. Child and Family 4:8, winter, 1965
23. Ibid, p 10
24. Montagu A[17]: p 225
25. Mead M, Macgregor FC: Growth and Culture. New York, Putnam's, 1951, pp 42–43
26. Ainsworth MD: Infancy in Uganda. Baltimore, Johns Hopkins University Press, 1967, p 451
27. Montagu A[17]: p 245
28. Ibid, p 238
29. Erikson EH: Childhood and Society. New York, Norton, 1950, pp 219–222
30. Brazelton TB: How babies learn about love. Redbook 149:101, 155–158, July, 1977
31. Bakwin H: Emotional deprivation in infants. Pediatr 35:512, October, 1949
32. Province S, Lipton RC: Infants in Institutions. New York, International Universities Press, 1962
33. Hollender MH: The wish to be held. Arch Gen Psychiatr 22:445–453, May, 1970
34. Hollender MH: Prostitution, the body, and human relations. Intern J Psychoanal 42:404–413, Parts 4–5, 1961
35. Bernard HW: Human Development in Western Culture, 3rd ed. Boston, Allyn and Bacon, 1970, p 238
36. Erikson EH[29]: pp 224–226
37. Barber JM, Stokes LG, Billings DM: Adult and Child Care. Saint Louis, Mosby, 1977, p 37
38. Lidz T: The Person. His Development Throughout the Life Cycle. New York, Basic Books, 1968, pp 54–62
39. Ibid, pp 48–54
40. Smart MS, Smart RC: Preschool Children: Development and Relationships. New York, Macmillan, 1973, pp 218
41. Breckenridge ME, Murphy MN: Growth and Development of the Young Child, 8th ed. Philadelphia, Saunders, 1969, pp 41–42
42. Ibid, p 442
43. Breckenridge ME, Murphy MN[41]: p 42
44. Erikson EH[29]: pp 226–227
45. Gesell AL, Ilg FL: The Child from 5–10. New York, Harper and Brothers, 1946, pp 131–158
46. Ibid, pp 159–187
47. Ibid, pp 188–211
48. Ibid, pp 212–223
49. Ibid, p 217
50. Bernard HW[35]: p 335
51. Ibid, p 335
52. Pillitteri A: Nursing Care of the Growing Family. Boston, Little, Brown, 1977, p 232
53. Maslow A[1]: p 43
54. Erikson EH[29]: pp 227–228
55. Lidz I[38]: p 303
56. Ibid, pp 304–308
57. Hollender MH[34]: pp 404–413
58. Montagu A[17]: p 164

59. Lidz T[38]: pp 308–321
60. Ibid, pp 321–342
61. Ibid, p 345
62. Ibid, p 342–359
63. Bernard HW[35]: p 343
64. Heilbrum AB Jr: Sex role identity in adolescent females, a theoretical paradox. Adolescence 3:79–88, spring, 1968
65. Becker WC: Consequences of different kinds of parental discipline. In Hoffman ML, Hoffman LW (eds): Review of Child Development Research, Vol 1. New York, Russell Sage Foundation, 1964, pp 169–208
66. Bernard HW[35]: p 364
67. Ibid, p 371
68. Maslow A[1]: p 44
69. Erikson EH[29]: pp 229–231
70. D'Arcy MC: The Mind and Heart of Love. New York, Holt, 1947, pp 39–73, 114–139
71. Sheehy G: Passages. New York, Dutton, 1974, pp 87–88
72. Kinsey AC et al: Sexual Behavior in the Human Female. Philadelphia, Saunders, 1953, pp 570–590
73. Montagu A[17]: p 246
74. Maslow A[1]: p 194
75. Sheehy G[71]: p 90
76. Ibid, pp 171–176
77. Montagu A[17]: p 173
78. Erikson EH[29]: p 231
79. Sheehy G[71]: p 272
80. Masters WH, Johnson VE: Counseling with sexually incompatible marriage partners. In Brecher R, Brecher E (eds): An Analysis of Human Sexual Response. New York, Signet, 1966, pp 210–213
81. Sheehy G[71]: pp 340–349
82. Maslow A[1]: p 199
83. Erikson EH[29]: pp 231–233
84. Maslow A[1]: pp 196–199
85. Duvall EM: Family Development, 4th ed. Philadelphia, Lippincott, 1971, p 220
86. Concept Formalization in Nursing: Process and Product. By the Nursing Development Conference Group. Boston, Little, Brown, 1973, pp 119–126
87. Ibid, p 117
88. Orem DE: Nursing: Concepts of Practice. New York, McGraw–Hill, 1971, pp 72–77
89. Ibid, p 79
90. Montagu A[17]: p 31
91. Rubin R[22]: pp 8, 10
92. Editorial[20], p 556
93. Cooke RE[21]: pp 334–340
94. Otto H: The human potentialities of nurses and patients. Nurs Outlook 13:32–35, August, 1965

Chapter Six •

The Need for Tenderness

Rita M. Carty

Maslow's[1] premise that tenderness is a need for human existence and growth is generally accepted and will provide the foundation for this chapter. That others, such as Sullivan[2] and Montagu,[3] support the position of tenderness as a basic need is reassuring but does little to clarify just what tenderness is. Maslow[1] treats tenderness as a part of his description of love, as have Fromm[4] and Adler.[5] In reviewing the literature it becomes clear that tenderness is seldom, if ever, considered as a definite concept in itself with particular attributes that are identifiable. Instead, it is usually considered within the broader aspect of love.

This chapter will concentrate on what can be behaviorally defined as tenderness within interpersonal relationships, specifically within the mother–child relationship.

The paucity of materials in the professional literature, as well as in the popular press, dealing with tenderness as a concept is disheartening. In trying to understand tenderness within interpersonal relationships, specifically the mother–child relationship, the concepts of love, caring, attachment, and bonding will be explored. The goal is to distill from these established concepts a description of tender behaviors that can then be identified within interpersonal relationships, thereby establishing the concept of tenderness.

Once this is established, it will then form the data base for assessing the fulfillment or deprivation of the tenderness need in interpersonal relationships, specifically in the mother–child relationship. The ability to assess the tenderness need will give health care providers the opportunity to work with a need that is actively involved in health maintenance for all age groups, for both sexes, and for people in different cultures. That this need is expressed differently in each age group and each male and female role in different cultures and socioeconomic groups only adds to its importance and to the importance of its assessment. If the tenderness need is being met and fulfilled in individuals together with the other basic needs pertinent to interpersonal relationships, it can be assumed that the individual will maintain health and avoid interruption in these same relationships.

Love

Maslow[1] describes love as consisting primarily of a feeling of tenderness and affection, with great enjoyment, happiness, satisfaction, elation, and even ecstasy in experiencing this feeling. He stresses further that psychologic health results from being loved rather than from being deprived of love and that the love need involves both the giving and the receiving of love. This statement supports Fromm's[4] position that genuine love is an experience of productiveness and implies care, respect, responsibility, and knowledge. In considering the mother–child relationship, Maslow[1] cites the example of the loving mother who would rather cough herself than hear her child cough.

Rollo May[6] defines love as experiencing delight in the presence of the other person and affirming his value and development as much as one's own. He states that love consists of two elements: (1) the worth and good of the other person, and (2) one's own joy and happiness in the relationship with the loved one. May[6] speaks of tenderness as that yeast without which love would be like unrisen bread. He believes that tenderness has been generally scorned and often separated out of the love experience because tenderness has been equated with weakness. May[6] rejects the notion that tenderness is weakness and stresses that tenderness is a part of strength, in that one can be as gentle as he is strong if he has the basis of strength within himself from which to give.

Fromm,[4] Adler,[5] and May[6] support the premise that tenderness is an element of love and support Maslow's[1] premise that it is a need for human growth and existence. Collectively, these authors seem to establish that tenderness is an element that, although needed within love relationships, is not automatically present. These authors do not specify exactly what tenderness is, but they imply that the ability to be tender depends on the individual's own concept of self and his ability to give of himself to another in a reciprocal relationship that includes care, responsibility, and respect for the other.

Caring

It appears obvious that human infants and young children need care to ensure that they survive and come to no harm. Bowlby[7] believes that despite variations there are patterns of human behavior that result in mating, in the care of babies and young children, and the attachment of the young to parents, that are found almost universally. Leininger[8] states that, from an anthropologic viewpoint, caring is one of the oldest and most universal expectations for human development and survival throughout man's long history and in different places in the world. She further emphasizes that caring for self and other individuals is a universal phenomenon producing important humanistic attributes that women tend to direct and monitor. This occurs in caring behaviors and roles cross-culturally. Leininger[8] identified seventeen major constructs related to care, caring behaviors, and the caring process, all of which relate to tenderness at some level. Leininger's[8] constructs include: (1) comfort, (2) support, (3) compassion, (4) empathy, (5) direct helping behaviors, (6) coping, (7) specific stress alleviations, (8) touching, (9) nurturance, (1)) succorance, (11) surveillance, (12) protection, (13) restoration, (14) stimulation, (15) health maintenance, (16) health instruction, and (17) health consultation.

Attachment and Bonding

According to Yarrow and Pedersen,[9] attachment refers to a relationship characterized by strong interdependence and intense affect. The development of this relationship is a reciprocal interactive process in which the infant elicits caretaking and other responses from the mother while the mother, in turn, evokes visual regard, vocalizations, smiles, and approach movements from the infant. These infant responses then stimulate further nurturant and affectionate behaviors in the mother. Klaus and Kennell[10] use the term "bonding" to describe the development of attachment from parent to infant and they state that this bonding is crucial to the survival and development of the infant. They also believe that the original mother–infant bond is the wellspring for all the infant's future attachments and that it is also the foundational relationship from which the child's sense of self is developed.

Ainsworth[11,12] and Bowlby[7] include crying, clinging, sucking, grasping, reaching, looking, and smiling among the attachment behaviors in young infants. The predictable outcome of these behaviors is bringing the mother into physical contact with or in close physical proximity of the infant. Klaus and Kennell[10] describe attachment behaviors on the part of the mother or father in the bonding process as fondling, kissing, cuddling, and prolonged gazing. These behaviors mandate contact and also allow for verbal or nonverbal expression of affection toward the infant or child. Yarrow and Pedersen[9] add another dimension to this process, stating that this process assumes a contingent relationship between mother and infant or young child. A contingent relationship includes a high degree of maternal responsiveness to the infant's signals followed by the mother's ability to engage the infant in stimulating interactions. Yarrow and Pedersen[9] maintain that contingent responsiveness and stimulation are qualities similar to warmth and nurturance, but, when applied to the mother–infant relationship, each can be analyzed differently. Essentially, the behaviors on the part of both the infant and the mother in the attachment and bonding process provide for an interactional and reciprocal relationship that is dependent on and affected by the continual interplay of both.

From the concepts of love, caring, attachment, and bonding several elements emerge as consistent threads in the interactional process of each. These threads include the reciprocal nature of the relationships, the specific behaviors and the commitment to the relationship on the part of the participants. From these elements the beginning of a concept of tenderness can be formulated consisting of specific behaviors that can be identified in interpersonal relationships, particularly within the mother–child relationship.

Maternal Tenderness

Clark defined maternal tenderness in terms that included cutaneous stimulation and vocalizations. Cutaneous stimulation includes gentle rocking, patting, caressing, cuddling or kissing, and exploration. Vocalizations include lulling, quiet chattering, or statements of affection. Clark's descriptions were based on observations of mother–infant interactions from three different cultures.[13]

Table 6.1 *Specific Tender Behaviors*

Categories	Mother		Infant to 1 Year		Child 1 Year to 5 Years	
	Initiating	*Responding*	*Initating*	*Responding*	*Initiating*	*Responding*
Physical Closeness	Holding →		Cuddles →		Cuddles →	
	Cuddling →		Seeks closeness →		Seeks closeness →	
	Moving →		Protests separation →		Displays separation anxiety	
	Rocking →		←	Holding	←	Holding
	←	Picking up				
			Reaches out →		Reaches out →	
Eye to Eye Contact	Gazing →		Gazing →		Smiling →	
	Smiling →		Smiling →		Seeks visual closeness	
	←	Gives visual approval			Seeks visual approval	
Vocalizations	Lulling →		Cooing →		Requests for affection →	
	Quiet chattering →		Mouth noises →		Statements of affection →	
	Statements of affection →		Babbling →			Acknowledgement of affection
	Request for affection →					
		Acknowledgement of affection				
Touching	Kissing →				Kissing →	
	Patting →		Kissing →		Caressing →	
	Exploring →		Caressing →			
	Caressing →					
	Hugging →		Exploring →			
					Exploring →	
					Hugging →	

Definition of Tenderness

In consideration of the common threads that emerged from the concepts of love, caring, attachment, and bonding and in view of the above description of maternal tenderness, an operational definition of tenderness in the mother–child relationship is postulated. *Tenderness in the mother–child relationship is a reciprocal interactional process involving positive feelings of affection, demonstrated by: physical closeness, eye to eye contact, vocalizations, and touching. This process is reciprocal in that it can be initiated by either the mother or the child by use of specific behaviors and that either mother or child will respond with other specific behaviors* (Table 6.1). *This process provides that the child's needs are met and also provides the mother with the satisfaction of being needed by her child at the same time that she is being successful in meeting the child's needs. The crucial aspect of this process is the intent of the actions (tender behaviors) by the participants (mother or child) that produces a tender response in either mother or child* (Figure 6.1).

The assumption that all mother–infant or mother–child interactions are tender ones is false. Tenderness may be lacking in some mother–child interactions at certain times, and in some it may be lacking all of the time. In accepting Maslow's[1] premise that tenderness is a need for human development and survival, we can assume that when tenderness is lacking both the mother's and the child's development and well-being will be threatened in some way and to some degree. Thus it is important for any health professional working with mother–child or mother–infant dyads to be able to identify the presence or absence of tenderness in that relationship.

The nursing process as presented by Yura and Walsh provides a framework for the beginning identification of tenderness or tender behaviors in mother–child relationships.[14] It allows for assessing the presence or absence of tender behaviors within mother–child relationships; it provides for planning strategies to maintain, increase, or initiate tender behaviors; it provides actions to maintain, increase, or initiate tender behaviors in the relationship; and it assures evaluation of the outcome of the tender behaviors to determine if the tenderness need has been fulfilled. In order to utilize this approach, mother–child relationships must first be analyzed.

Analysis of Tenderness

Much of the research on attachment and bonding has focused on the neonate or infants in the first year of life. Many of the attachment and bonding behaviors are interchangeable with the tender behaviors as previously described. The intent

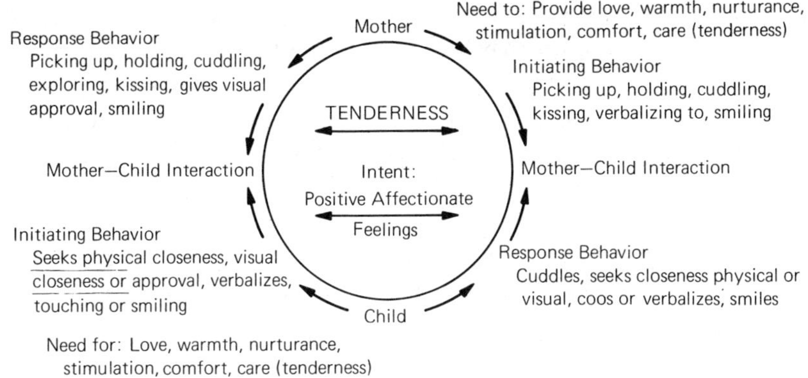

Fig. 6.1: *The interactional process of tenderness.*

factor will be considered as the difference between the behaviors; that is, tender behaviors are always initiated with or responded to with positive affectionate feelings on the part of the mother or the child. For this reason, the mother–child relationship with regard to the older child, who should be showing continuity in the mother–child attachment and has the ability to express himself verbally or position himself physically, will be considered.[15]

The client studies that follow will focus on the need for tenderness in the mother–child relationship. Drawing on the tenderness concept as a data base for analyzing tenderness need fulfillment or need deprivation, assessment actions, planning strategies, implementation methods, and evaluation results will be indicated for each mother–child relationship. In order for the nurse or other health care professional to meet the needs of health maintenance or those imposed by health deficit for their clients, each step in the nursing process must be explicit. Considerations such as age differences and response differences based on sex, culture, or socioeconomic level are all important factors that influence the various steps of the process. Especially important for nurses is the identification of a nursing diagnosis.

The concept of tenderness developed herein specifies several criteria that must be considered in implementing the nursing process. Both mother and child have the need for tenderness. Tenderness is reciprocal and can be initiated by either the mother or the child by use of specific behaviors. The intent of these behaviors is always the communication of positive feelings of affection. Because of the intent of the initiating behaviors, the response behaviors, if the need is met, will also be specific and provide for the mother's or the child's needs as indicated.

For example, a child's tenderness need may be for physical closeness, so he sits on his mother's lap and hugs her. The mother's tenderness need may be to provide the child with safety and comfort in a strange environment, so she holds the child on her lap, cuddling and patting him. The reverse also holds true, in that the mother's tenderness need may be to know that her child has not rejected her, so she reaches out to the child. The child responds by running to the mother and hugging her, thus meeting her need for tenderness. Within the four sets of actions are positive feelings of affection that motivate the tender actions and are evident in the child's hugs of the mother and the mother's cuddling and patting of the child.

These examples illustrate how the criteria of the tenderness concept provide the data base for use of the nursing process in determining tenderness need fulfillment or deprivation.

Client Situations

Five mother–child relationships were observed during a six-month period. All of the children were admitted to the pediatric unit of a large medical center. They spent at least 24 hours in the pediatric intensive care unit. The mother–child relationship was observed on admission, while the child was in intensive care, and one month after the child was discharged from the hospital to the home. The five children were preschoolers ranging in age from 27 months to 63 months. They were all within the norms for age-appropriate behaviors according to growth and development theory.[16,17] Three of the children had surgical procedures and two of the children had medical conditions. All of the children had living parents. The parents of three children were married and living together; the parents of one child were not married and living together whereas the parents of the remaining child were neither married nor living together. Four of the five mothers held fulltime jobs and one mother had six other children at home. Mothers spent more time with the children than did the fathers. As Leininger has pointed out, women tend to monitor and direct caring roles in most cultures of the world.[8]

Situation: A 3-Year-Old Girl

The first mother–child relationship involved a 3-year, 3-month-old female with a diagnosis of brain tumor of the cerebellum. She was the second child of a 22-year-old mother who worked as a salesclerk. The family was Caucasian, and although the father was very involved with the child, it was the mother who stayed with her on a 24 hour basis. The mother stayed in the hospital from the time of admission until the child's second postoperative night—a total of 62 consecutive hours.

On admission, observations of this mother–child relationship revealed several behaviors. They included the mother's constant presence with the child and the child's needs for physical closeness to her mother as demonstrated by her sitting on her mother's lap and holding her hands. The mother, in turn, cuddled the child on her lap. The child constantly looked to her mother when staff members approached. The mother responded with verbal reassurances as: "Now that's just a temperature; it won't hurt," and "I'm here with you."

At this time, prior to surgery, the mother has a need to be with her ill child. This need is demonstrated by her constant presence for the first 62 hours of the child's hospitalization. The child's need is for physical closeness to her mother in a strange and frightening environment. That the tenderness need is also present and that tenderness is present in the mother–child relationship is demonstrated by the child holding her mother's hands while sitting on her lap and by the mother cuddling the child on her lap. Other observable behaviors include the child looking to her mother when hospital staff members enter to perform nursing activities. The child's need for safety is probably basic here. The mother's response not only meets that need with verbal reassurances and her physical presence, but conveys that her intent is tenderness by the words she uses and in her attitude toward the child.

Even though other basic needs in addition to the tenderness need are involved in this situation, the tender behaviors of physical closeness, gazing, holding, and cuddling are very evident in the assessment of this relationship. That the intent of these behaviors was tenderness seems obvious in the way in which both mother and child initiated and/or responded to the behaviors. Identification of the tenderness need helps the nurse to make a nursing diagnosis and plan strategies for implementation. The need at this time is for physical closeness between mother and child.

Planning strategies for intervention at this time include maintenance of a tender mother–child relationship by recognition, encouragement, and support of the present tender behaviors.

Implementation of these strategies in a hospital situation involves allowing the mother to be present with the child at all times. To accomplish this, both mother and child should be prepared for various nursing activities to be performed and the mother's assistance will be requested and utilized if possible. If the mother feels she cannot handle the situation, or if certain activities mandate exclusion of the mother from the room, this should be determined ahead of time and both mother and child prepared as indicated. If a mother feels she is able to stay with the child, she should be allowed to do so. If she feels she is not able to be with the child, she should be supported in this decision and should not feel guilty about being absent.

Evaluation at this time indicated that the present tender mother–child relationship was maintained. Mother was able to remain constantly with the child, and the child went into surgery without protest.

Following surgery, observations of this mother–child relationship included mother being constantly present, speaking softly and reassuringly to the child, stroking the child's body, and kissing her hand. At first the child refused to look at or speak to her mother. She also refused to take liquids or void on request although she never regressed in bowel or bladder control throughout the hospitalization. The child also hid her eyes and spent time playing with her lips with her one free hand. Her mother continued to stay near, to touch the child, and to speak to her. Finally the child began to respond by laughing at baby pictures of herself and then desperately clung to her mother when she was allowed to be up and out of bed.

Following surgery the mother has a need to be near the child and to touch the child. These needs soon include the need to be recognized and responded to by the child. That tenderness is involved is evident in the form of touch. The mother strokes and kisses the child, speaking softly and reassuringly to her. These are all tender behaviors.

Tenderness is reciprocal and assessment includes the observation of the child responding to these behaviors. In effect it appeared as if she were unable to communicate tender feelings. This may have been due to the trauma of the surgery itself, her recovery from anesthesia and surgery, or to her feelings about surgery. At this time the nurse may conclude that the mother has a need for physical closeness and the child is unable to respond to this need. Planning should include support for the mother, whose tender behaviors were not being responded to, and encouragement of the mother to continue expressing her own tender behaviors even though the child is unable to reciprocate at this time.

Implementation of these strategies included allowing the mother to remain with the child and encouraging her to read to her and show her familiar objects and toys, together with encouraging her to continue to kiss and touch the child. These actions on the part of the mother were eventually responded to by the child.

Evaluation at this time stems from the fact that some basic needs of the child at the time immediately following surgery were not being met. There is speculation that the child's immediate response was based on physiologic need deficit rather than psychologic need deficit. The child was able to respond to the mother's continued tender behaviors. This stress situation illustrates that the more basic physiologic needs have priority over the higher needs of love and tenderness. However, an unanswered question is: Would the child have responded rapidly physiologically, if the mother's constant love and tenderness had not been present?

One month after discharge from the hospital the home observation of the mother–child relationship revealed some different behaviors for the dyad. The child moved quickly away from the mother in the observer's presence. She was physically active and getting into verbal disagreements with her older brother. She had periods of crying or pouting easily and running off by herself and refusing to be either calmed down or cheered up by mother. Her mother cuddled and held the child after these episodes. The child verbally expressed that she did not like her mother anymore and that she wished her mother would go away. Her mother responded to this by expressing her love for the child and saying that she would miss the child if she, the mother, went away.

Assessment of the mother–child relationship in the home setting provided data about the tenderness ingredient. Although the mother's tender behaviors appeared appropriate and consistent with her past actions, the child was not reciprocating. The child's behavior probably reflected her inner feelings about the total hospitalization and surgery experience as well as her mother's very recent return to fulltime employment. Although the child's lack of response was distressing to the mother, her own strength and belief in the relationship allowed her to express continued positive tender feelings toward the child.

The nursing diagnosis at this time is disturbance of the tender mother–child relationship. Planning strategies for intervention focused on support for the mother and her continued tender approach to her child and recognition that the child's need for tenderness continues. Implementation of strategies encouraged the mother to believe that her continued tender approach would eventually bring about a tender response in the child as it had in the past.

Evaluation of this total relationship supports the need for tenderness in the mother–child relationship. When the tenderness need of the mother was not being met by the child, the mother was distressed. Fortunately this mother's own inner strength allowed her to continue to be tender, even though the child was unable to respond. The child's need for tenderness continues despite an inability to reciprocate appropriately.

Situation: A 3-Year-Old Boy

This mother–child relationship involved a 3-year, 3-month-old male and his mother who was 45 years old and had recently come to the United States from South America. She was a domestic by trade. The child's parents were not married, but had lived together for several years. Both mother and child spoke English and Spanish. The child was admitted for elective chest surgery. The mother stayed with the child constantly from the time of admission until the first postoperative night.

Observations of this mother–child relationship during the admission process revealed a child who stayed physically close to his mother and looked to her before responding to any questions or engaging in any activity. He often hugged her. His mother responded to him by staying close, reaching out to him, and holding him briefly. His mother also verbally reassured him that "It was o.k."

Assessment of this relationship revealed that both the mother and child had a need for physical closeness. The mother's need is to be with her child, who is about to have a surgical procedure. The child's need is for safety and protection in a strange and frightening environment. The need for tenderness from his mother is demonstrated by his closeness to her and his looking to her and hugging her. The mother's need is to stay close to the child, to reach out to him, and to hold him. She also speaks reassuringly to him. These behaviors on the part of the mother and the child indicate that tenderness is present in their relationship.

The nursing diagnosis is an increased need for physical closeness between the mother and the child within the present stress situation. Planning strategies include providing for physical closeness and support and maintenance of the present tender mother–child relationship. Implementation strategies include those measures necessary to maintain physical closeness in the hospital situation. Recognition and support of the mother–child relationship is also provided by the nurse by verbal acknowledgment that mother and child have a close loving relationship.

Evaluation at this time indicates that the present tender mother–child relationship was maintained. The mother was able to remain constantly with the child, and the child went to surgery without protest.

Observations following surgery noted that the child returned from the recovery room to the intensive care unit crying and asking for his mother. Mother responded by crying also and wanting to touch the child. This action was interfered with by the father who spoke sharply to the mother while he physically moved her from the bedside.

Later it was learned that the father thought it would be harmful to the child to look at or touch him at this time. His actions were based on old cultural beliefs and adherence to cultural customs, to which his wife apparently was not responding at the time. One can speculate that the mother no longer held these beliefs or that her need to know the child was all right, to touch him for reassurance was greater than her belief in traditional cultural customs. The cultural implications in this situation also raise questions about the male and female role in the expression of tenderness. Although the mother did speak to and touch and stroke the child with encouragement, the father remained apart from these interactions. It was not until the child was removed from the intensive care unit that the father held and hugged and spoke to the child. Another interesting factor in this situation was the child's response to the nurse's touch. When the child became anxious about the nurse's actions or any activity related to care, he was able to be calmed by the nurse speaking to him and stroking his arm and hair and holding his hand when his mother was not present to do this.

Assessment at this time included identification of the need for touch and expression of feelings within a different cultural framework. Also included was the identification of the different expressions of feelings based on sex roles within a given culture. That the tenderness need is involved at this level is evident in the form the touch takes and the child's response to it. Touch in this situation consisted primarily of stroking the child's arms and hair and holding his hands. When these tender behaviors were used, either by his mother or the nurse, the child became calm.

The nursing diagnosis was the need for touch in this stress situation within cultural limits and sex role differences. The child's need to be touched, the mother's need to touch and the father's need to remain apart from the interactions—actions based on sex role and cultural beliefs—were all considered in this diagnosis. Planning strategies for intervention based on the nursing diagnosis included encouragement for the mother to touch and be close. It was also determined that the complexity of the setting, or expectations of the staff, or fear were not the basis for the apparent need of the father to be apart from the tender relationship. His seemingly aloof behavior may have been based on his sex role and cultural beliefs. In this case, recognition and support for the father's need to be apart is necessary. Implementation of strategies allowed the mother to be with the child and encouraged her to speak to, touch, and stroke the child. These same strategies reassured the father, as they had the mother, that it was all right to speak to and touch the child, but acknowledged to the father that he may decide when he wants to do this. These same strategies presented the nurse with a calming approach to the child to which he responded readily.

Evaluation of these strategies was very positive in that the mother did meet her needs to speak to and touch the child. The child's need for this was evident in his response. It was further evident in his response to the nurse's use of touch. Also, the father was able to show his feelings and hold and hug the child once the child was out of the intensive care unit.

One month after the child's discharge from the hospital to the home, the mother–child relationship consisted of many tender behaviors. A very happy and healthy child moved freely to and from his mother, touching and speaking to her. He was eager to play and show off his toys with his mother's approval. An interesting factor in this situation was that the father had quit his job and had stayed home with the child during the recovery period. The father spoke warmly and proudly of his son and of how well the child had recovered. Although there was not the touching that occurred between mother and child, there seemed to be a very loving relationship between father and child.

At this time tenderness needs were identified and were being met within the mother–child and father–child relationship. Healthy and tender mother–child and father–child relationships were being maintained. Recognition and support were provided for the relationships. Evaluation revealed that tenderness was given and received by mother, father, and child throughout the interactions that were observed.

Situation: A 5-Year-Old Girl

The third mother–child relationship studied was that of a 5-year, 3-month-old Black female, and her 28-year-old, presently unmarried mother. The child was the youngest of three children. The child had a diagnosis of brain abscess which was made after a 3-month history of illness that began with the aspiration of a sunflower seed. The child was transferred to the medical center from a suburban hospital for a brain and a bone scan and subsequent surgery. The child's mother was with her the day prior to surgery and the day of surgery. Following that, the mother came to see the child periodically. The mother occasionally stayed the night during the course of the hospitalization. The mother worked fulltime and also held a second job in the evenings. It should be noted that the child's father visited, but his visits were few in number and short in duration.

On admission the child was crying, fussy, and very demanding, constantly ordering her mother to do various things. Her mother responded by sitting in a chair at the child's bedside, apparently watching television, or by leaving the room. In assessing this relationship there was a conspicuous absence of touching, gazing, or verbal expressions between the two. Physical closeness was not maintained as the mother left the room, and the child, who was confined to bed with intravenous fluids running, could not follow. That the tenderness need is not being met is evident but that other need deficits are also in operation is also evident. The child is very ill and has been so for some period of time. Basic physiologic needs, such as electrolyte balance, are threatened in this situation. Basic psychologic needs, such as safety needs, and love and belonging needs are also threatened. The combination of these needs in the child and the mother's need for withdrawal from the situation prevent tender feelings and behaviors on the part of both mother and child.

The nursing diagnosis in this situation is total lack of tenderness in the mother–child relationship. Planning strategies were aimed at meeting the child's basic physiologic needs, and basic needs of safety, love, belonging, and tenderness as well as the mother's needs. Strategies were developed to promote the establishment of some beginning expression of tenderness in the mother–child relationship. Implementation included nursing actions to meet physiologic needs of the child while helping the child feel safe in her present environment. Only those nurses who were known by the child were assigned to care for her.

The child's fussy, demanding, and apparently unreasonable behavior soon frustrated these nurses. Attempts at establishing a relationship with the child were very difficult. The child screamed and cried and physically resisted all staff members and all nursing activities.

The mother continued to withdraw from the child and the staff and was resistant to any attempts at discussing her relationship with the child.

Evaluation of behaviors indicated that some of the mother's and the child's needs are still not being met. Although the child's physiologic needs were met, the unsuccessful attempt at working with the mother to help her in her relationship with the child left the child's needs for love, belonging, and tenderness unmet. The child's behavior was so frustrating to the nurses that they were unable to provide love and tenderness to her. When the child went to surgery, she was screaming.

Evaluation of the mother's behavior is based on speculation that the mother had many personal needs that had not been recognized or worked with throughout the course of her daughter's illness. There was an indication from the child's history that the mother had been slow in seeking proper medical attention for the child and finally did so at the insistence of the child's kindergarten teacher. Hospitalization for the child followed a grand mal seizure. What degree of responsibility the mother felt in regard to this is unknown, as she refused to share her feelings at the time. Just how difficult the child had been during the prior 3-month period and what type of stress that placed on a mother with two jobs and two other daughters and no other immediate support systems is also unknown.

Immediately following surgery the mother–child relationship continued to be stressful. When the child returned from surgery, her mother became upset and could not enter the intensive care unit. She was supported in her decision to leave the hospital while she was encouraged to come back later or to call. She did neither; when she returned to the hospital late the next afternoon, the child screamed at her, "Go away; I don't want you here." Following this interaction the mother's visits were short, lasting about one hour, and occurring on the average of every other day. The mother was called at home and informed of the child's progress and encouraged to visit.

The absence of tender behaviors is very obvious in this mother–child relationship. The lack of physical closeness, touching, holding, or kissing prevailed even after the child was allowed out of bed. Verbal interactions consisted primarily of demands on the part of the child and rebuffs on the part of the mother. When they were together, both mother and child spent their time watching television.

Since the mother had been resistive to all attempts at intervention and continued to withdraw from the situation, a decision was made to concentrate on working with the child. The child had been critically ill, and the first several postoperative days had been very difficult ones for her. She had been a difficult child to care for and a difficult child to like. The nursing diagnosis at this time was the lack of tenderness need fulfillment.

Planning strategies focused on the need to establish a tender nurse–client relationship.

Implementation focused on staff nurses approaching the child with tender behaviors. One approach was for the nurses to touch the child at times other than when they were doing required treatments. The nurses also held the child's hands or stroked her hair or face while looking at her and speaking to her. This approach, together with telling the child that she was getting better, brought about a subsequent decrease in the child's demanding behavior and a decrease in the amount of crying and whining on the part of the child.

Evaluation of these actions demonstrated that some positive results followed these actions as described above. The child also began calling the nurses by name and wanted to sit in the wheelchair in the nurse's station. She began to show some interest in activities and would color and draw with encouragement. She began smiling at and talking to the nurses, but never initiated touch with them, although she accepted their touching her.

One month following the child's discharge, a home visit was made. Although mother and child were observed in their own home and the child was physically healthy and very active, their relationship did not appear different than it had been in the hospital. There was no touching, looking to each other, or verbal exchanges. The mother reported that the child had been difficult to deal with since returning home from the hospital.

Although the mother was committed to continuing with the child's follow-up medical care, she remained resistant to intervention aimed at the relationship. It was evident that mother and child were continuing to have difficulty in their relationship and the nurse's concern was that future difficulty might occur. Continued efforts with the mother were planned that it was hoped, would be helpful to her and the child as individuals and in their relationship with each other.

Situation: A 2-Year-Old Boy

The fourth mother–child relationship consisted of a 2-year, 3-month old white male and his 42-year old mother. There were six other children in the family ranging in age from 8 to 17 years. His mother was a registered nurse who had not worked professionally for a number of years. The child's diagnosis was seizure disorder following a gastrointestinal viral infection. The child was admitted from the emergency room and then placed on intensive care unit status every six hours when phenobarbital was administered intravenously. His mother was constantly at his bedside for his entire stay in the hospital. Touching was very obvious in this relationship. The mother stroked either the child's arms or legs and he responded by frequently reaching out to her. The child looked to his mother whenever he was approached by hospital staff, and she responded by reassuring him throughout required treatments and by distracting him from the activity by pointing out interesting things like the smiling faces on the electrodes.

Assessment of this relationship identifies the tender behaviors of physical closeness, touching, gazing, and verbalizations. That these were tender behaviors seems very evident by their intent of positive feelings of affection. The mother's touching of the child was responded to by the child reaching out to her. The child's looking to her was responded to by touch, verbalizations and contingent stimulations. The nurse concluded there was a tender mother–child relationship. Planning strategies focused on support of the tender mother–child relationship and implementation focused on encouragement of a continued tender relationship.

Evaluation was positive in that the child responded extremely well to his mother and the nursing staff throughout the course of hospitalization.

Throughout the child's stay in the hospital and at the time of the home visit, the above behaviors remained evident. The child responded almost immediately to his mother's presence and reassurance. His mother also stimulated him by reading to him or playing games using small toys. These interactions appear to be a continuation of what Yarrow and Pedersen[9] have called contingent responsiveness to the child and the mother's ability to stimulate the child. These interactions also represent tenderness.

It is interesting to note that in both of the relationships involving mothers and male children, tender behaviors have been readily observable. In particular, the behaviors of physical closeness, touching, and verbalizing have been very evident. These observations are somewhat contrary to the findings of Goldberg and

Lewis[18] and Brooks and Lewis,[19] who have found that mothers touch and vocalize more to girls than boys.

Situation: A 2-Year-Old Girl

The fifth mother–child relationship involved a 2-year, 9-month old Black female and a 26-year-old mother. The child had a diagnosis of ventricular septal defect, but was admitted to the hospital following a self-administered overdose of her digitalis. The child was the youngest of three children. Her mother worked fulltime, and the child stayed with a babysitter during the day. Both mother and father were with the child on admission, but it was the mother who the child wanted by her bedside. The child looked to and reached out to her mother during admission procedures. Her mother responded by touching the child and speaking to her. Her mother stayed with the child by her bedside the remainder of the day, talking to her and touching her. Once the child was allowed out of bed, she spent a great deal of time visiting about the unit. She hugged and kissed staff members, who, in return, spent a great deal of time holding her and hugging and kissing her.

Assessment of this relationship identifies the child's need for safety in a strange and frightening environment. This is demonstrated by her wanting her mother at her bedside. She looked to and reached out to her mother during procedures, and her mother responded with touching and speaking to the child. The child's needs and behaviors evoked a tender response in the mother. With the mother's support, this child was admitted and treated without crying or resistance. One interesting development in this situation was the observation of the child's ability to transfer and initiate tender behaviors with staff members who certainly responded to them.

Of all the children observed, this was the only child who displayed tender behaviors to staff in such a demonstrative manner. She was the least ill of all the children observed and the only child who had had prior hospitalizations. One can speculate that her past hospitalization experiences had been positive ones, and that her positive relationship with her mother allowed her to transfer positive feelings to staff members. This example illustrates one factor in the tenderness concept: that is, the mother–child relationship is the basic relationship in which tender behaviors are learned. The strength of that relationship is also the base from which the child is then able to transfer tender feelings and behaviors to others.

The nursing diagnosis for this situation was an established tender mother–child relationship. Planning strategies focused on maintenance of the present relationship within the hospital situation. Implementation included allowing the mother to be present during the admitting process and subsequent treatments. Evaluation was positive in that the child was cooperative and responded quickly to treatments. She was soon out of danger and up and about the unit.

One month following discharge from the hospital in the home situation, the above relationship continued to be evident. Tenderness was certainly an ingredient in this relationship. This child was the only one observed who had a congenital defect that was known since birth. It would be an interesting study to investigate the relationship, if any, between known congenital defects in the child and the mother–child tenderness factor. Is there a difference in these mother–child relationships in comparison to mother–child relationships involving healthy children?

Conclusion

It appears that tender behaviors, as identified herein, can be observed in mother–child relationships. The presence or absence of these behaviors is the most obvious factor. The degree of tenderness in these behaviors or a means of measuring tenderness is not easy and is another question. It would appear from this small sample that the degree of tenderness is an important variable. For instance, in the first mother–child relationship tender behaviors were readily observable, but following surgery and one month after discharge, some conflict was evident in the relationship.

The nursing process as outlined by Yura and Walsh does provide a means for the beginning identification of tenderness in the mother–child relationship.[14] At present there are no specific tools to measure tenderness in the assessment phase of this process. The development of a tool to identify specific tender behaviors and the degree of these behaviors is a necessary next step in the development of the concept of tenderness. That this is a task relevant to nursing is evident from the presentations. Until such tools are available, the nurse will need to rely on her own sensitivity, observation, and judgment to assess tenderness. The tenderness need is a need for growth and development and a deficit in this need produces disturbances in mother–child relationships. Nurses are actively involved with mothers and children in a variety of settings with all age groups, and during most major developmental phases in the child's and the mother's life. Nurses, therefore, are a primary group of health care providers to be involved with the identification of tenderness and concerned with methods of intervention that would maintain, increase, or initiate tender mother–child relationships.

In this chapter, children who had been hospitalized and who spent some time in a specialty unit, the intensive care unit, and their mothers were the population observed. Hospitalization must be considered a variable that was present in the interactions that were observed. There is speculation that other variables such as the child's condition, the type of surgery, the child's length of stay in the hospital, the child's age, the mother's preparedness for the hospitalization, and her ability to cope with the total situation, may all have affected the mother–child relationship. Essentially, these are questions that cannot be answered at this time but provide areas to be explored in the future.

To be able to observe mother–child relationships in their own regular and routine environment for tender behaviors is also an essential step in confirming the existence and degree of tenderness in the mother–child relationship.

References

1. Maslow A: Motivation and Personality, 2nd ed. New York, Harper & Row, 1970
2. Sullivan HS: Interpersonal Theory of Psychiatry. New York, Norton, 1953
3. Montagu, A: Touching, the Human Significance of the Skin. New York, Columbia University Press, 1971
4. Fromm E: Man for Himself. New York, Holt, 1947
5. Adler A: Superiority and Social Interest: A Collection of Later Writings. Edited by HL and RR Ansbacher. Evanston, Northwestern University Press, 1964
6. May R: Man's Search for Himself. New York, Norton, 1953
7. Bowlby J: Attachment and Loss, Volume I (Attachment). New York, Basic Books, 1969
8. Leininger M: The phenomenon of caring. Am Nurse Found 12:2, 14, February, 1977
9. Yarrow L, Pedersen F: Attachment: Its origins and cause. Young Children 27:302–312, June, 1972
10. Klaus M, Kennell JH: Maternal-Infant Bonding. St. Louis, Mosby, 1976
11. Ainsworth MDS: Object relations, dependency and attachment: A theoretical reunion of the infant-mother relationship. Child Dev 40: 969–1025, 1969
12. Ainsworth MDS: Attachment and Dependency: A Comparison In Attachment and Dependency. Edited by J. L. Geruerty. Washington, DC, Winston, 1972
13. Clark, AL: Maternal tenderness—cultural generation implications. In American Nurses' Association Clinical Conference Papers. Kansas City, Mo, American Nurses Association, 1973, pp 98–123
14. Yura H, Walsh M: The Nursing Process: Assessing, Planning, Implementing, Evaluating, 2nd ed. New York, Appleton-Century-Crofts, 1973
15. Carr S, Dobbs JM, Carr T: Mother-infant attachment: The importance of the mother's visual field. Child Dev 46:331–338, 1975
16. Papolia D, Olds S: A Child's World. New York, McGraw-Hill, 1975
17. Stone LJ, Church J: Childhood and Adolescence, 3rd ed., New York, Random House, 1975
18. Goldberg S, Lewis M: Play behavior in the year old infant: Early sex differences. Child Dev 40:21–31, 1969
19. Brooks J, Lewis M: Attachment behaviors in thirteen-month old opposite-sex twins. Child Dev 45:243–247, 1974

Chapter Seven •

The Need for Activity

Cynthia D. Sculco

Maslow, in developing the hierarchy of basic human needs, emphasized that physical needs are met before psychosocial needs.[1] One of man's basic needs is activity, and in this chapter the dimensions of activity optimal for maintaining health will be considered, particularly the importance of exercise in the maintenance of psychologic and physical wellness.

The significance of exercise in promoting physical and mental well-being has only recently been explored. Exercise as therapy, as a means to improve self-concept, and as an aid to coping with stress is currently being studied.[2,3] Robert Butler has stated that "Substantial evidence supports the value of exercise in maintaining health, improved circulation and respiration, better sleep and diminished stress. Exercise reduces the risk of heart attack and enhances survival following an attack."[4]

The hazards of inactivity are all too well known to the practicing health professional. Mary Francis Borgman stated that the development of a sound, well-conditioned body through the use of proper exercise is the keystone of health maintenance.[5] She continues by stating that the concept of body development for the purpose of health maintenance in the well client has largely been ignored in the nursing curriculum. As a result, most nurses simply overlook this aspect of health even though in many instances it is the single most important factor in preventing disability.

The implications of these statements affect all age groups, particularly the older population, as stressed by Butler in his extensive study of the aging population in America.[6] He emphasizes such activities as swimming, walking, running, and bicycling as especially good and inexpensive forms of exercise because they actively improve circulatory and respiratory function. "Exercise is the closest thing to an anti-aging pill now available. It acts like a miracle drug and it is free for the doing."[7] It is interesting that Butler also identifies dancing as an excellent activity for the older population because it combines social, interpersonal, and physical pleasure.[8] This premise is reinforced by a recent article in the *Washington Post:* "Senior citizens say dancing puts them on top of the world."[9] The article relates the responses of senior citizens to a weekly modern dance class. The article quotes a senior citizen: "Dancing has brought me back to life again." Both a mental and a physical awakening in this population has been attributed to dance.

What is meant by the frequently discussed term, physical fitness? The concept of physical fitness is aptly defined by Kilborn as a state in which there are sufficient physical reserves to perform the activities of daily living without fatigue and other symptoms.[10] Most authorities agree that regular exercise is the method whereby physical fitness is achieved.[11] The increase in physical reserves appears to result in man's overall feeling of well-being. Mann has attributed this well feeling to physiologic changes in the cardiovascular system that include bradycardia during rest and submaximal exercises, increased cardiac output, increased resting stroke volume, decreased systemic arterial pressure, longer diastolic period available for coronary perfusion, and a redistribution of blood flow to active muscles.[12] The psychologic changes are not so conclusive or well defined, but some studies indicate that exercise modifies the individual's emotional stress level.[13]

Support for the positive effects of exercise has been well documented.[14,15] Many studies support exercise training for the geriatric population because of the positive effects on both physical and mental status.[16,17,18] Powell studied the psychologic effects of exercise therapy on institutionalized geriatric mental patients and concluded that exercise therapy was more successful than social therapy treatment.[19] He conjectured that social therapy may not be so successful because patients can shut out these therapeutic activities through disinterest. In physical activities the neurologic system, the musculoskeletal system and other body systems are stimulated and lack of participation is more difficult.

Folkins attempted to explain the relationship between physical and psychologic fitness.[20] He stated that psychologic fitness may be the result of feedback from skeletal and/or cardiac musculature. It has been demonstrated that muscles in good tone do not send out so many electrical impulses and this reduced electrical activity in the muscle may be a significant feedback cue for the individual to rate himself as less anxious. A study by Chapman and Mitchell demonstrated that a trained jogger responded to stress with greater stroke volume rather than with increased heart rate.[21] They proposed that the increased stroke volume method of accomodating stress is not only more efficient, because it is associated with the release of smaller amounts of adrenalin than occurs with increased heart rate, but also produces fewer anxiety associated cues, e.g., the racing heart. These studies point to a definite physiologic relationship where exercise is an adjunct to physical and mental health.

When addressing the question of optimum activity to maintain health, one must consider several variables, of which age and sex are prominent. Aging has been described as a gradual and continued irreversible diffusion of energy that results in structural and functional alterations.[22] Butler, however, focuses on the myth of aging, especially the concept of chronologic aging.[23] He notes that there are great differences in the rates of physiologic, chronologic, psychologic, and social aging within the person and from individual to individual. Physiologic indicators show a greater range of mean values in old age than in any other age category. Chronologic age is therefore a convenient but imprecise indicator of physical, mental, and emotional status. Although age is a variable, one should be reluctant to draw conclusions regarding physical ability in the absence of other information. Sex is another significant factor in considering activity. Skills that require great muscular strength are usually performed better by males than by females at all ages. The following variables have been studied extensively: body build, personality, racial and social groups, sensory perception, ability, attitudes toward the body, and movement and emotional states. However, the evidence is too conflicting to permit general conclusions at this time.[24]

Kenneth Cooper has probably contributed the most of all investigators toward emphasizing the importance of a well-conditioned body for both psychologic and physical well-being.[25] In his numerous volumes on aerobics he has developed norms for the average individual according to age and sex. It is obvious from simple observation that people of all ages are exercising on a regular basis more than ever before. The focus of exercise is also being increasingly shifted toward the concept of prevention, a system far more prevalent in European countries than in the United States. In 1961 Raab reported that during the period 1954–1961 a system of preventive mass reconditioning was developed in West Germany.[26] At that time 2000 such training facilities existed in Russia, where exercise programs were available for citizens within their occupational settings.

For many years the American Medical Association has advocated the importance of physical fitness and stressed the need for health professionals to encourage and participate in fitness programs.[27] The Committee on Exercise and Physical Fitness of the American Medical Association has defined physical fitness in the following manner: "Physical fitness is the general capacity to adapt and respond favorably to physical effort."[28] The degree of physical fitness depends on the individual's state of health, constitution, and present and previous activity.

It is essential for a nurse to be able to assess the physical fitness status of a client. The nurse should be able to establish whether or not the client is physically fit and, if not, what variables should be considered in suggesting strategies toward improvement. Determining a client's fitness begins with a history of his reaction to physical stress. The following questions can be used to assist with the assessment:

What are his current activities?
What were his activities in the past?
How do his past activities differ from his present ones?
Does he have any symptoms suggesting untoward reactions to exercise?
How long does it take him to recover from strenuous exercise?[29]

The Harvard Step Test is suggested to provide a reasonably reliable determination of physiologic reserve.[30] The client is asked to step up and down on a bench at a rate of 30 times per minute for 4 minutes unless fatigue causes him to stop prematurely. The pulse is then measured after 1 minute, 2 minutes, and 3 minutes for 30 seconds and a recovery index is established. Because it does not result in an increased utilization of oxygen, this is an anaerobic measure of fitness. Dr. Cooper feels that a minimum of 12 minutes of exercise is necessary to adequately measure a client's ability to use oxygen effectively.[31] One's aerobic capacity is dependent on the ability to rapidly breathe large amounts of air, forcefully delivery large amounts of blood and effectively deliver oxygen to all parts of the body. "In short, it depends upon efficient lungs, a powerful heart and a good vascular system. Because it reflects the conditions of these vital organs, the aerobic* capacity is the best index of overall physical fitness."[32]

As previously discussed, age and sex must be taken into consideration when assessing the client. Lange-Andersen has developed a table for maximum allowable physical exertion as determined by age.[33] Unless physical condition is excellent, the initial program should be limited to exercise achieving no more than 70 percent of the maximum allowable heart rate listed for the client's age.[34]

*Physical exertion requires that a supply of oxygen be available to body organs and tissues (muscles). This supply is obtained by the extraction of oxygen from the bloodstream. The maximum uptake of oxygen during exercise is referred to as "aerobic capacity." When a person is in good health, a greater amount of oxygen can be delivered to the body organs and tissues.

In further assessing the client a routine examination should include a thorough family and client history, a general physical examination, determination of resting blood pressure, standard 12 lead electrocardiogram (ECG) and measurement of blood lipid levels. This information is helpful in establishing a total chronic heart disease risk profile for the individual.[35] All medications should be carefully reviewed because the taking of certain medications is a definite contraindication to exercise testing or training. It has been recommended by Wilmore that anyone over 35 years of age have a stress test as part of the routine physical examination prior to beginning any exercise program.[36] The exercise stress test can also be included as a helpful diagnostic tool. In a recent study Cumming reported that 27 percent of 510 male subjects exhibited an abnormal ECG response to exercise.[37] It is interesting to note that if the test had not exceeded 85 percent of those subjects' predicted maximal heart rate, one-half of the abnormal findings would have been missed.

There are three basic types of exercise stress testing: the Master Two Step test, bicycle ergometers, and the motor driven treadmill. All of these tests usually include electrocardiogram readings. The motor driven treadmill is a particularly good test that is widely used in America for obtaining measurements of a client's cardiovascular response to strenuous exercise. It is a versatile testing device that allows variation in the intensity of the test by increasing the slope and the speed of the treadmill. The client may walk or jog. Naughton has developed a standardized treadmill test in which slope and speed are varied in set increments.[38] Energy expenditure in his test is calibrated and at each incremental change an additional amount of work equal to a Met is added. A Met is defined as the metabolic equivalent of one's resting rate of oxygen consumption, normally approximately 3.5 ml oxygen/kg/minute. The heart rate and blood pressure are monitored during the test. The heart rate is a good indicator of metabolic activity in an individual. Wilmore states that a heart rate equal to 140 beats/minute is roughly equivalent to 23 or 24 ml of oxygen per kg body weight per minute for that individual.[39] If the examiner wishes the client to exercise at six Mets or six times his resting metabolic rate, then a heart rate of 140 beats per minute should be achieved with the test.

Naughton states that, in his experience, most cardiac clients, symptomatic or asymptomatic, will achieve their limitations at seven Mets or less and most sedentary subjects at ten Mets or less, whereas physically active middle-aged subjects can attain thresholds between ten and sixteen Mets.[40] The test results can be used to rate persons according to physiologic functional classes (FC): Persons limited to two Mets or less are rated FC IV, three to four Mets, FC III; five to six Mets, FC II; and seven Mets or greater, FC I.

Another parameter that can be evaluated by stress testing is endurance. The oxygen uptake can be assessed at various levels of exercise. "The highest value attained, if the test is truly a maximal test to exhaustion is referred to as the maximal oxygen uptake (V O_2 max)."[41] Oxygen uptake is related to one's body weight and is expressed as ml oxygen/body weight/minute. "While highly conditioned athletes may have values greater than 80 ml/kg/min, post myocardial infarction clients typically have values of less than 20 ml/kg/min."[42] Fortunately, V O_2 max is highly responsive to physical conditioning and can increase by 10 percent to 25 percent after six months or less of formal physical activity. The V O_2 max can be estimated from the duration of the standardized exercise test if the equipment is not available for actual measurement.[42]

Kenneth Cooper assesses an individual's fitness and categorizes it depending on oxygen consumption in ml/kg/minute into one of five fitness categories ranging from very poor to excellent.[43] The 12-minute field test, in which an individual is asked to walk or run as far as possible in 12 minutes, is used to assess an individual's fitness. It has been demonstrated by Cooper[44] that distance covered correlates very closely with treadmill measurements of oxygen consumption and aerobic capacity.[44] "The basic physiologic response to exercise is an increase in total body oxygen consumption made possible by increases in pulmonary ventilation, cardiac output, and oxygen extraction by the tissues."[45]

Dr. Cooper's aerobic program emphasizes the importance of duration of exercise in order for a training effect to occur. He uses a point system based on the energy expended to perform an activity to rate an exercise and advocates a minimum of 30 points per week to maintain a state of physical fitness. Variables of age and sex are accounted for by varying the time required to accomplish the activity. An example of Cooper's point system for the walking exercise program for a woman between the ages of 30 to 39 years would be as follows: 0 points for walking a mile in more than 19 minutes, and 2 points for walking a mile in 14 minutes, 15 seconds.

Therefore, it is important for the nurse to know what physical fitness is and how it can be assessed. The need for specific knowledge about exercise that can be applied to the average normal individual so as to maximize his health potential is paramount. To assist the nurse in advising a client about achieving his maximum health potential, the nursing process will be used in the following situation.

Client Situation

T.D., a 27-year-old white female graduate student, has no specific complaints for a general physical examination. She is not overweight but states that she tires easily. The nurse practitioner in the student health clinic is the primary care provider for this client. A complete physical examination is done including a thorough family and client history, supine and standing blood pressure, standard 12 lead electrocardiogram, routine urinanalysis, complete blood count, blood lipid levels, and an assessment of the level of the client's stress and anxiety. T.D. is presently taking no medications regularly. After the general assessment the nurse concludes that there are no apparent physical abnormalities.

Another aspect of this practitioner's physical examination includes an assessment of the individual's level of physical fitness. The utilization of the specific steps of the nursing process focusing on the basic need for exercise provides the general framework. The specific data are collected according to the four phases of the nursing process: assessing, planning, implementing, and evaluating. Several questions were asked to assist in the collection of appropriate data needed to assess the level of physical fitness.

First, T.D. was asked about her current level of activity. She responded that she was a graduate student and spent most of her time in the library studying. She would go to class and study 8 to 10 hours per day, and was taking 18 credits in an attempt to finish her course work as soon as possible. Her main type of physical activity consisted of an occasional set of tennis.

The second question referred to her activities in the past. T.D. responded that she had been very athletic in high school, especially in water sports such as long distance swimming, which she did at least twice a week.

The third question was about how her present activity level differed from her past activity level. In response T.D. noted that the opportunity to participate in regular exercise was very limited and that she had not been active in sports for at least six years.

The next inquiry focused on whether or not T.D. had any symptoms that inferred an untoward response to physical exercise. The answer to this question was negative.

The next question focused on the assessment of the client's current status in terms of physical fitness, asking specifically how long it takes the client to recover from strenuous exercise. The Harvard Step Test was used as a simple way of indicating physical fitness capacity. T.D.'s recovery index was 58. That is, after 4 minutes of strenuous exercise her total pulse rate taken after 1 minute, 2 minutes, and 3 minutes for 30 seconds was a cumulative 205. The recovery index (RI) is calculated[46]:

$$\text{RI} = \frac{\text{duration of exercise in seconds} \times 100}{\text{sum of 30 second pulse counts in recovery} \times 2}$$

The lower the recovery index, the poorer the physical fitness status of the client. This is a convenient measure of fitness and is easily performed. It is also an excellent measure of progress made by participation in conditioning exercises.

Nursing Diagnosis

After a review of the data and the recovery index, it was concluded that T.D. was deconditioned and that this might explain her easy fatiguability.

According to the American Medical Association's Committee on Exercise and Physical Fitness, persons under 40 years of age who have not participated in any extensive physical exercise since their high school and college days and who have employment that does not require moderately heavy physical activity on a regular basis have been characterized as deconditioned.[47]

In order to obtain additional information the nurse explained how T.D. could evaluate herself by running for 12 minutes and checking the distance covered, using the aerobic or fitness test as recommended by Cooper.[48] In performing the 12-minute field test, T.D. covered 1 mile or the equivalent of 25.0 ml/kg/min oxygen consumption. For a female in the 30 to 39 year age range a level of greater than 48 ml/kg/minute is necessary to be considered in the excellent fitness category (approximately 1.75 miles covered in 12 minutes).

Planning

Since a beginning level of fitness had been established and a tentative diagnosis had been made, it was appropriate that an individual prescription for an exercise program be developed for T.D. According to Wilmore, four major considerations must be taken into account before prescribing an exercise regimen for apparently healthy individuals[49]: mode, frequency, duration, and intensity of exercise. Mode refers to the specific type of exercise; it is important that it be a form of exercise that an individual enjoys if he is to follow through with an exercise program. From T.D.'s history it was evident that the majority of her exercise in the past had been in the form of swimming but because of lack of facilities in her area she preferred to begin a jogging program. The practitioner versed in Cooper's aerobic program advised T.D. that during the first 5 weeks of the training program she should limit herself to walking at increasing rates until she was able to walk 1½ miles in 22 minutes. Dr. Cooper's book was recommended to T.D. for a more extensive analysis of the total program. The specifics were then explained in terms of the point system as delineated by Cooper.

After the mode of exercise had been determined, the frequency was discussed with T.D. It was suggested that the optimal frequency for a conditioning program was participation three to five times per week.[50] In terms of duration it has been concluded that 20 to 30 minutes is the ideal period once the individual has become conditioned to maximize the training effect.[51] The intensity of the exercise was also discussed with the client. It has been demonstrated that exercising to 70 to 80 percent of the individual's maximal effort will achieve a reasonable level of fitness.[52] The ability to carry on a conversation with a jogging companion is a good measure of the appropriate intensity in a running program. In some programs exertion level is measured in terms of heart rate; for example, the YMCA's program of fitness uses target heart rates that are age dependent (e.g., the 155–160 range for individuals 30 to 40 years of age).[53]

During assessment, the nurse considered numerous variables before developing a plan for the client, including age, sex, present state of physical fitness, present living situation, the time available for active exercise, and past physical activity history.

Implementation

The aerobic program focusing on jogging as the activity of choice was begun by T.D. The implementation of the plan was completely dependent on the client because she had only a limited amount of time to participate in group activities. T.D. was to return in six weeks, i.e., one week after the jogging phase of her program had begun. T.D.'s return proved that the assessment of the need for exercise was correct and the program was beginning to show some results. Her recovery index was now 80 and she stated that she felt much better both psychologically and physically. She claimed to have more energy and ability to concentrate more effectively. She was encouraged to continue her program, with periodic follow-up by the nurse and showed continued improvement.

In this first client situation the nursing process was used to help an apparently healthy individual to improve her level of wellness by means of activity modification. The baseline data presented were for the apparently healthy individual. In the second client situation, attention will be focused on a client who is convalescing from a myocardial infarction. Again, the nursing process provides the framework for evaluation of the client. To assist the nurse in the assessment of this client's level of activity and to ascertain whether or not a desirable level is being maintained, four general questions developed by Marjorie Byrne relating to levels of wellness will be utilized[54]:

1. What are the limitations with which the individual must cope?
2. To what degree is he utilizing the potential of which he is capable?
3. How does the individual view or evaluate his situation?
4. What are the environmental resources available to him and how can they be utilized more effectively?

Client Situation

R.K., a 55-year-old business executive, experienced persistent left-sided chest pain while attending a fund-raising dinner six months prior to this report. He was admitted to a local hospital, where an electrocardiogram confirmed an anterior wall myocardial infarction. He was admitted to the coronary care unit and three days later was transferred to the progressive care unit. He had no complications and followed the expected course of recovery. He was discharged to his home eight days after admission and returned to work two months after the infarction. During a routine six month follow-up visit, R.K. complained to the progressive care unit nurse that he tired easily and had voluntarily curtailed much of his previous activities. He felt particularly fatigued at the end of the day.

Byrne's questions regarding levels of wellness are useful in assessing this client's activity level and needs. First is: What are the limitations, if any, regarding physical activity and exercise with which he must cope? More specifically, does the client have the cardiac reserve to perform the activities of daily living and work and maintain social and community relationships? As Zohman and Tobis have noted, most activities of daily living and work do not require maintenance of cardiac output greater than three to four times the resting level.[55] It is normal for all persons to borrow oxygen from the tissues during heavy exercise. This oxygen debt, however, must be repaid at the end of the exercise. The cardiac client has a decreased ability to deliver oxygen to the tissues by way of the circulatory system and thus has a greater oxygen debt than the normal person. Therefore, the recovery period after exercise or activity for a cardiac person will be longer. A slow pulse rate at the end of the working day is a good indicator that the client is able to meet the demands of his working situation.

It is possible to evaluate a client's energy reserve within a controlled environment. This can be correlated with specific energy expenditures related to different types of work activities. The energy levels of different activities have been standardized and correlated with the four functional classifications (FC I–IV). For example, desk work requires 1½ to 2 Mets, although metabolic increases can occur due to anxiety or excitement. In contrast, a man digging ditches requires 7 to 8 Mets.

Fatigue, according to Zohman and Tobis, is often a symptom of impaired cardiac reserve and may result from low or inadequate cardiac output for the task at hand.[56] Therefore, it is important for the nurse to know whether or not the client has an adequate cardiac reserve to meet the demands of his regular day-to-day activities at home and at work. One method of establishing R.K.'s cardiac reserve is with a stress test, a routine procedure that can be done prior to the client's returning to work.

R.K. was given a stress test before he returned to work to evaluate his response to strenuous exercise and work. The stress test was performed on a treadmill and was submaximal in nature.

The target heart rate was specified as the end point of the test rather than the subject's determination of when a state of complete exhaustion had been reached.

The end points in most submaximal stress tests are the target heart rates. Target heart rates have been established for clients of different ages by the Committee on Exercise of the American Heart Association. According to Lange-

Andersen, by the time a man reaches 70 years of age his maximum aerobic power is 50 percent of what it was at 20 years of age.[57] Therefore, it is important that the heart rate be adjusted for age. The client continues with the treadmill test as long as he shows no signs of ischemia, arrhythmia, or chest pain. The speed and the grade are gradually increased until the target heart rate is reached. As the slope and the speed of the treadmill increase, the unconditioned person reaches his maximum heart rate and is forced to stop at a lower level than the conditioned client. "The well-conditioned person will be able to do work at much higher intensities than the poorly conditioned one and will have a much higher oxygen uptake when he reaches the point of exhaustion."[58] The physical fitness is expressed by the work level at which he attains the target heart rate. Blood pressure, pulse, and electrocardiogram are monitored throughout the test and recovery period.

Both the blood pressure and the pulse rate are good indicators of cardiac work load. "An efficient cardiovascular adaptation to muscular exercise is achieved when the systolic pressure remains numerically greater than the heart beat per minute."[59]

It has been noted by Fox that individuals who have had a favorable recovery from myocardial infarction should not undertake high levels of exercise for at least three months and probably more.[60] This recommendation is reinforced by Cooper, who states that rehabilitative exercise programs for cardiac clients must remain quite mild.[61] For this reason he recommends that cardiac clients exercise at a level that does not cause their heart rate to exceed specific age-adjusted rates.

The benefits of exercise programs for cardiac clients have been widely documented. Detry states that the major benefit of exercise in persons with coronary artery disease was a significant reduction in heart rates achieved at submaximal workloads, although little change in maximally achieved heart rates was noted.[62] In work on the physiology of exercise it has been observed that myocardial oxygen demand is closely linked to the product of the heart rate and systolic blood pressure, known as the double product (D.P.). Robinson found that because exercise training results in lower heart rates and blood pressures for a given workload, oxygen requirements are decreased and angina and/or electrocardiogram ST depressions are reduced for a given workload.[63] Clinically, the improved relationship between oxygen supply and demand is reflected in a higher workload capacity and higher heart rates, at which angina and ST segment depression appear.

Assessment

Because R. K.'s stress test was completed prior to his return to work, the data were helpful for the nurse in assessing any apparent physical limitations. The stress test results classified R. K. in poor physical condition. He reached his target heart rate after only six minutes of exercise walking at a rate of 2 miles per hour, with a 10 percent grade to the treadmill. The oxygen consumption was 23 ml/kg/minute. After the initial stress testing R. K. was advised to enter a supervised exercise program and lose weight from his 190-pound, 5-foot 9-inch frame. At the time of the initial testing there were no other medical contraindications to beginning the exercise program. R. K. told the nurse that the reason he had not participated in the exercise program was that he just could not afford the time. He reiterated that he had a very high-powered job, rarely had time for lunch, and often returned home from work after 8 P.M.

The nurse listened and continued to collect data about the client. She was aware of the research studies that stated that the quality of life for the cardiovascular client is improved by exercise. Minnesota Multiphasic Psychological Institute (MMPI) psychologic tests given during an exercise training program have shown a decrease in scores related to depression, an increase in extroversion, and an increase in a sense of well-being.[64]

The second question asked in the assessment phase was: To what extent is R. K. utilizing the potential of which he is capable? It appears that he is in a poorly conditioned state with potential to be in a much better physical state. The description of his present life style gave the nurse reason to believe that he was taxing his cardiac reserve and apparently had not provided for sufficient rest periods during his working hours to prevent an oxygen debt from occurring.

As discussed earlier, the need for adequate rest periods is based on the cardiac client's requiring a longer recovery period in which to repay his oxygen debt than a normal person because of decreased cardiac reserve. Many cardiac clients can sustain activities for short periods of time if they have a sufficiently long recovery period. They can also perform a sustained activity provided there are opportunities for prolonged recovery periods. Zohman and Tobis noted that if an individual has the cardiac reserve necessary for the job he is to perform he should allow his pulse rate to return to normal or close to normal levels between each period of peak work.[65] There may be three basic reasons why the pulse rate does not return to normal: disease, lack of physical fitness, or environmental conditions, such as extreme heat. The major benefits of exercise for the cardiac client have already been mentioned, the most important of which is the decrease of myocardial oxygen demands. This would in turn lower the oxygen debt for a client such as R. K.

A review of R. K.'s past life style revealed an overweight person, working long hours, without exercise and with limited time for any form of relaxation; this resulted in a very high anxiety state that he himself identified.

The third question that the nurse asked R. K. was: how does he review or evaluate his own situation? As noted earlier he was apparently very displeased with his present life style. He stated that he was ready to look at his total life pattern and make changes as needed, since he was having difficulty coping with all of the responsibilities that he had at the present time.

When asked the fourth question during the assessment, which referred to the specific environmental resources available to him for exercise, he answered that there was a YMCA within a 15-minute walk from his home that offered a variety of exercise programs.

The data regarding R. K.'s status were reviewed by the nurse. The recommendation to enroll in an exercise program was well received and he selected an early morning routine that he felt would be more conducive to his daily routine. The data concerning his stress test were reviewed with R. K. It was noted that his metabolic rate of oxygen consumption was 23 ml/kg/minute, or 6 Mets. R. K. was, therefore, classified in functional category 2. He was not taking any medications that would be contraindicated in an exercise program.

Nursing Diagnosis

The following nursing diagnoses were made. The client: (1) was overweight as a result of consuming excess calories and inactivity; (2) was deconditioned as a result of lack of exercise and a slight decrease in cardiac reserve as a result of a myocardial infarction six months ago; and (3) suffered from mild anxiety as a result of work-related tension.

Planning

The short- and long-term goals were established between the nurse and the client. For the short-term goals R. K. was to (1) lose one pound per week; (2) enroll in the YMCA physical conditioning program and participate in the program three times per week; (3) review his working schedule and organize the day so that high-energy periods are followed by a recovery (or low-energy) period; and (4) keep a log of daily activities to be reviewed with the nurse at the end of one month for the purpose of evaluating the work and rest pattern.

According to the long-term goals identified at the same time, R. K. was to: (1) lose 20 pounds within six months; (2) improve the deconditioned state as evidenced by an improved stress test at six months; and (3) provide documented evidence that there were adequate rest periods during the daily working schedule.

An exercise prescription given to a cardiac client should observe the following principles:

1. The exercise should be isotonic rather than isometric. The rationale for this is that there is greater myocardial oxygen consumption with static work as well as an increased incidence of premature ventricular contractions because the valsalva maneuver is often utilized.
2. The exercise should be definitely aerobic in nature, which will allow for

adequate transportation of oxygen. A steady state can be obtained in 2 to 5 minutes, after which oxygen intake and utilization are in equilibrium. Short episodes of exercise result in anaerobic activity that results in an increase in lactic acid and a large oxygen debt. This can produce a feeling of fatigue and lead to a cessation of exercising; therefore no training effect can occur.

3. The exercise should alternate with rest periods.
4. Exercise should be submaximal (a percentage of the maximum value for the individual). Sixty to eighty percent of a measured predicted maximal V O_2 value for the individual is recommended by Zohman and Tobis.[66]

It is essential in all exercise programs that there is a warming-up and a cooling-down period in each exercise session. During the exercise program the target heart rate should not be exceeded. According to Hellerstein, whenever the target heart rate levels are exceeded by a prescribed activity the intensity of the activity should be decreased and the subject reevaluated if functional capacity appears to be deteriorating.[67] It is important for the client to be an active participant in the evaluation of the exercise program by his routinely evaluating and recording his heart rate and any symptoms during exercise. He should be able to determine whether or not his heart rate is within the prescribed range. Dr. Cooper recommends that cardiac clients who are 55 years of age and older should not exceed 125 heartbeats per minute when they first begin their exercise program.[68] This is in keeping with the belief that the cardiac client should begin with a submaximal heart rate that is approximately 20 beats below that which was achieved on the treadmill test.

Implementation and Evaluation

The exercise program prescribed for R. K. consisted of 7 minutes of warm-up, or calisthenic, type of exercises followed by approximately 30 minutes of exercise and then by a 5- to 10-minute period of slow rhythmic exercises performed during the cooling-down period. The exercise period consisted of a combination of jogging and walking. The run–walk sequences are gradually increased until the client can run one mile. R. K.'s training intensity at average and peak expenditures during the training session were 16 to 22 ml O_2/kg/minute and heart rates of 120 to 144. Walking 3.5 miles per hour is an example of this average expenditure and jogging at 5 miles per hour is the peak level expenditure. Obviously these activities will not be continued for one hour but will be divided into smaller units, with an active exercise period of approximately 30 minutes. In the beginning the program consisted mainly of walking and then proceeded to slow jogging, using the target pulse rate as a guide.

Because the exercise prescription was reviewed with the client, R. K. was well informed as to the specifics of the program in which he was to participate. At his one-month return visit he noted the following changes: he had lost five pounds, his resting pulse was 70 (down from 82), his blood pressure was 150/70, and his respirations were 14 per minute. He reported that he was progressing very well with the exercise program and was now walking 1 mile in 13 minutes and jogging 1 mile in 11 minutes 10 seconds. In addition to the physical benefits that R. K. reported, he observed that he felt as if he had more energy now than prior to beginning the program. He was able to schedule his activities in a more realistic fashion and stated that he no longer became fatigued at the conclusion of a work day. R. K. realized the benefits he had already achieved within this very short period of time and looked forward to more improvement as he continued in the program. Long-term follow-up of R. K. will be done; however, the evidence indicates that at this time he has satisfactorily met the short-term goals that were established and the plan that was developed was appropriate to meet the objectives outlined.

The nurse intervened appropriately in assisting R. K. to achieve a higher level of wellness and, as he stated, the exercise program had contributed to an improvement in his quality of life.

The importance of nurses truly understanding the benefits of exercise and exercise regimens cannot be overemphasized. The presentation of this second client situation has applied the basic principles required for an understanding of exercise training for therapeutic purposes. The final client situation will take on another dimension and look at a client in whom the basic need for activity and exercise is unattainable.

Client Situation

J. B., a 63-year-old married woman with osteoarthritis of the hip, underwent a Charnley right total hip replacement. She did extremely well after surgery and progressed to crutch walking and returned to her home with her wound well healed five weeks after surgery. She was quite pleased with her pain-free hip and ambulated well. However, six months after the surgery she again experienced pain in the right hip and developed a very pronounced limp. A seropurulent discharge drained from the wound and cultures from it grew *Staphylococcus aureus*. A sinogram showed the presence of dye around the prosthetic components. J. B. was hospitalized and the total hip replacement and cement (methyl methacrylate) in the acetabulum and femoral canal were removed. Postoperatively closed tube irrigation was employed and continued for 7 days, at which time the cultures were negative. Balanced skeletal traction was applied using a Steinman pin through the tibial tubercle; this was maintained for six weeks.

The wound healed and no further drainage occurred. J. B. required a 2-inch heel and sole lift on her right shoe and forearm crutches to ambulate. Six months after discharge she had good motion and no pain in her right hip, but she had a severe limp and continued to need crutches for walking.

Assessment

To further explore the activity level, J. B. was assessed two weeks after removal of the infected hip replacement. One of the major nursing concerns for a client such as J. B. is the prevention of the potential hazards, both physical and psychologic, that may result from her state of inactivity. Alteration in activity alone may produce various levels of illness that can be identified.

To assist in the assessment of J. B.'s activity level during this period of skeletal traction, questions based on Carnevali and Brueckner's concept of immobilization will be used.[69] Their definition of immobility is broad and includes prescribed or unavoidable restriction of movement in any area of the client's life. Carnevali lists seven variables to be considered when assessing the immobilized client: area, cause, extent, direction, duration, sequelae, and volition.

According to Carnevali, movement restriction can occur in any one of the following areas: physical, intellectual, emotional, and social. J. B. is obviously in a state of prescribed physical restriction of movement. Nurses are well informed about the major complications of inactivity, including decubitus ulcers, resulting from prolonged pressure on a bony prominence, contractures due to prolonged inactivity of the joints, atrophy of the muscles, thrombus formation resulting from inactivity, and hypostatic pneumonia resulting from stasis of secretions. In a comprehensive study Olsen has reviewed the effects of physical immobility on the various systems of the body, that is, on cardiovascular function, respiratory function, gastrointestinal function, motor function, urinary function, metabolic equilibrium, and psychosocial equilibrium.[70]

It was essential that a total system assessment be completed for J. B., seeking potential effects of inactivity. The assessment included documentation as to whether or not there were any alterations in the cardiovascular or respiratory systems. The baseline data that were gathered included pulse rate (88), blood pressure (160/80), peripheral pulses that were excellent, and auscultation of the heart and lungs, which revealed no abnormality.

It has been well documented that cardiac workload is increased with bedrest. According to Coe there is a 30 percent increase in the heart's workload when a person is in the recumbent position.[71] He also noted a progressive increase in the resting heart rate and tachycardia during moderate work after a client had been immobilized for only three weeks. Taylor documented that after only three weeks of bedrest the ability of healthy young men to walk 3.5 miles per hour on a 10 percent incline was decreased by 75 percent due to decreased cardiac reserve.[72]

In a longitudinal study on the effects of bedrest on training in submaximal and maximal performance, Bengt noted that the most striking effect of prolonged bedrest was a pronounced impairment of circulatory adaptation to exercise.[73] The strongest evidence in his study was the decrease in maximal oxygen uptake at the end of immobilization, the average decrease being 28 percent. These changes cannot be induced solely by a diminished venomotor response to the upright position and Bengt theorized that bedrest does impair circulatory adaptation to muscular exercise by an unidentified myocardial effect. Recovery from these physiologic changes in the study subjects did occur, but in some instances recovery required 5 to 10 weeks.

The gastrointestinal system was then assessed. J. B. was asked about her appetite, her oral intake, and her pattern of elimination. The nurse was cognizant of the fact that immobilized clients have an accelerated catabolic activity and may suffer from anorexia.

Hulley has attributed the symptoms of anorexia, malaise, nausea, vomiting, abdominal cramps, constipation, weight loss, and lethargy to the polydypsia and polyuria that result from the hypercalcemia of immobilization.[74] In 1948 Deitrick conducted a comprehensive study of immobilization of four normal healthy young men.[75] The subjects were immobilized for 6 weeks. The study was so well controlled and documented that there has been minimal refutation of the major findings. This study confirmed that hypercalciuria was present in these immobilized subjects as well as nitrogen loss, with negative nitrogen and calcium metabolic balances. It was noted that nitrogen excretion begins to increase in the fifth or sixth day of immobilization. There was an associated decline in the basic metabolic rate of 6.9 percent. Miller reported that when healthy immobilized young people were given an adequate diet they retained less than 20 percent of their protein and calcium intake.[76] Protein and bone mineral loss in clients with fractures and in hemiplegic clients were three to four times greater than that for other clients. Therefore, the importance of a diet that is well-balanced, appetizing, attractive, and high in protein is an integral aspect of the total rehabilitation plan for any immobilized person. When interviewed by the nurse, J. B. stated that she enjoyed her meals, drank at least 6 glasses of fluids per day and had no problems with constipation or diarrhea.

The nurse was also aware of the importance of fluids in the prevention of renal calculi, which are not uncommon in clients on prolonged bedrest as a result of the associated hypercalciuria. The risk of urinary tract infections is also decreased by an adequate fluid intake. The complications of renal calculi and urinary infections are not uncommon with this client population; therefore assessment of the genitourinary system, with frequent urinanalyses, is important.

The nurse continued the assessment with concentration on the musculoskeletal system. The assessment up to this point had not produced any abnormal physical findings. The nurse was well aware of the three major complications resulting from immobility that lead to musculoskeletal deterioration: osteoporosis, contractures, and decubitus ulcers.

Arnstein discussed the problem of disuse osteoporosis and noted that radiographic osteoporosis appears with an average loss of 2 percent of the total body calcium.[77] It was noted that osteoporosis is a result of bone absorption resulting from the restriction of movement. Abramson claimed that the force applied to bone by contracting muscle is the most effective means of preventing osteoporosis due to disuse. "It would seem that the evidence is in favor of muscle contraction and against weight bearing in terms of their ability to prevent osteoporosis."[78] The importance of maintaining activity (taking into consideration the limitations of the medical problems) cannot be emphasized enough. It is interesting that weightlessness or zero gravity is a new area in which bone loss and hypercalciuria have been observed. The astronauts in Gemini 4, 5, and 7 flights showed mild but definite bone loss in the calcaneus and the phalanges of the hands. On the Gemini 7 flight an exercise program was initiated and the problems appeared to decrease.[79]

J. B.'s nurse was well-informed about how contractures occur when muscles are inactive and lose their full range of motion and how decubiti will result from pressure. The nurse found on examination that J. B.'s skin, although dry, showed no evidence of pressure areas.

Since the first postoperative day, passive and active range of motion exercises of all unaffected limbs were carried out. From the first postoperative day, exercises of the affected limb included active and passive flexion and extension of the foot and ankle and quadriceps and gluteal isometric exercises. This exercise program prevented J. B.'s joint contracture and probably, as pointed out earlier, lessened her development of osteoporosis. J. B. had a full range of motion of both upper extremities and had been feeding herself and washing her upper torso with the aid of a trapeze. There were full ranges of motion in the unaffected limbs and very mild evidence of atrophy of the quadriceps. The affected limb had a full range of motion in the foot and ankle with noticeable atrophy of the quadriceps and abductors. There was a 60-degree hip flexion and a 45-degree abduction possible when in the traction apparatus.

After a complete review of the area of physical immobilization, the nurse reviewed the areas of emotional, intellectual, and social immobilization. The relationship between physical activity and a sense of psychologic well-being has been established. In some instances the psychologic manifestations may be the result of the biochemical changes. Miller noted that hypercalcemia, with its resultant biochemical and metabolic disorders, may indeed influence behavior.[80] The psychologic state of the client can become an immobilizing factor just as a stiff knee or a painful hip can. Intellectually speaking, the client must be well informed if she is to participate and carry out the exercises that are recommended. It is important for the nurse to prepare the client for ambulation emotionally as well as physically. The fact that her affected limb is now two inches shorter than the other leg and that she will have a pronounced limp in spite of the raises on her shoe may result in an inability for her to accept this altered body image. This lack of acceptance of herself may be interpreted by the client as a lack of acceptance by others, which could result in a self-imposed social immobilization. Miller observed in a study of nursing home residents that the major psychobiologic effects of inactivity were: increasing depression, fear and panic, and exacerbation of preexisting paranoia and organic brain syndrome. Depression and a sense of being overwhelmed were the main components of this immobilization syndrome. In addition, he observed a bizarre physical behavior that he refers to as the kinesiopathologic sequela of prolonged immobilization. Once the elderly person became inactive for a period of time he appeared to develop regressive behavior and an inability to coordinate muscular activities necessary for walking. Within minutes or hours of retraining, this bizarre clinical syndrome disappeared.

Some of the major effects of mobility loss have been reviewed. This information needs to be integrated into nursing practice for the purpose of developing strategies to prevent and to deal with these problems if they occur.

J. B. did not evidence any major complications related to immobilization and therefore the focus of the nursing care was on the rehabilitative aspects of the musculoskeletal system. After the assessment was completed the nurse reviewed the findings according to Carnevali's seven aspects of immobility.[82] The area, cause, and extent of the immobility were described as follows: J. B.'s immobilization is of a predominantly physical nature as a result of an infection of a total hip replacement involving the right hip area only. The nurse described the direction, duration, sequelae, and volition of J. B.'s immobilization as follows: She consulted the orthopedic surgeon for his interpretation of J. B.'s potential for improvement and future direction. It was noted that once traction is removed J. B. will ambulate with a walker without weight bearing, and then gradually progress to crutches with weight bearing as tolerated. Because the limb has been shortened, a shoe with an appropriate raise must be ready when J. B. is ready to begin ambulation. In terms of duration, there was a specific time limit of six weeks set for J. B.'s immobilization. In terms of the sequelae, the nurse was aware that after six weeks of traction due to the removal of a hip prothesis the hip flexors, extensors, adductors, and especially the abductors are weakened and a vigorous exercise program is needed. The last aspect was that of volition, which addresses the question of whether the inactive state was prescribed or voluntary. In J. B.'s situation of course it was prescribed.

Nursing Diagnosis

The data having been collected and reviewed, the nurse is now ready to state the nursing diagnoses. The following diagnoses were made. There was: (1) limited range of motion of the right hip due to removal of an infected total hip replacement; (2) atrophy of the right quadricep muscles due to limitation caused by the previously painful and infected hip; and (3) weakness of the abductor muscles of the right hip as a result of removal of the infected total hip replacement and disuse and muscle shortening.

Planning and Implementation

The short-range goals were then established for J. B. J. B. will be able to: (1) demonstrate full range of motion of all unaffected joints at the end of six weeks; (2) perform flexion and extension of the right hip joint to 50 to 60 degrees after removal of the traction at the end of six weeks; (3) perform isometric quadriceps setting exercises of 100 repetitions 3 to 4 times per day at the end of six weeks; (4) abduct the hip joint to 30 degrees passively at the end of six weeks; and (5) perform isometric abduction exercises four times per day without assistance at the end of six weeks. The long-term goals were also established. J. B. will be able to: (1) walk one mile with forearm crutches at the end of six months; (2) perform 100 hip antigravity flexion and extension exercises at least two times per day at the end of six months; (3) perform 100 antigravity abductor exercises at least two times a day at the end of six months; and (4) perform independently all activities of daily living at the end of six months. After the establishment of the short- and long-term goals a plan was developed with J. B. outlining the specific exercises that she would be doing in bed for the first six weeks. Initially passive range of motion exercises to all joints was performed. It was explained to J. B. that the reason skeletal traction was used with the Pearson attachment was to allow her to flex and extend her affected knee and ankle joints. From the first day after surgery J. B. was taught how to do the quadricep, gluteal, and abductor exercises which she was encouraged to do by herself four times a day, at least five repetitions of three sets each.

The nurse worked closely with J. B. for the first two weeks to ensure her understanding of the exercises and to monitor her ability to perform the exercises correctly. During the last four weeks of traction, the nurse worked with J. B. on a more independent basis and monitored her progress.

Evaluation

At the end of six weeks, J. B. was evaluated prior to beginning ambulation. The following goals had been achieved. The client: (1) demonstrated full range of motion of all unaffected joints; (2) performed flexion and extension of the right hip to 50 degrees; (3) demonstrated increased strength in the quadriceps and gluteal muscles of the affected hip; and (4) demonstrated abduction ability of the right hip passively to 10 degrees. At this point, J. B. achieved most of her short-term goals, which would be necessary to begin ambulation. If the abductors are weak the client's limp will be more pronounced and there will be an increase in the energy expenditure needed to perform ambulation. J. B. began to ambulate with the assistance of a walker and a raised shoe lift of two inches. She did experience mild pain. An intensive program of exercises to strengthen the hip flexors, extensors, adductors, and especially the abductors was continued. J. B. was discharged to her home after being ambulatory with crutches for one week. She was to return to clinic three times a week to continue her exercise training.

J. B. returned to clinic for a reevaluation at the end of six months. The following data were collected at that time. J. B. was walking without pain with forearm crutches. The maximum distance covered was one quarter mile due to fatigue. Hip flexors and extensors were in good condition, with strong abductors noted. J. B. had achieved most of the objectives that had been mutually established and she reported on her ability to carry out all activities of daily living without difficulty. A walking program to increase overall fitness was developed for J. B. Although her limitations will never allow her to be active in a "normal" manner, her situation highlights the fact that with the proper rehabilitation program complete independence is a realistic and achieveable goal even for a client with prolonged and profound activity deprivation.

The client situations presented have demonstrated how the nursing process can be utilized as a framework for providing care to clients with various alterations in their level of activity. The first client situation focused on an apparently healthy young woman whose goal was to achieve a higher level of wellness. The collected data provided the foundation on which the strategies for improvement of this person's deconditioned state were developed. This study highlighted the benefits of exercise and how a higher level of wellness can be achieved by a program to increase an individual's state of physical fitness. The discussion centered on what was necessary, expected, and required for the specific need to be met, and strategies that would meet the need for exercise.

The second client situation illustrated the care provided to a person who had a myocardial infarction and demonstrated limitations in activity as a result of a deconditioned state and a diminished cardiac reserve. His physical condition was aggravated by a variety of work-related stressors. Definitive improvement was noted after a program of therapeutic exercises. This study provided an example of a client whose deconditioned state interfered with his ability to achieve the activity level of which he was capable. The nursing process was utilized to assist the client in the elimination of the deficit and return the client to a higher level of wellness.

The third client situation demonstrated a definitive need violation and the nursing process again provided the framework for meeting the client's needs. Once the nursing diagnoses were made, strategies were developed for the successful achievement of the goals that were established. This elderly client developed an infected total hip replacement that was removed and resulted in permanent limitations in her activity. Improvement was noted with an extensive exercise therapy program and the client was able to become ambulatory and independent in her activities of daily living. It was through the establishment of short- and long-term goals and the evaluation of these goals that the decision was made that nursing interventions had been appropriate.

Activity is a basic need of all men and women and it is important for nurses to be well informed in the area of activity and exercise. Nurses should become involved in studying the relationship of activity to the maintenance of health, physical as well as psychologic. During the last one hundred years, as a result of increased mechanization and refined transportation, the need for activity has been lessened. The impact on man is now being scientifically documented. Today it is observed that there is a resurgence of a commitment by many to be physically fit regardless of their age.

The client situations have demonstrated various levels of wellness and the problems that occur when the need for activity is not met. This chapter is an attempt to increase the knowledge of the nurse regarding the need for activity, with the hope that the principles that have been discussed will be incorporated into the nurse's professional practice.

References

1. Maslow A: Motivation and Personality, 2nd ed. New York, Harper & Row, 1970
2. Stamford BA: Physiological effects of training upon institutionalized geriatric men. J Gerontol 27:451–455, 1972
3. Folkins CH, Lynch S, et al.: Psychological fitness as a function of physical fitness. Arch Phys Med Rehabil 42:503–508, 1972
4. Butler R: Why Survive? Being Old in America. New York, Harper & Row, 1975, p 367
5. Borgman MF: Exercise and health maintenance. J Nurs Ed 16:7, January, 1977
6. Butler R[4]: p 367
7. Butler R[4]: p 366
8. Butler R[4]: p 368
9. Krucoff C: Senior citizens say dancing puts them on top of the world. In Washington Post, Thursday May 26, 1977 DC4
10. Kilbom A: How to Obtain Physical Fitness. In Larsen GA, Malmbay RO (eds): Coronary Heart Disease and Physical Fitness. Baltimore, University Park Press, 1971, p 175

11. Kneittgen HG: Programs of Exercise, Physiological Considerations. In Morse RL (ed): Exercise and the Heart. Illinois, Charles C Thomas, 1972, pp 53–56
12. Mann GV, Garett HL, et al.: Exercise to prevent coronary heart disease. Am J Med 46:12–27, January, 1969
13. Fox SM: Exercise today to prevent a coronary tomorrow. Med Opinion 4:42, June, 1975
14. deVries HA: Physiological effects of an exercise training regimen upon men fifty two-eighty eight. J Gerontol 25:325–336, 1970
15. Stamford BA[2]: pp 451–455
16. Barry J, Daly J, et al.: The effects of physical conditioning on older individuals, I: Work capacity, circulatory respiratory function, and work electrocardiogram. J Gerontol 21:182–191, 1966
17. Smith J, Fink S: The relationship between physical improvement and psychological factors in chronically ill patients. J Clin Psychol 19:289–292, 1963
18. Barry J, Steinmetz JR, et al.: The effects of physical conditioning on older individuals, II: Motor performance and cognitive function. J Gerontol 21:192–199, 1966
19. Powell R: Psychological effects of exercise therapy upon institutionalized geriatric mental patients. J Gerontol 29:160, 1974
20. Folkins C, Lynch S: Psychological fitness as a function of physical fitness. Arch Phys Med Rehabil 53:508, 1972
21. Chapman CB, Mitchell JH: Physiology of exercise. Sci Am 212:88–96, 1965
22. Bortz EL: Stress and aging. Geriatrics 10:93, 1956
23. Butler R[4]: p 7
24. Morehouse L, Miller A: Physiology of Exercise. St. Louis, Mosby, 1967, p 39
25. Cooper K: The New Aerobics. New York, Bantam, 1970
26. Raab W: Preventive medical mass reconditioning abroad, Why Not in the USA? Ann Inter Med 54:1191, 1961
27. AMA Committee on Exercise and Physical Fitness: Is Your Patient Fit? JAMA 201:131–132, July 10, 1967
28. Ibid: p 131
29. Ibid: p 131
30. Ibid: p 131
31. Cooper K[25]: p 28
32. Ibid: p 16
33. Lange-Andersen: The determinants of physical performance capacity in health and disease. In Naughton JP, Hellerstein HK (eds): Exercise Testing and Exercise Training in Coronary Heart Disease. New York, Academic, 1973, p 36
34. The Committee on Exercise: Exercise Testing and Training of Individuals with Heart Disease or at High Risk for its Development: A Handbook for Physicians. New York, American Heart Association, 1975, p 24
35. Wilmore J: Exercise prescription: role of the physiatrist and allied health professional. Arch Phys Med Rehabil 57:315–319, July, 1976
36. Ibid: pp 315–319
37. Cumming GR: Yield of ischemic exercise electrocardiograms in relation to exercise intensity in normal population. Br Heart J 34:919–23, 1972
38. Naughton J, Haider R: Methods of exercise testing. In Naughton JP, Hellerstein HK (eds): Exercise Testing and Exercise Training in Coronary Heart Disease. New York, Academic, p 89

39. Wilmore J: Exercise control, heart rate. In Wilson P (ed): Adult Fitness and Cardiac Rehabilitation. Baltimore, University Park Press, 1975, p 289
40. Naughton J, Haider R[38]: p 90
41. Wilmore J[39]: op cit: p 315
42. Ibid: p 315
43. Cooper K[25]: p 28
44. Ibid: p 29
45. The Committee on Exercise: Exercise Testing and Training of Apparently Healthy Individuals: A Handbook for Physicians. New York, American Heart Association, 1972, p 8
46. AMA Committee on Exercise and Physical Fitness [27]: p 131
47. AMA Committee on Exercise and Physical Fitness: Evaluation for exercise participation in the apparantly healthy individual. JAMA 219:900, February 14, 1972
48. Cooper K[25]: pp 28–29
49. Wilmore J: Prescribing exercise for healthy adults. In Wilson P (ed): Adult Fitness and Cardiac Rehabilitation. Baltimore, University Park Press, 1975, p 147
50. Ibid: p 147
51. Ibid: p 147
52. AMA Committee on Exercise and Physical Fitness: Evaluation of exercise participation in apparently healthy individuals[47]: p. 901
53. Nagle F: A YMCA-university fitness program. In Wilson P: Adult Fitness and Cardiac Rehabilitation. Baltimore, University Park Press, 1975, p 244
54. Byrne M, Thompson L: Key Concepts for the Study and Practice of Nursing. St. Louis, Mosby, 1972, p 40
55. Zohman L, Tobis J: Cardiac Rehabilitation. New York, Grune & Stratton, 1970, p 8
56. Ibid: p 10
57. Lange-Andersen K: The determinants of physical performance capacity in health and disease. In Naughton JP, Hellerstein HK (eds): Exercise Testing and Exercise Training in Coronary Heart Disease. New York, Academic, 1973, p 37
58. The Committee on Exercise: Exercise Testing and Training of Apparently Healthy Individuals: A Handbook for Physicians. New York, American Heart Association, 1972, p 8
59. Zohman L, Tobis J[55]: p 97
60. Fox S, Naughton J: Physical activity and the prevention of coronary heart disease. Prevent Med 1:105, 1972
61. Cooper K[25]: p 123
62. Detry JM: Increased arteriovenous oxygen difference after physical training in coronary heart disease. Circulation 44:109, 1971
63. Robinson B: Relation of heart rate and systolic blood pressure to the onset of pain and angina pectoris. Circulation 35:1073–83, 1967
64. Hellerstein HK: Exercise therapy in coronary disease. Bull N Y Acad Med 44:1028, 1968
65. Zohman L, Tobis J[55]: p 101
66. Zohman L, Tobis J[55]: p 160
67. Hellerstein HK, Hirsch EZ, et al.: Principles of exercise prescription for normals and cardiac subjects. In Naughton JP, Hellerstein HK (eds): Exercise Testing and Exercise Training in Coronary Heart Disease. New York, Academic, 1973, p 161

68. Cooper K[25]: p 124
69. Carnevali D, Brueckner S: Immobilization—reassessment of a concept. Am J Nurs 70:1502–1507, July, 1970
70. Olsen E, Johnson B, et al.: The hazards of immobility. Am J Nurs 67:781–797, April, 1967
71. Coe SW: Cardiac work and the chair treatment of acute coronary thrombus. Ann Intern Med 40:42–47, January, 1954
72. Taylor HL: Effects of bedrest on cardiovascular functions and work performance. J Applied Psychol 2:223–239, November, 1949
73. Bengt, S: Response to exercise after bedrest and after training: A longitudinal study of adaptive changes in oxygen transport and body composition. Circulation 37–38 (suppl):1–78, 1968
74. Hulley SB, Vogle JM, et al.: The effects of supplemental oral phosphate on the bone mineral changes during prolonged bed rest. J Clin Invest 50:2506, 1971
75. Deitrick JE, Whedon GD, et al.: Effects of immobilization upon various metabolic and physiologic functions of normal men. Am J Med 4:3–32, 1948
76. Miller M: Iatrogenic and nurisgenic effects of prolonged immobilization of the ill aged. J Am Geriatr Soc 23:362, August, 1975
77. Arnstein AR: Regional osteoporosis. Orthoped Clin North Am 3:586, November, 1972
78. Abramson AS, Delagi EF: Influence of weight bearing in muscle contraction on disuse osteoporosis. Arch Phys Med Rehabil 42:149, 1961
79. Lutwak L, Whedon GD, et al.: Mineral, electrolyte and nitrogen balance studies of the Gemini VII fourteen day orbital space flight. J Clin Endocrinol 29:1140, 1969
80. Miller M[76]: p 367
81. Ibid: p 367
82. Carnevali D, Brueckner S[69]: pp 1502–1507

Chapter Eight •

The Need for Sleep

Helen Yura

Perhaps one of the most interesting states in which man finds himself is sleep. Although sleep is not new to man and animals, interest in the subject has mounted in recent years, particularly since the discovery of rapid eye movement (REM) sleep in 1954. Research aimed at studying the sleep state in man and in animals is extensive, and the descriptive reports are plentiful. The research related to sleep received an added boost from the space program, for it had to be calculated just how much sleep an astronaut needed to assure health and top level performance. Sleep is involved in personal growth and development; it affects health and well-being, moods, behavior, energy, and emotions. Sleep shapes our very life style. It is necessary for attention, happiness, for learning, and work.

The importance of sleep to each person hardly needs mentioning. For those suffering deprivation of sleep, the overwhelming wish to get "a good night's sleep" lends support to the compelling nature of this human need. A large portion (approximately one-third) of our existence occurs in this slumber state. Sleep researchers and physiologists are not apt to indicate that death will occur from lack of sleep; however, most of us can relate personal experiences that support efforts to fulfill this need as well as show the impact of lack of sleep. Some of us exert our efforts to get to sleep or at least try to get as much as needed after a pressing day whereas others expend energy to fight off sleep—to capture as much of wakefulness as possible—and look at the need to sleep as a bother and nuisance.

It is the author's opinion that the need for sleep for herself as well as for the client has largely been ignored by the nurse. Complaints about difficulty in getting to sleep have largely been handled by the periodic, even automatic, dispensing of drugs with little application of the art and the science of nursing (inherent in the nursing process) to assure a safe and wholesome approach to the scope of the need as well as to determine the most feasible nursing strategies based on a fully assessed state of sleep for an individual client.

The theoretical framework for the presentation on sleep will be drawn from a variety of existing physiologic theories. These theories will support the development of the data base for the state of sleep in wellness or need satisfaction as well as for alterations in sleep. Scientific studies have supplied data about the sleep center of the brain and have shed some light on the waking state. Because the purpose of a theory is to give focus and direction to a course of research, it is subject to change as fruits of results are realized. One theoretician and researcher of sleep is Hernandez-Peon, whose sleep theory is summarized in the following paragraphs.

Activators and Inhibitors

The brain is composed of neural teams of activators and inhibitors, the dominance of each alternating like the motion of an interlocked balance scale. While they are active in their roles they are also antagonistic. The inhibitor must suppress the activator in order to be dominant, or vice versa. Neither activators nor inhibitors remain dominant over an extended period of time. When the censor becomes dominant, alertness diminishes and sleep reigns. Wakefulness returns when the activator dominates.[1]

Balance between Systems

"The balance between the sleep and arousal systems must be delicate, permitting the sleeping person to receive relevant warnings from his senses, permitting volition, enforcing needed rest yet maintaining communication with the outside environment for survival." A rhythmicity among attention, alertness, drowsiness, sleep, and wakefulness persists lifelong. The muscular relaxation attending sleep may come from an inhibition imposed on the muscles by the hypnogenic circuit in the brain. After a period of intense and continuous discharge by nerve cells, cell fatigue sets in, causing a slowdown of inhibitory neurons. "Even during sleep a person will move, change position, turn over—suggesting the delicacy of a balance in which there is a never utter inhibition, nor ever total lack of inhibition."[2]

The Filtering System

A subcortical inhibiting system may be at work to filter out sensory inflow during acts of concentration. This inhibiting or filtering system permits attention changes as a person slips from wakefulness into sleep. Without such a system, one would expect the sleeping person to be aware of the "pressure of bedclothes and sheets, the slight wind caused by exhalation of breath, the sounds of the night, and the beating of the heart."[3] To understand this mechanism, it is useful to first consider some aspects of the operation of the vigilance system. It is speculated that a set of neurons that have no direct, active role in causing alertness may be located within the reticular formation and distributed along the vigilance system. They might function as the registrars of conscious experience. If such neurons exist they would have to be active at times when we have conscious experience such as in waking and in dreaming, but inactive when we do not. This would act in phase with the vigilance system during waking. At this time the severe and active filtering system prevents a bombardment of irrelevant stimuli. Similarly, during REM or desynchronized sleep the filtering system is operative, but during this period, when the vigilance system is largely inhibited, the neurons that register conscious experience might be out of phase with the arousal system, although they may manifest an active role (i.e., in dreaming). During the synchronized period of sleep, when the vigilance system is partly dominated by the sleep system, conscious experience neurons would be almost totally inactive. The absence of sensory filtering due to their inactivity would mean that the brain receives incoming impulses, but does not perceive and respond in a focused manner without consciousness. The assumption that there may be conscious experience mediators tied in with the vigilance system may help to explain some strange phenomenon like somnambulism (sleepwalking), which occurs during the synchronized slow wave period.[4]

The Motivational System

James Olds discovered that there is a certain overlapping between the hypnogenic pathway and the reinforcement area. This region includes septal and hypothalamic areas now known to produce signs of pleasure when stimulated to a certain extent, but punishment if overstimulated. Both the sleep system and this reward, or motivation, system appear to send fibers through a bundle in the medial forebrain. Areas in another portion of the brain that have been found to produce negative or aversive reaction when stimulated overlap anatomically with arousal regions. The balance of motivational factors (positive and negative reinforcement) may be linked to balance of the sleep and wakefulness systems. Pleasant and unpleasant sensations can be elicited directly by the senses, or indirectly by memories and thoughts. Like sleep and wakefulness, they are subject to the impulses coming from the environment and from the body via the spinal cord and are subject to descending impulses expressing the will of the cortex. It would be plausible for the motivational system to work in an antagonistic balance, like sleep and arousal, and to be subject to the inhibitory system of sleep and the arousing vigilance system.[5]

Anatomic Considerations

Sleep is not a consequence of an arousal system that has been turned off. It is not mere absence of activity in the nervous system, but an actively inhibiting process. In approximately the middle of the human brain, about three inches behind the bridge of the nose and just above the palate lies a dense cluster of nuclei—the hypothalamus. It is a concentrated mass of gray matter that regulates such fundamental life functions as eating, drinking, and essential emotional reactions such as rapid heartbeat, body temperature, and sexual activity. This part of the brain is fully developed at birth.[6] In the midpart of the brain a bundle of nerve fibers connects the neocortex with the limbic system, a group of nuclei that have probably not experienced very many evolutionary changes in 100 million years, and are basically similar in anatomy, if not function, in all mammals. This ancient cortex—the rhinoencephalon—contains concentric folds and blobs and four fiber systems connecting it with the neocortex and the brainstem. A delimited pathway of nerve cells, extending downward along the spinal cord, must transmit neural messages downward from higher brain areas to subjugate the vigilance system and let sleep prevail. Thus, projecting pathways from the cortex might transmit the order for a sleep of volition along a pathway that would finally enter the spinal cord, causing the relaxation of body functioning and relative inertia of the muscles. More areas need to be probed, as many gaps still exist in our knowledge of the chain of command in sleep.

Sleep has been produced experimentally by cholinergic stimulation in an area near the temples, the pyriform cortex within the temporal lobes, and studies are now planned that would determine the anatomic route of sleep. This would be accomplished by inducing neurons as they lead to the preoptic region of the hypothalamus and the bundle of fibers joining the neocortex and limbic systems in the middle of the brain. Cholinergic stimulation has produced sleep from a nub of tissue on the surface of the hemisphere at the center of the forehead and in the olfactory tubercle that is connected with a fiber bundle in the preoptic area. This pathway of descending sleep messages, like tributaries to a river, seems to curve down from the forward part of the brain, a little below the temples, to the brainstem. Converging on the pons in the brainstem are the messages transmitted from the curving pathway and from a sleep-evoking area just recently discovered in the cerebellum, the hindpart of the brain.[7]

The small, pine cone-shaped pineal gland is attached to the top of the brainstem and is thought to be a regulator of rhythmicity for the body.[8] In acting as a clock that establishes day–night rhythms (as has been theoretically proposed), it does not abruptly switch the brain from one activity or level of consciousness to another. Rather, it informs the brain that the appropriate moment for switching is at hand. The brain then makes up its mind—it may choose to ignore bedtime and stay awake long past the sleep hour fixed by habit and the earth's revolutions. With a bit more difficulty, it awakens at a time chosen consciously rather than because of any secretions of the pineal gland. The actual change in consciousness is accomplished in a different part of the brain, by a network of nerve cells rooted in one small part of the brainstem. This master switch of awareness, about the size of the little finger, is the reticular activating system (RAS). "It alerts the brain to incoming information from the senses, and from the centers of thought, memory and feeling. More than that, it adjudicates the relative importance of that information permitting the mind to focus in a single stimulus."[9]

The primary function of the reticular activating system is self-preservation. It unfailingly triggers an awareness of danger or the threat of danger. Signals from such internal functions as breathing and heartbeat bombard the brain constantly, yet the brain pays little attention to them unless the RAS alerts it that something is wrong. Similarly, a mother will sleep through loud stereo noise coming from the neighbors' home, but will waken at the faintest cry from her baby. A sleeping father may not hear a child crying, but is likely to be immediately aroused by a whiff of smoke.[10]

The RAS normally switches back and forth at regular intervals between the day dreaming alpha rhythm and the alert beta rhythm, and at least twice a day it switches between sleep and wakefulness. It was once thought that sleep was produced simply by switching off the RAS. It was discovered that damage to the RAS caused complete loss of consciousness instead of induction of sleep in the individual, it caused a coma.[11] Later it was found that a second mechanism modulated the RAS. This is the raphe system, located in the middle of the RAS, and is believed to suppress the RAS. It is speculated that the raphe system is the chief supplier of the sleep-inducing chemical serotonin.[12]

The theory that sleep serves a synthetic anabolic function has been gaining ground recently. It has been found that the secretion of human growth hormone is sleep dependent and the quantity secreted is related (except in the obese) to the amount of Stage 3 or 4 sleep. This hormone is known to promote protein synthesis and peaks of mitotic activity on skin, in bone marrow, the liver, the reticuloendothelial system, and the pineal gland have been shown.[13]

Knowledge accumulated to date has led to a formulation of the sequence of the states and stages of sleep as follows. There are two states: non-rapid eye movement (NREM) and rapid eye movement (REM). The REM state is comprised of four stages. Stage 1 NREM occurs first at the onset of the sleep cycle for a brief period, followed by Stage 2 (another brief period), and then Stages 3 and 4, which are stages of deep sleep. NREM Stages 1 through 4 last a total of about one hour followed by NREM Stages 3 and 2, then the first REM state (lasting approximately ten minutes). This completes the first sleep cycle. After this the second sleep cycle begins, with first brief NREM sleep stages 1 and 2, then the longer NREM Stages 3 and 4, which are followed by REM sleep. Throughout the night (approximately 8 hours), NREM alternates with REM sleep, the length of REM state increasing to approximately one-half hour with each subsequent occurrence, NREM stages 3 and 4 decreasing, and NREM Stage 2 increasing as the night passes. *Ninety minutes* constitutes the usual periodicity of the sleep cycle. The duration of first cycle averages 70 to 80 minutes, the second and third average 100 to 110 minutes, and the later cycles are somewhat shorter (Fig. 8.1).[14,15]

Dreaming

The first and shortest dream is usually set in the present and focuses on a problem occupying the mind prior to sleep. This sets the theme for the dreams to follow. The next two dreams usually deal with situations from the past while incorporating some feelings from the present. The fourth dream is often set in the future and concerns some kind of wish fulfillment. The fifth and final dream of the night incorporates material from all previous dreams, but particularly from the preceding one.

Sleep as a Vital Human Need

Need theory, especially that of Maslow and Montagu, makes a contribution by supporting the valuing of vital human needs, one of which is sleep. Fulfilling or satisfying vital human needs is the goal of human beings. The manner and extent of satisfaction or disatisfaction have important implications for human behavior and personality development.[16] Maslow believes that gratification of basic human needs leads to consequences labeled at times as desirable, good, healthy, self-actualizing. "The requiredness of basic need gratifiers differentiates them from all other need gratifiers. The organism itself, out of its own nature, points to an intrinsic range of satisfiers for which no substitute is possible as is the case, for instance, with habitual needs, or even with many neurotic needs."[17]

Nursing practitioners must be particularly mindful of providing an environment (internal and external) that will assure normal sleep for a client. This is postulated on the acceptance of sleep as a vital human need that requires satisfaction in order for mental and physical health to be maintained and for a recovery

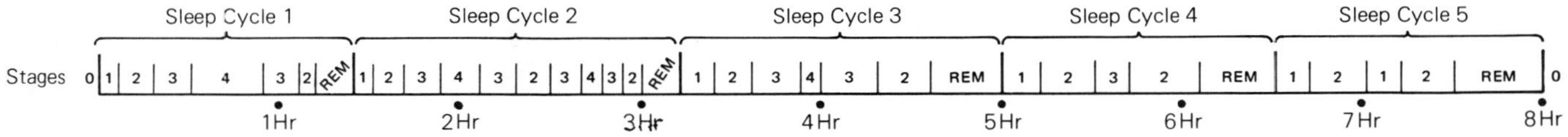

Fig. 8.1: Sleep Cycle Schema.

from illness to be facilitated in the sick client. In helping the sick client, it seems easy to be preoccupied with applying the medical plan and selecting nursing strategies while failing to assume responsibility for the maintenance and integrity of all vital human needs, whether or not they are the focus for pathophysiologic and psychopathologic events. These vital needs must be sustained to maintain wellness and to prevent the occurrence of illness.

Thus, the nurse must master the data that are part of the wellness model for sleep for human beings. In other words, what is the data base gathered by the nurse from the client, his family, and his environment by means of a complete health assessment (including a physical examination) that support the conclusion that normal sleep is evident for the client? The following data base has been developed to gather descriptive evidence and provide a framework for decision making by the nurse regarding sleep. Normal sleep and the healthy client will be discussed first.

General Data Base for Normal Sleep

Multiple parameters will be considered in the development of the data base for sleep. Among these will be age, sex, lifestyle, socioethnocultural factors, and level of growth and development of the client.

Onset of Sleep

Sleep is an organized behavior that is performed repeatedly day after day and is an integral part of the rhythm of our daily lives. At the onset of sleep, there is a general feeling of lassitude, lagging attention, and a loss of interest in surroundings. This state is associated with the approach of sleep based on our past experience with sleep. Fatigue and lack of stimulation or monotony favor a feeling of drowsiness. An expression of this feeling is yawning, a paroximal respiratory movement lasting about 5 to 7 seconds that is described as something intermediate between a reflex and an expressive movement. Yawning is often associated with stretching, transient cardiac acceleration, and digital vasoconstriction. This cardiovascular response is thought to be an indirect vasomotor adjustment furthering the circulation in the lungs and brain.[18]

With drowsiness there is nonintentional closure of eyelids, and brain waves begin to assume a regular pattern known as an alpha rhythm. The person experiences a state of relaxed wakefulness or serenity called Stage 0. A moment of tension or attempt at problem solving will disrupt this pattern and return the person to wakefulness. If eyelids are open, eyes have a dull expression that is suggestive of sleepiness. The sleepy person may develop diplopia or have difficulty or complete inability in fixating both eyes on a point in spite of extreme effort to do so. There is an outward divergence of the eyeballs that is characterized by double vision and is brought on by the absence of centrifugal influences from the central nervous system. This divergence can also occur in the waking state as a result of alcohol intoxification or prolonged wakefulness.[19] There is a fall in muscle tonus, a decrease in knee jerk, a slowing of heart rate, and a lowering of blood pressure. Some persons experience a floating feeling; others see a flash of light or hear a musical note. This frequently ends in a jerk or start, called a myoclonia, that may briefly bring the person back to complete wakefulness. Most persons have experienced this just before falling asleep. It has been demonstrated scientifically that it occurs when the alpha rhythm has been absent for a few seconds and small, slow brain waves begin. Myoclonias generally occur during the first five minutes of sleep and are considered normal. Muscular contractions may take place in one or in a group of muscles—in arms, legs, or even in the entire body, throughout the sleep cycle. These contractions usually do not interfere with sleep during the remainder of the night and are more likely to occur in adults than in children, and in those who are nervous, in a state of fatigue, or who are in an emotional state, whether it is agreeable or disagreeable.[20]

With further relaxation, alpha brain waves become smaller, decreasing in amplitude, and the person drifts between drowsiness and sleep.[21] The act of falling asleep is influenced by what we do, think, and feel, by what happens to us, and by environmental factors. Changes in barometric pressure may increase sleepiness, as will heat, tedium, a repetitive task, and certain hours of the day. One is more likely to fall asleep when barometric pressure is low. Exercise has little or no effect on sleep patterns although excessive and strenuous exercise immediately before going to bed may delay sleep onset in some persons. No exercise or limited exercise (as in bedrest conditions) shows no effect.

Sleep researchers have shown that 95 percent of well persons between the ages of 15 and 50 fall asleep before 30 minutes have passed. It is impossible, even with an electroencephalogram reading, to pinpoint the exact moment of sleep onset. It is not gradual, but happens in an instant. In the infant, an indication that it has happened may be closed eyelids and an absence of crying. The essential difference between sleep and wakefulness is the loss of awareness. Sleep onset is the moment when a meaningful stimulus fails to elicit its accustomed response. However, a stimulus of sufficient magnitude or significance (e.g., loud noise, soft calling of one's name) will bring about arousal.[22]

Sleep Stages

At the beginning of Stage 1 sleep, there is a floating sensation with drifting idle images. At this point the person may not think that he is asleep. This stage lasts only a few moments. At the time when visual perception ceases, eyes begin to slowly roll from side to side (synchronously or asynchronously); this is one of the most reliable signs of the onset of sleep. From this point in the sleep cycle, the person progresses through the stages described earlier (beginning with NREM sleep) before the first REM period occurs. As a rule, pupillary reflexes are preserved in sleep. The pupils are small and can be made smaller by shining a light into the eyes after carefully separating the eyelids.

As the person enters Stage 2, he is soundly asleep, but can be awakened with little difficulty. He usually cannot be disturbed by turning on a light in the room.[23] Brain wave tracings grow larger, displaying quick bursts of rapid waves called spindles.

In Stage 3 sleep, the EEG shows spindle bursts and irregular brain waves interspersed with large slow waves occurring about every second. It would take a loud noise to awaken the sleeper. Muscles are totally relaxed, breathing is even, blood pressure is falling, and temperature is dropping.

In Stage 4, the deepest sleep of all, the sleeper rarely moves and muscles are completely relaxed. It is difficult to awaken the person. A child is virtually unreachable and it may take several minutes for him to return to full arousal, if he can be aroused at all. If awakened, the sleeper begins to focus slowly and may report no experience of mental activity. The EEG tracing shows slow synchronized high amplitude waves. It reports brain response to stimuli such as sounds, but these do not seem to reach the conscious level. In Stage 4 sleep, which occurs about 30 to 40 minutes following sleep onset, a series of body movements mark the start of the reascent through the NREM stages to the first REM period.

REM sleep marks the beginning of vivid dreaming. It will take a loud extraneous noise (e.g., honking horns, sirens) to awaken the person. However, it is important to note that even a slight noise with personal significance (e.g., the whimpering of a child) will cause the person to awaken.[24] Throughout the night this cyclic variation between NREM and REM sleep takes place. For the adult who sleeps 7.5 to 8 hours per night, 1 to 1.5 to 2 hours of the total is spent in REM sleep.[25]

Sleep Requirements

The determination of individual sleep requirements is a critical variable in the development of a data base for normal sleep for a person. People sleep different lengths of time and the character and quality of sleep within these varying lengths also differs. There is a broad range of normality in sleep patterns and this range does not seem to be directly related to major differences in physiology and personality.[26]

Physiologic Changes During Sleep

There is a sharp reduction in the formation of urine and the pH of the urine is decreased during sleep. Likewise, the rate of metabolism of the body and the body temperature are decreased. "The cerebral circulation has been found to increase during sleep. Also, the volume of the blood in the brain is increased and it is interesting to note that external stimulation may cause the volume to decrease even though the subject does not awaken."[27] During sleep, the heart rate is slowed and blood pressure is slightly decreased; at the same time the pulse is increased. The blood pressure is likely to reach its lowest point during the first half hour of sleep and it does not necessarily coincide with the lowest heart rate during sleep. It was discovered that stomach acid has an increased flow during REM dreams, occasionally awakening the person by giving him a stomachache. Less air is breathed during sleep and it is expected that there is a correlation between the depth of sleep and the degree of decrease in ventilation.

In terms of physical activity, much activity is noted in light sleep, whereas there is very little movement in deep sleep. In the NREM state, called quiet sleep, there is slow, regular breathing, the general absence of body movement, and slow regular brain activity. The body can move, but does not move during NREM sleep; it is not paralyzed. Perception ends and the sleeper has lost contact with his environment. The five senses no longer gather information and communicate stimuli to the brain. There is EEG evidence of a transient intrusion of wakefulness when gross body movements occur during NREM (such as rolling over), yet the individual may not be responsive at the time nor recall having moved if awakened immediately after. It is during NREM sleep that snoring occurs—thus it is not necessarily "quiet" sleep.[28]

REM sleep, called active sleep, is a complete contrast. With the onset of REM sleep, the sleeper's body is still immobile, but small, convulsive twitches of the face and fingertips are noted. Snoring ceases and breathing becomes irregular. It is first very fast, then slow, and then appears to stop for a few seconds. An observer will note the corneal bulges of the sleeper's eyes darting around back and forth under the eyelids. "Cerebral blood flow and brain temperature soar to new heights, but the large muscles of the body are completely paralized; arms, legs, and trunk cannot move. Throbbing penile erections occur in adult—and newborn—males."[29] Short-lived contractions of the middle ear occur that are identical to those seen in wakefulness as a response to various intensities and pitches of sound. The sleeptalker can also hear what someone in the waking state says. The content is often incorporated into his dreams and answers may be given to the outsider. This person usually never remembers talking in his sleep even though he may be awakened immediately after the episode. Disconnected and incoherent sleeptalking usually occurs in deep sleep whereas talk of a more intelligent pattern arises during REM sleep.[30] Any vocalizations that were noted in children occurred in association with NREM sleep; this is the general pattern for adults. In like manner, enuresis usually occurs during NREM sleep in children.[31]

The immobility of the body and the abolition of the usual upright posture are indicative of sleep due to inoperative tonic reflexes of proprioceptive, labyrinthine, and visual origin that are responsible for righting the body and maintaining the normal standing position. The body is allowed to assume a dorsal or lateral position (even before the onset of sleep) that depends almost entirely on gravity for its preservation. Muscular relaxation, as a concomitant of sleep, leads to decreased metabolic activity and recovery from muscular fatigue.[32] There is a powerful contraction (or at least resistance from internal forcing) of the anal and vesicular sphincters.

No normal person "sleeps like a log." The sleeper changes positions 20 to 60 times during the night while utilizing no more than a total of 3 to 5 minutes of rest time. The nose makes the person turn over at night because it serves as a monitor of body rest and fatigue levels. It causes a shift in the body position during sleep so that the person can get the maximum body relaxation. When sleeping on the left side, the right side of the body continues to perform most of the body functions. When the right side gets tired, the person turns and the left side takes over. Body movement is the mechanism that differentiates sleep from unconsciousness. Gross body movements during REM sleep demarcate separate episodes of a dream. Sleepwalking is usually related to what a person is dreaming.[33] It has been noted that some sleepers move 50 percent more during certain seasons of the year than others. Temporary paralysis may result when a sleeper fails to change his position often enough (for whatever reason) or when he sleeps in such a way as to produce continuous pressure on certain nerves. Motility research findings suggest that the normal person is not entirely oblivious to the feelings of discomfort from lying too long in one position in wakefulness and in sleep.[34]

It is believed that every normal person awakens several times during a single night. Toward the end of the night, sleep is considerably lighter, with movements and awakenings more frequent than in earlier sleep. There is a gradual increase in the number of afferent impulses from such situations as a distended bladder, a contracting empty stomach, and perhaps from the muscles as the body temperature rises. These, aided by morning noises and daylight, bring the sleeper to lighter sleep and then to actual awakening.[35]

Another characteristic of sleep in healthy adults that appears only during sleep or anesthesia is the toe extension response. It is elicited by scratching the sole of the foot and denotes a positive Babinski sign. The person must be deeply asleep before the curling up of the big toe can be noted.[36]

A decrease in the ventilation of the lungs and in irritability of the respiratory center is noted during sleep. A cycle of recurring respiratory acceleration has been demonstrated in relation to dreaming during the REM state. Snoring sounds are made by vibrations in the soft palate and posterior faucial pillars during sleep. Snoring occurs in both sexes and in all age groups, but is more common in older persons. It is believed that the palate muscles of older persons have a lower tonus. Factors favoring snoring include a dorsal position and an open mouth. However, there may be organic causes of snoring, resulting from nasal obstruction and edematous changes in the pharynx and larynx.

There is no evidence that digestion is affected in any way. X-rays indicate peristaltic movements of the colon during sleep whereas the sigmoid colon remains quiet, becoming active on waking.[37]

Body temperature drops during sleep. It is believed that the drop is due to rest in the horizontal position and to muscular relaxation. It is a fact that within a typical 24-hour course a person's temperature begins to fall before bedtime even if he chooses to forego sleep and stay awake all night. Some researchers interpreted this as proof that the sleep state itself may not be directly responsible for the lowered temperature observed during sleep. However, the establishment and maintenance of the normal 24-hour temperature curve for a person depends on the regular alternation between sleep and wakefulness. A temperature drop has been demonstrated in persons who lie down after standing up for an hour.[38] There seems to be no demonstrable connection between body temperature and the frequency of body movement during sleep.

Muscular relaxation is thought to be responsible for the increase in phosphate excretion while lying down either awake or asleep. Most changes in excretion of urine can be traced to one or another concomitant of sleep; namely, horizontal posture, relaxation, low temperature, fasting, and darkness. It is estimated that a person burns about 800 calories during 8 hours of sleep. In the majority of sleepers studied by researchers, at the time of going to bed the red blood count and hemoglobin were lower than they were in the morning of the same day.[39] Hormone secretion is active during sleep. There is strong release of adrenal cortical hormone, cortisol, and growth hormone. Our bodies continue to grow, replace worn out cells, and store energy. Skin does most of its growing at night.[40]

Sleep Patterns

The average person experiences approximately 35 sleep stage changes during a typical night.[41] Stage 2 is associated with REM sleep in 85 percent of occurrences. A person experiences many different types of sleep, each functioning at a different depth of consciousness. Most remembered dreaming takes place in the REM period. REM sleep is sometimes called paradoxical sleep because the brain activity at that time resembles that of waking.

Deep sleep (Stages 3 to 4) occurs primarily during the early part of the night. Most of the middle and late parts of the night are spent in REM sleep and Stage 2. If sleep has been lost, considerably more time is spent in Stage 4. REM sleep occurs during daytime naps. Stages 0–1–3 are relatively short and transient. REM is less frequent but lasts longer. REM rarely occurs more than 4 or 5 times a night, whereas Stage 2 may occur as often as 15 or more times.[42]

There are definite differences in sleep patterns based on age. Changes are primarily developmental in nature. Webb suggests that we fully recognize these developmental differences, be awed by them and provide the best environment for their unfolding.[43] The amount of Stage 4 sleep is greatest in childhood and decreases with age. As a person grows older, the amount of Stage 4 sleep decreases, sometimes dropping to one-sixth of its original level. In some instances, it may disappear altogether. Aging leads to decrease in Stage 4 and an increase in Stage 1 sleep, as well as to more broken sleep, awakenings during the night, and surfacing to Stage 0. An elderly person's sleep reverts to a broken pattern of naps commonly noted in infancy. For the infant, about 50 percent of sleep is in the REM state (8 or 9 hours of the total). For some infants, this could reach 85 percent. In premature infants of 32 to 36 weeks gestation, the percent of REM sleep is higher, approximately 75 percent of the total. This is suggestive of the early intrauterine life of the child, when REM sleep is the all-encompassing mode of existence. It is speculated that perhaps the real function of REM sleep is fulfilled early in life. REM sleep is necessary for normal pre- and postnatal maturation of the brain.[44] Within a year a baby's REM rate drops to 25 percent of his total sleep and it remains at this percentage for most of his life.[45]

Newborn infants sleep an average of 16½ hours daily. Gradually, the baby begins to give up some sleeping time and by the 26th week, he averages 14 hours of sleep, with three-fourths of this occurring at night. As the person passes to age 2, sleep time averages 12½ hours plus a nap of 1½ hours. At age 6, the nap is given up with 11 hours of night sleep being the average. At age 10, 10 hours of sleep is evident, 9 at age 15 and 8½–8¾ for 15 to 19 year olds. It is noted that American children sleep about 1½ hours longer than German or English children.[46] It has been shown that younger children with higher IQ's sleep less on the average than children who are not so bright.[47] As the person grows older there is more control over sleeping and waking, with some flexibility allowed. But we are born with sleep needs and it is futile to change this.

The content of dreams differs with age. The dreams of small children relate to animals—lions, spiders, gorillas, bears, etc., and older children dream of being victims of others—frequent dream emotions are fear and apprehension.

It is known (especially by parents) that children become quiet much less promptly on going to bed than do adults.

There is an incredible consistency in the total amount of sleep and the amount of each type of sleep a particular person gets when averaged over a week or month. In the forties changes in the substructure are most prominent, with the diminishing of Stage 4 deep sleep and increases in awakening (Stage 0) and light sleep (Stage 1). In the late ages, naps are resurgent and nighttime awakenings are more frequent.[48]

In quiet sleep the infant lies without movement except for an occasional startlelike movement resembling the Moro reflex that does not awaken or disturb the infant. During active sleep, the infant has frequent and continuous movements, fine twitches, and tremors, with head moving from side to side; there is irregular and fast rapid respiration and heart rate; there are smiles, grimaces, sucking movements, and easily observable frequent and rapid eye movements. Eyes may even be partially open. Occasionally, vocalization may occur. REM sleep appears rhythmically every 60 minutes rather than every 90 minutes, as in the adult cycle.[49]

Major changes in the substructure of sleep occur during the first year. The spindles that identify Stage 2 sleep appear in the second month and are fully developed in the second half of the first year. Throughout all life stages, the most striking dimension remains the *individuality of differences*. The stabilized range of sleep for the adult is about 8 hours.

The two significant differences between two- and four-year-olds are that four-year-olds have less Stage 1 sleep and longer REM cycles. The sleep substructure seems to have become organized and stabilized before the second year. Youngsters tend to go to bed later, take fewer naps, and sleep less as childhood passes. Problems during this period may relate to the maintenance of a nap period when the child does not need one due to the natural maturation process. An important difference between the sleep pattern of the 4 to 5-year-olds in comparison with 2 to 3-year-olds is that the 2 to 3-year-olds show their first REM period within an hour after sleep onset whereas the 4 to 5-year-olds' first REM period does not appear until three hours after sleep onset.[50] It appears that the initial REM of a typical cycle is missed.

The amount of Stage 1 REM sleep declines from about 30 to 25 percent by the age of 12. Except for the differences in total sleep amounts, "most of the variations appear to be our own creations imposed upon a largely stable system."[51]

From age thirty to the late years, the substructure of sleep assumes a course of accelerating changes that clearly break through the patterns of sleeping and waking, with resultant diminishing control of the sleep process. The amount of time spent awake after sleep onset (Stage 0) increases ninefold for the 60-year-old, with the number of awakenings increasing from an average of one per night to six per night. Light sleep (Stage 1) is 2½ times as great in the 60-year-old as in young adults under 30. REM sleep and Stage 2 sleep show little change, but there is a 15 to 30 percent drop in deep sleep (Stage 4).

A slight rise in the amount of sleep within 24 hours has been demonstrated in persons over the age of 60. The overall amounts of sleep show small changes whereas the range of individual differences clearly increased.[52] Naps also show a consistent increase with age. However, overall there remains a greater evidence of the maintenance of the integrity of sleep with age.

Webb summarizes the established facts about sleep and aging as: (1) the patterns of sleep follow natural and inherent changes; (2) wide individual differences are noted in the pace and timing of these changes; and (3) problems result more from our expectations about sleep and our social needs than from sleep itself.[53]

Body movements during Stage 1 in 5 to 13-year-olds, while less frequent than in young children, are generally more frequent than in the postpuberty population and much more than in adults.[54] The delay is thought to be related to the fact that children at this age have acquired a highly developed waking–sleeping diurnal pattern, and also to the fact that they are at a very active age, having achieved full mobility and great curiosity. It is expected that they endure considerable muscular fatigue that affects their sleep pattern. They spend as much as two hours in Stage 4 sleep soon after onset of sleep, in contrast to 40 to 60 minutes spent by adults. Fatigue is an important factor and accounts for the fact that most of Stage 4 sleep occurs in the first half of the night. Adults may show a missed initial REM sleep period when excessively fatigued or sleep deprived.[55]

It is thought that as perception and memory functions develop in the growing infant, dreaming develops in parallel fashion. Perhaps sometime during or after vision has been gained by the infant, a correspondence develops between the spatial pattern of REMs and the visual imagery of a dream. "This correlation is probably effected by the cortex."[56]

It is interesting to note that as the person grows older, the time of awakening remains fairly constant while the time at which to retire for sleep is a later hour, so that the transition from sleeping on an average of 16 hours per day to the average of 8 demonstrates a loss of hours at bedtime more than at the time of awakening. These changes show a relationship to the increasing periods of wakefulness during the day. Metabolism, weather, season, health, amount of stress, and type of work do have an impact on the pattern and amount of sleep for a person. Whether a person sleeps much or little, the amount of dreaming time, and of Stage 4 and REM sleep is always proportionally the same.

There is a remarkably consistent lack of difference between the sleep of male and of female persons. In the pre-liberation era, there were quite different day-to-day differences in the physical activities of men and women and varying attitudinal, situational, and emotional reactions to life. Of course, many differences still exist together with various physiologic differences. However, researchers have been able to demonstrate that these day-to-day activities and responses have little or no effect on sleep differences between men and women. Studies do show a difference between men and women in the relationship of the aging process and sleep. The sleep patterns of women are generally more resistant to age changes. In one study, it was demonstrated that the sleep of a 60-year-old woman showed a pattern more akin to that of a man at age 50 rather than 60.[57] As noted earlier, male persons usually experience erections at regular intervals during the night. This is true for infants and for those in their late 80s. Even men who complain of impotence on waking are subject to erections during sleep. Little data are available about sleep and women. It has been noted that there is an increase in nipple size and the blood supply to the vaginal area. This occurs at intervals during the night, but there seems to be no connection to REM sleep. Differences have been noted in the dream content of male and female persons. Linde indicates that women dream of indoors, facial details, jewelry, and conversations whereas men dream of tools, weapons, money, and physical aggression. Boys dream of tools, implements, and things whereas girls' dreams are longer and portray more people. The dreams of pregnant women are characterized by imagery, seeds, and fertility. Dreams of menstruating women relate to anatomy, rooms, babies, and mother. Regarding sex dreams, 98 percent of men experience orgasm in dream content. Forty percent of women describe dreams with more romantic overtones, of which a greater amount of such content is reported in women over the age of 40.[58]

Hartmann reports that women have more Stage 4 sleep during progestational periods, especially during the premenstrual phase of the menstrual cycle and that the physiologic components of premenstrual tension may be partly related to this requirement. Women have reported that allowing more sleep during the week before menses improved their mood considerably.[59]

Karacan and Williams report that the overall sleep pattern observed during gestation is characterized by a longer sleep latency, frequent awakenings, shorter sleep time, and a marked reduction in Stage 4 sleep. There was a marked reduction in Stage 4 sleep in the last trimester of pregnancy. A suppression of Stage 1 and REM sleep was noted immediately after delivery. However, by the second postpartum week, these profound sleep changes dissipated and normal sleep pattern ensued.[60] In a study of college women's REM dreams, dream content was found to be unpleasant during the menstrual cycle phase, when they felt most depressed.[61]

Different people sleep for different lengths of time. A normal healthy person may sleep longer one night than another and, as noted earlier, he has a sleep pattern that changes as he progresses in age.

The quality of dream content varies in REM sleep and is different in NREM sleep. It has been observed that more detail and more emotion comprise REM dreams that occur later in the night than those which occur earlier. The first dream of the night tends to be related to current problems whereas later dreams include incidents from childhood and adolescence which appear as flashbacks. Early morning NREM dreaming has been described as wandering aimlessly, feeling lost or floating. There is evidence of thinking of things, logical reasoning, and experiencing strange, shadowy, and mysterious feelings.[62] Nonrecallers of dreams have been found to have fewer eye movements per unit time than those with recall.[63]

Another interesting finding relates to the lack of difference in sleep patterns of persons who lead very different lives. For example, the sleep patterns of healthy persons differ little or not at all from the patterns of institutionalized schizophrenic persons. Though these persons live in an almost desocialized world and act in bizarre ways, their sleep patterns follow those of healthy persons of comparable age. This holds true for those who are mentally retarded, whose learning or reading capacity is very different from that of the average person.[64]

As noted earlier, sleep differences are surprisingly small when individual sleep patterns are averaged over a period of a week to a month. Although there may be individual variations among healthy individuals—ranging from normals of 4½ to 5 to 10 to 12 hours of sleep needed, each individual sleep pattern is consistent with little variation over a period of time. When variations in sleep lengths occur by choice or circumstance, an adjustment in the differential temporal distribution of sleep stages within sleep period occurs. Webb calculates that "a reduction of sleep by 25 percent . . . results in a 36 percent reduction of REM sleep, a 25 percent reduction in Stage 2 . . . and only a 1 percent reduction in Stage 4 sleep. A 50 percent reduction in sleep . . . results in a differential 'deprivation' or loss of 70 percent REM sleep, 50 percent Stage 2 sleep, and 2 percent Stage 4 sleep."[65] When sleep is prolonged, that is, increased 25 or more percent, REM sleep and Stage 2 sleep increase, but no increase in Stage 4 sleep is noted. Webb speculates on the determinants of stable sleep length differences. He believes that stable biophysical dimension genetically and environmentally derived (metabolism, central nervous system states, biochemical conditions, and temperature) is influenced, as are transient biophysical state variables such as malnutrition, alcohol and drug consumption, and chronic low grade infections. Early environmental conditioning resulting from, for example, parental attitude and control, economic and cultural determinants, personally and environmentally induced stress or the lack of stress over a period of time, task demands or the lack of these demands, and voluntarily imposed regimens constitute sleep length determinants.[66]

Healthy persons are subject to sleep time changes resulting from shift work and jet travel. Clear differences have been shown for persons who sleep during the day and work during the night. For those who had not fully adapted to day sleep, it was found that sleep during the day was different from regular sleep, and the timing of sleep stages within sleep was radically altered. REM sleep occupied the sleep period early in day sleep and diminished toward the usual sleep time. The opposite effect was noted for Stage 4 sleep. Day sleep is more broken, with a sharp increase in the number of arousals and Stage 1 sleep. The length of the sleep period is reduced. Likewise, performance during what is usually the sleep period sharply deteriorates. Webb stresses that tasks sensitive to sleep loss that are performed after midnight show reduced efficiency during the time even though no sleep deprivation exists. Errors increase and long-term and low-motivation tasks show decreases. Sleep patterns reorganize themselves into their usual, original form when the new sleep–work schedule is maintained for a period of time, and performance gradually improves.

Rhythmicity is the rule when considering sleep and wakefulness. Even when the timing is modified willfully or in response to external or internal circumstances, the original rhythm persists. There is a time for sleep and a time to be awake and our bodies follow this schedule; adaptation to major schedule variations takes time. Occasional variations, like one trip to the west or the east coast, will have only a subtle, short, limited, disturbing effect on the basic sleep and waking rhythm, but there is an effect on rhythm and performance.

In a survey of major cities to determine the percentage of the population working on a night shift, the range was 13 to 33 percent within manufacturing industrial complexes. These figures do not include the large numbers involved in providing health and nursing care, law enforcement, transporation, sanitation, the military and the entertainment and communication industries. The solution to human problems related to reversal of sleep and waking rhythms is permanent shifts to allow rhythmic adaptation over a period of time. In all situations, however, there is a systematic nature to sleep. It is a sensitive and a self-protection system, responding to variations in format and geared to the maintenance of its integrity in the event of imposed variations in the individual form.[68]

Kleitman found that both right- and left-handed persons assumed a right-sided sleep position in slightly more than one half of the times, but that for persons in whom handedness was well developed it was more likely that a sleep position was assumed that would allow the preferred hand to be free.[69]

Data about the dreams of the healthy person are prevalent in the literature. These data lend support to the need for dreams in order to maintain the healthy state and they eliminate some of the aura and mystery associated with dreaming. There is a difference in the amount and the type of recall from REM and NREM sleep; recall rates are higher for the former than for the latter. In recall, NREM mental activity is described as more like thinking and less like dreaming. It is less vivid, less visual, more conceptual, more plausible, under greater volitional control and more concerned with our contemporary lives than REM sleep. It generally occurs in lighter sleep, and is more pleasant. It more closely resembles "that large portion of our waking thought that wanders in a seemingly disorganized, drifting, nondirected fashion whenever we are not attending to external stimuli or actively working out a problem or daydream." Dement points out that investigations reveal that REM sleep can no longer exclusively be considered synonymous with dreaming and NREM a mental void.[70] It is significant that there is a total inability to exercise control over events of the dream and that everyone dreams, regardless of whether dreams are remembered or not. Most are not. Mental activity at the onset of sleep was found to influence dream content. The later in the night the dream occurs, the less relationship there is to the events of the previous day and the more closely it relates to events in childhood, with more evidence of dependence on stored images. It has been shown that the dreams of persons blind from birth are totally lacking in visual imagery and no scanning eye movements are present during the REM sleep periods. Auditory dreams have been reported by healthy blind persons during REM periods when awakened at that time. For those who became blind later in life, eye movements were observed and dreams had visual imagery.[71]

Awakening is a characteristic of sleep that distinguishes it from sleeplike states brought on by anesthesia or coma. On awakening, a person can be just as drowsy as before going to sleep and overall performance may be as poor or poorer for a short period than it was at bedtime.[72] The person reports feeling well on rising after a good sleep.

Specific Data Base for Normal Sleep

In addition to the general data base relating to the sleep patterns for the healthy person, specific data about the sleep patterns, the sleep environment, and the manner of maintaining sleep integrity of the healthy person must be determined by the nurse. The following data are applicable.

1. Determine the type of immediate territorial environment conducive to sleep. Consider the place for sleeping.
   A. Sleep-related furnishings: bed (single, double, queen-size, king-size, waterbed); loft; mat; carpet; youth bed; sleeping bag; crib; cradle; tent; trailer
   B. With whom: alone; with another; with others
   C. Bedding: none; mattress (type, firmness, size); pillows (none, one, more than one, large or small, feathers, dacron, foam-filled); sheets; pillow cases; bedspread; blankets (number, light or heavy, electric); quilts (number, light or heavy, down or feather); combination of coverings
2. Determine the preferred level of darkness, room temperature, humidity, and amount of noise tolerated in order for sleep to commence.
3. Determine the larger scope of the environment where sleep takes place.
   A. Where: room in private home in the city, the suburbs, the country; room in a hotel, motel, hospital, tenement, apartment; in large city, small town, village, planned community, retirement community, dormitory, college campus, camp (military, mining, leisure); outdoors (protected, unprotected)
   B. Type: small; large; garden; high rise
4. Determine the personal preference of dress for sleep: no clothing; underwear; diaper; pajamas; nightgown (light, heavy); daytime clothes; bed socks; bunting
5. Determine the presleep rituals of the person.
   A. Bathing: warm bath; warm shower; cool bath; cool shower; sponge bath; no bathing
   B. Personal care: emptying bladder; diaper change; brushing teeth; combing hair; curling hair
   C. Snacks: glass of warm milk, cup of tea, cocoa, coffee, soft drink, alcohol; light snack; heavy snack; evening meal
   D. Habits: pulling down bed covers; hot water bottle placed in bed; teddy bear, doll, favorite blanket or toy; locking doors; checking windows; checking the environment for security purposes; water turned off; winding clock; setting alarm; putting children to bed; feeding and providing for any pets; watering plants
6. Determine the presleep activities of the person: reading; writing; listening to the radio or records; watching television; light conversation; counting sheep; arguing; playing table games; light exercise regimen; heavy exercise; office work; homework, studying, cleaning, washing dishes or clothes; rocking, being rocked, cuddled, scolded; lovemaking; walking the dog.
7. Determine the presleep religious activities of the person: absence of religious activities; hymn singing (alone, with family, with others); reciting traditional

prayers, personal prayers; reading Bible (Old and New Testaments), Koran; meditating, kneeling to pray; praying while in bed; use of associated items (incense, candles, rosary beads, Holy water, prayer books).

8. Determine the personal sleep patterns of the person. Consider a one- (or preferably two-) week period from which to establish an average or norm for a person rather than the experience of one or two nights. Determine the time the person goes to bed; the amount of time in bed before falling asleep; number of times awakened during night; what time of night awakenings occur; purpose of awakenings; activities of the person during awakenings (if any); are awakenings associated with external happenings such as arrival of newspaper, sirens, baby crying, being crowded out of bed, loss of bed coverings, too cold or too warm, heavy rain, lightning, etc., or internal happenings such as full bladder, hunger, numbness of limbs; time in morning awakened, awakening by self, awakened by alarm, by children, parent, spouse, other; person's estimate of quality of sleep; person's ability to remember and convey data (excellent, good, fair, poor) by self estimate, by estimate of significant others; what recollection, if any, is there of dreams; does the person feel refreshed when fully awake; were naps taken during the day (when, how long, how many); were naps planned, prescribed, self-determined.

From this broad data base, the nurse determines the specific individualized data base for the client. She may then conclude that she and/or the client follow an individual pattern of sleeping–awaking that is appropriate to the person of the nurse and the client and within the biologic rhythms that prevail for each person. The results are a feeling of well-being, useful level of energy, the ability to think, decide, concentrate, and to perform one's life responsibilities, as it stems from the maintenance of the integrity of the sleep–awake cycle and the fulfillment of the need for sleep.

When the nurse has mastered the data base appropriate to the healthy or wellness state as it relates to sleep for herself and/or the client, a series of strategies are available to preserve the integrity of the sleep–awake cycle for the individual nurse and the client. These strategies comprise the art and the science of nursing and take into account the personal aspects of a particular person—his sleep pattern and methods used on a day-to-day basis to preserve the integrity of his sleep system.

Nursing strategies to maintain the integrity of the sleep system include both internal and external strategies and those discussed herein will also include a survey of the various modalities used by people to assure sleep–awake rhythmicity. External strategies relate to the environmental (atmospheric, geographic, and territorial), social, and cultural dimensions that promote sleep integrity. Internal strategies relate to personal, intellectual, physiologic, emotional, and spiritual factors that have a bearing on the promotion and maintenance of sleep integrity.

Nursing Strategies to Maintain Sleep Integrity

The nurse has access to a broad range of strategies to promote the maintenance of the integrity of the sleep–awake cycles for herself and for the healthy client. When the particular sleep need and sleep pattern for a person have been established and the need for sleep for this person has been diagnosed as having been effectually met, the nurse and the client will plan to continue and enhance the meeting of the need for sleep, designating and supporting those strategies most acceptable and useful to the client.

Provide the type of immediate territorial environment conducive to sleep. In the event that the client is in a different territory, an environment that most closely simulates the usual client environment would be most useful. Eliminate loud noises, ringing of telephones, and strong odors. Rhythmic and monotonous stimuli from the environment are aids to sleep, particularly for children. There are records of rain on tin roofs just for this purpose. Rocking and lullabies are examples of such acts. Although radio and television may foster sleep for the adult, the sounds of these may well negate sleep for the child who is put to bed straining to hear the sounds, who feels deprived of watching or hearing programs allowed for older brothers and sisters and adults.[73] As a highly adaptive process, sleep is sensitive to the surroundings in which it occurs and is self-protective as a continuing process. A sleeping person is not completely independent of his surroundings. It is interesting to note that sounds, including conversation, in the presence of the sleeping person will evoke a response based on the meaning of the sounds. A sleeping person may be oblivious to conversation held in his midst, but might be awakened at the sound of his name. Webb summarizes four major general findings relating to environmental influences on sleep that would be particularly helpful to the nurse. (1) The sleep stage the person is in will make a difference in terms of its bringing on arousal. Less stimulation is needed for Stage 1 sleep and increasingly more is needed as the sleeper progresses to Stages 2, 3 and 4. (2) Low intensity noises are less likely to arouse a sleeping person than loud noises. Older sleeping persons are more responsive to noise than young sleepers and the level of arousal in sleep is an issue in deciding the effect of sleep. It is possible to have no behavioral arousal, yet brain arousal may be recorded by the EEG. (It has been found that a burst of 55 decible noise—mild enough not to wake the average sleeper—jolts the nervous system in the same manner as in the awake state. (3) The relevant meaning attached to the noise as well as a person's adaptability to the sound are significant as are sound patterns. Continuous noises have little effect whereas sharp changes or variant patterns have a greater effect. (4) The degree of disruption of sleep will depend on the type of sleeper response and the nature of the environmental requirements. Some sounds or noises may momentarily arouse a sleeper whereas others will require protective action such as the sound of someone breaking into one's home, an intruder, a fire alarm, etc.[74] Thus, a sleeper ignores environmental changes that are routine, limited in intensity, or deemed irrelevant.

Noise abatement can be fostered by soundproofing the sleeping room or home, by using draperies—the thicker the better, as most outside noise enters through windows. The use of an airconditioner or fan opposite the source of a noise will help to mask it. Carpeting is a relatively inexpensive, but highly effective, sound absorber. A light cut pile rug with a layer of rubberized hairfelt or open cell foam beneath it will cut down more noise than a single layer ankle deep carpet. Acoustic tile with grooves or perforations will subdue inside clatter, particularly if the tiles are hung or placed a few inches below an existing ceiling. Smooth tiles should be avoided because they have less absorbency potential. Select tiles that can be easily cleaned. Other acoustical tips include the use of one-inch thick cork tiles on walls and ceilings or as insulation for electrical appliances—under and around such appliances as dishwashers, ice making machines, and air conditioners. Walls lined with bookshelves or closets help, as do sofas and chairs unholstered with soft materials rather than those with contemporary designs using exposed wood, glass, and metal which bounce noise around a room.

There are a few other alternatives, such as the use of small machines designed to produce so-called white sound that masks nearby clamor by pleasantly monopolizing one's ear. Earplugs are available, but only the reusable synthetic foam plugs have been shown to have value. Cotton or rubber ones are virtually worthless and should be avoided. Persons prone to ear infections or who do not use earplugs properly should avoid their use. For selected clients, a sleep sanctuary complete with lights and ventilation can be custom built over one's bed. These sanctuaries are made of a soundproof glass and wood structure and, depending on specifications, may range in price from $1500 to $5000. Prefabricated sound-controlled environments are also available in a variety of sizes and prices for those inclined to make such a purchase. The services of an acoustical engineer may be useful for noises that do not yield to techniques mentioned.[75]

Provide for appropriate security, such as locked doors, security personnel for buildings and grounds, and frequent observation to check the safety of the persons. Night lights for hallways, railings, institutional and noninstitutional sleeping rooms away from noise areas as kitchens, garbage disposal mechanisms, shipping and unloading, busy entrances, elevators and escalators, heavy traffic, ambulance entrances, etc.

Provide for the level of darkness, humidity, temperature, controlled tolerable noise level, and freedom from noxious odors, to facilitate sleep. It is known that lower atmospheric pressure favors the onset of sleep whereas an increasing pressure has the opposite effect. Repetitive light or sound stimuli have been found to be conducive to sleep. Adjust room temperature to suit the needs of the sleeper. Generally, cooler temperatures are desired at night with humidity at about 40 percent for comfort. In very dry rooms, a pan of water on a radiator or at selected spots in the room may be helpful. High humidity is much more difficult to control and adjustments to clothing and amount of activity might be all that is available. The use of humidifiers and dehumidifiers can be particularly useful if available.

Facilitate the personal preference of dress for sleep for the person. Provide opportunity to and encourage client to wear own bedtime clothing. Accept the variation of bedtime dress or lack of it based on client preference. Facilitate the laundering and repair of this clothing. Have available additional sets of bedtime clothing in case of accidental soiling, particularly for infants and young children.

Facilitate the presleep rituals of the person that have been determined to be needed and effective in fostering sleep. Rocking and lullabies by a loving parent or significant other person are soothing and relaxing and predispose the child to sleep. The telling of bedtime stories may help.

Foster the development of sleep habits. Gently caressing and mildly restraining the physical movements of infants and young children may foster the onset of sleep. Facilitate the use of beds and bedding preferred by the client that used to free the full weight of the body. Provide protection from falls from beds, cribs, and cradles.

Sitting in front of a fire talking over events and accomplishments of the day with a significant person, particularly someone you love, is a good preparation for sleep. Luxuriating in a warm bath with the tub filled with water, gently massaging and washing away all muscular and joint kinks is also good before sleep. Washing should be done slowly, with gentle stretching of limbs and trunk as the bath proceeds.

Tryptophan is an amino acid found in many foods (such as milk) that helps to induce a healthy, normal slumber and accounts for the fact that results are noted from a glass of warm milk—an age-old prescription thought to have mainly a psychologic effect. Tryptophan is found in meats, milk, cheese, peanuts, peanut butter, eggs, spinach, lima beans, puffed rice, liver, and chicken, to mention a few sources. The amount of tryptophan per 4-ounce serving ranges from .2 to .5 grams in the foods mentioned. It is estimated that one gram of tryptophan at least one-half hour (not to exceed one hour) prior to going to bed has a natural sleep-promoting effect. The exact mechanism by which tryptophan promotes sleep is not yet known.[76] It is expected that the amino acid affects the production of serotonin, which in turn affects the sleep center. Any of the above mentioned foods should be avoided if the person demonstrates an allergy to any or all of them. Beverages and products that have a stimulating effect on the person (including smoking of tobacco) should be avoided. Great individuality is noted in the ability to tolerate coffee, tea, cola, and cocoa—ranging from no tolerance to unlimited tolerance.

Heeding the signs of sleep and falling asleep at the crest of sleepiness are appropriate. Fighting or resenting the need to sleep to get a few more things done may precipitate sleep problems that are easier to prevent than to cure. It is not helpful to go to bed if one is not sleepy or even to stay in bed whiling away hours and tensing up at the fact that one still has not fallen asleep. Yoga is helpful in bringing about relaxation for some by promoting tranquility and repose. Untensing muscles by using established relaxation techniques can be helpful in inducing sleep.

Following a routine for sleep is recommended. Little harm will come from an occasional disruption to do something special that requires a later sleeptime. If hungry at bedtime, a light snack utilizing some foods containing tryptophan may be helpful. Weight watchers will need to be particularly selective in foods taken to assure calorie and weight control endeavors. For some persons, eating or drinking anything at bedtime is a sure way to stay awake; for these persons, food and fluids should be omitted, taking care that a balanced nutritional diet with appropriate amounts of fluids has been taken in during the day.

The client should be taught to practice breathing exercises—deep breathing helps relaxation. McKim recommends that a person seeking deep muscle relaxation in preparation for sleep should initially lie down in a comfortable, quiet place. He should then do the following: First, systematically tense, experience the tension, then relax specific muscle groups such as fists—clench, hold, and relax. Then flex, hold, and relax wrists, followed by tensing the biceps by bringing hands to shoulders, experiencing the tension and then relaxing. Shrug shoulders and touch ears with shoulders, hold, then relax. Wrinkle the forehead up, hold, and relax; then frown, hold, and relax. Close eyes tightly, hold, then relax. Push tongue against the roof of the mouth, relax, then follow by pressing lips together, hold, and relax. After this push the head back, hold, and relax, then take a deep breath and hold it—exhale. Suck in the abdomen, tensing the abdominal muscles, hold, and relax. Tense buttocks, feel the tension, then relax. Lift legs, tensing thighs, hold, and relax. Point toes toward head, tensing arches, hold tension, then relax. Repeat the tensing, holding, and relaxing of each muscle group again with more intensity. A positive and deeply relaxed feeling should prevail.[77]

Alternatively, the client can be instructed to follow a round of relaxation efforts directed toward putting his body to sleep gradually from toes to head. He should be told to: take a few deep breaths, slowly. Begin by tensing then fully relaxing ("putting to sleep") the toes, then the ankles, calves, thighs, pelvis, abdomen, fingers, wrists, shoulders, neck, jaw—unclench the teeth, relax facial muscles, forehead, and scalp. Proceed slowly and calmly. Repeat as often as necessary.

Support the presleep activities of the client that contribute to the onset of sleep. A person will fall asleep faster in a monotonous situation than when exposed to complete silence and darkness. There needs to be a disengagement from the ongoing activities of the day and a cooling down and separation from excitement as well as a need to sleep in order to foster onset of sleep. It is important to exclude the inflow of afferent impulses from the sense organs as much as possible.[78] The simple standbys of counting the ticks of the clock or counting sheep evoke sleep due to the rhythmic input to the central nervous system. By concentrating on a particular subject or stimulus, a person is less likely to attend to thoughts about the day or to be distracted by sounds that are known to keep the person awake. If a person believes that concentrating on a monotonous activity while lying in bed with eyes closed is likely to bring on sleep, then sleep is more likely to occur. If falling asleep is associated with this behavior, a sleep habit may be promoted. Refraining from any form of strenuous mental activity, particularly problem solving, will discourage wakefulness.

Webb states that the most direct route to sleep would be to amplify aspects of the sleep pattern through various forms of muscular relaxation. This includes progressive relaxation of the body beginning with the toes and proceeding upwards through biofeedback systems to facilitate the achievement of a signaled particular physiologic state, by arranging oneself in a sleep position most helpful in getting to sleep, and by selecting sleep inducing mechanisms that foster distraction, suggestion, and habit formation. A warm bath or shower may create a peripheral vascular response with blood going to the outer parts of the body, perhaps simulating what happens at sleep onset and forcing a quicker recurrence of sleep onset.[79] A gentle back rub may afford a considerable measure of relaxation.

Provide the opportunity and privacy for the client to fulfill presleep religious obligations as personally designated and/or required of him. Provide appropriate aids such as lighting to facilitate reading of prayers and religious passages, particularly by older persons. Adjust the environment to provide privacy for moments of personal prayer or meditation, if requested. Read religious passages selected and preferred by the client. Help children say prayers as determined by the parents. Have available copies of commonly utilized prayers and passages reflecting the major religions of the world.

Foster the overall sleep pattern of the person in accordance with his established norm. Sleep consistently raises its signals of need for children and adults. This holds true for naps as well as for nighttime sleep. Webb suggests that the length of time the child needs to sleep can be determined by waking the child up at the same time every morning, then watching the child for sleepiness at night. Nurses and parents should refrain from forcing a fully awake child to sleep at a predetermined time, whereas a sleepy child will need help in his struggle to stay awake. It is strategic that any gap between the nurse's or the parent's determination of the child's need to sleep and the child's *actual* need to sleep must be bridged to offset the creation of a problem related to sleep. It is important that the nurse respect her own and the client's sleep pattern, allowing for changes based on age, growth, and development.

Eliminate or reduce incompatible stimuli and behavior that negate sleep. Relieve worry, tension, and need for information. Allow the client to talk and solve problems that preoccupy him so that sleep can occur. Exclude as much as possible the inflow of afferent impulses from the sense organs by making adjustments in the environment, refraining from imparting bad news at bedtime or bringing up problems related to work, finances, etc., that usually bring with them the need for resolution. Provide time to "wind down" through small talk, designating a plan to solve problems or selecting one or many problems that could be solved easily, leaving the rest for tomorrow. If a strange environment serves as an incompatible stimulus, the use of familiar objects, clothing, etc., may diminish the strangeness to some extent—perhaps enough to allow sleep to occur. The presence of parents, family, significant others, and the nurse may have a calming and protective effect.

Repeated, monotonous, irrelevant, noninterfering stimuli decrease the effect of stimuli that distract from sleep. If the sleep inducing stimuli annoy or frighten the person, however, the probability of sleep induction is considerably reduced.

Use suggestion as a mechanism to bring about sleep. The suggestion that sleep will ensue to accompany the many strategies previously mentioned can in itself be effective in facilitating sleep. The expectations of sleep and the acceptance and trust in the sleep outcome may prevent the intrusion of arousal stimuli for the person. This suggestion may be made by the nurse or may be suggested by the client himself.

With the determination of the data base for sleep of the healthy person, particularly a specific healthy person, and the designation of the available multiple strategies to maintain sleep need integrity, strategies are selected by the client and/or the nurse for implementation on a day-to-day basis. The nurse applies a selection of strategies for herself, as does the client. Periodic evaluation is conducted by the nurse and by the client utilizing the data base presented earlier as the model against which sleep pattern data should be compared. Alterations that are inconsistent or incompatible for the wellness state require a reassessment for diagnostic purposes. The client returns to see the nurse who may verify the alteration, reassess the client circumstance, make a nursing diagnosis, prescribe a strategy or strategies that the client or nurse or both implement, then reevaluate to assure problem resolution. If the nursing diagnosis requires nursing therapy as well as intervention by other members of the health care team, appropriate referrals are made and additional strategies are prescribed in conjunction with nursing strategies. The plan of action and the participants (client, family, nurse, other nursing team and health team members) are designated. Implementation and evaluation follow, with reassessment and replanning as needed until the problem is resolved or diminished. If such activity is not possible or is delayed, action by the client, the family, the nurse, and others will be continued and determined accordingly.

Nursing Diagnoses: Alteration in Sleep Integrity

With a firm command of the healthy or wellness model for sleep, the nurse has a framework for subsequent nursing action and goal determination for the client who experiences an alteration in sleep integrity (the need for sleep is unmet, poorly met, or partially met).

When the need for sleep is unmet or poorly met, the client data reflect the alteration in the integrity of sleep—its pattern, its length, and its quality. Subnursing diagnoses stemming from the overall alteration include *excessive sleep, disturbed sleep,* and *insufficient* or *lack of sleep (sleep deprivation).* These diagnoses can be further qualified as acute, chronic, prolonged, intermittent, externally induced, or internally induced. In addition, the causative agent or state (the "due to") may be designated and has considerable bearing on the kind of nursing and other health care strategies planned as well as the expected outcome resulting from the implementation of these strategies. For example, sleep alterations due to excessive use of alcohol may be resolved by elimination of the causative agent (alcohol) in contrast to sleep alterations due to, for example, cancer of the brain, which may or may not respond to current available nursing, medical (including pharmacologic and radiologic), and surgical therapies.

Data Base for Sleep Deprivation and Disturbed Sleep

The data base assessed by the nurse for the client will be within the following *general data* for diagnoses of sleep deprivation and disturbed sleep. It is estimated that 30 million Americans suffer from sleep deprivation at one time or another for a variety of reasons. Evidence includes fatigue, depression, malaise, poor power of concentration, itchy eyes, increased irritability, increased sensitivity to pain, nervousness, loss of muscle tone, dizziness, reddened eyes, burning eyes, yawning, physical discomfort, anxiousness, behavioral changes, bizarre behavior, hallucinations, disorientation, confusion, suspicion, inability to derive support from others, difficulty staying awake during the day, tiredness, lack of appetite, digestion–elimination problems, exhaustion, extreme muscular weakness, difficulty in sustaining intellectual effort or attention span, and impairment of disposition. Kleitman indicates that these symptoms suggest a fatigue of the higher levels of the cerebral cortex—the levels that are responsible for the critical analysis of incoming impulses and the elaboration of adequate and appropriate responses based on a person's previous experience.[80]

Extremely sleepy persons and persons intoxicated with alcohol manifest dramatically opposite changes, despite similar outward behavioral appearance, in their ability to receive noxious cutaneous stimuli without experiencing pain. Extremely sleepy persons are particularly sensitive to pain.[81]

A higher level of physical effort is required to maintain mental performance. Sleep-deprived persons have more than their share of small accidents, lack coordination (particularly noticeable in sports), and feel less efficient than usual. They are mentally foggy, ineffectual, dull, depressed, dissatisfied without reason, hyperirritable, and respond sluggishly when swift action is needed. They are short-tempered and impatient with others over trifles. They appear a little older than age, look tense and strained, and are always tired. They lapse in performance efficiency, especially with tasks viewed as boring or unduly complex, and lack perseverance. They are subject to perceptual (visual, temporal, cognitive) distortions; their hearing may not be as keen as usual, and they misjudge distances when driving. After long deprivation (100 hours or more), there is disordered behavior resembling paranoid psychosis;[82] sleep gaps, early awakenings, long time (beyond 30 minutes) getting to sleep, excessive amounts of Stage 1 sleep (inappropriate to age), difficulty staying asleep, alteration in sleep stages (absence of REM, suppression of REM, excessive REM, absence of Stage 4 deep sleep, minimal Stage 4 sleep, excessive Stages 1 and 2 sleep), prolonged respiratory apnea during sleep, double vision, and a feeling of unreality are common.

Without sleep, skin is deprived of the rejuvenation that occurs during sleep such as replacement of dying cells, elimination of waste products, and circulation of essential ingredients such as minerals, vitamins and hormones. This results in sagging skin tissues; collagen (dark protein of tissues) becomes increasingly visible. Visible collagen accounts for dark circles under a person's eyes. Other tissues hold fluids (puffiness) and prolonged deprivation may result in these changes being irreversible.[83]

The person is able to perform most tasks that do not require sustained attention and that are not repetitive, low demand or uninteresting tasks; there is little evidence of physiologic deterioration. Higher cortical functions are depressed. The person can remain awake longer when engaged in muscular activity such as walking. If there is a history of sleep loss, the transition from one sleep stage to another may be uneven and erratic; body temperature does not fall in the same manner as for the average person; the client may experience a phase shift in circadian rhythms, she may have associated symptoms of premenstrual tension when more dreamtime is needed due to hormonal changes to alleviate irritability and other tension symptoms.[84] There may be disorientation, confusion, loss of train of thought, general apathy, a feeling of being spaced out, misperceptions, overresponsiveness to problems,[85] evidence of worry, fear, anger or excitement, and lack of interest; the client may be preoccupied with the need or desire to sleep.

Causes of Sleep Deprivation

Voluntary Control by Client (Self-imposed)

1. Unwillingness to heed signs of onset of sleep and to follow through by going to sleep.
2. Effort to complete a task—finish a project, study for examination, or continue work or play.
3. Continuation of presleep rituals that knowingly interfere with sleep onset and diminish quality of sleep—drinking alcohol or coffee, partaking of excessive exercise, and bathing or showering in water too hot or too cold.
4. Active involvement in problem solving and other intellectual efforts.

Additional Data Base By choice the client follows interests and needs rather than body rhythms; he ignores rhythmic cues for sleep or staying asleep; there is a strong need to sleep that is opposed to staying awake, resulting in conflict. The consequences of conflict can take the forms of irritability, aggressiveness, anxiety, or compromise making (rationalizations, conversations)[86]; he may believe that lack of sleep is indicative of a forceful, hardworking personality trait and that one must claim to have sleep trouble to be viewed as highly motivated and hardworking.[87] He may show evidence of hyperactivity; he is a high owered, driven person who has difficulty lying down and relaxing for sleep; and he has heavy energy output fueled with a great deal of drinking and smoking.[88]

Nursing Strategies

1. Provide information about the physiology of sleep, the need for sleep, and the impact (physiologic, intellectual, and emotional) of deprivation, and about what promotes and what interferes with sleep.
2. Provide assistance in planning the waking hours to allow the work of the day to be completed prior to bedtime.
3. Assist the client in determining his need for sleep in keeping with his biologic rhythms and establish a sleep rhythm with the client.
4. With the assistance of the client determine wholesome and effective presleep rituals that will be implemented.
5. Accept an occasional night or two of less sleep resulting from participating in personal, family, social, and religious holidays and celebrations.
6. Assist the client in finding ways to offset an occasional night of less sleep, such as sleeping longer on a subsequent night or taking a nap, and avoiding use of drugs (prescription and over the counter) to induce sleep or to induce wakefulness.
7. Teach the client relaxation and diversional exercises and methods to reduce problem solving at bedtime. Plan time and mode for practice of relaxation and clearing his mind of occupation and project-related details prior to bedtime until a new pattern is established.
8. Make plans and efforts with the client to change behavior and beliefs regarding self and the need for sleep. Consult with health care colleagues (clinical psychologist, psychiatrist, and clergyman) and make referrals as needed.

Personal and Situational Occurrences (Temporary and Prolonged)

These include separation from a family member or significant other person through illness, hospitalization, death, divorcc, and other separation; worry; concern about work; finances; nightmares and sleepwalking of family members (particularly children); snoring sleep partner; loss of job; and driving late at night.

Additional Data Base The absence of regular sleep is noted; even changing a pattern of bed position such as sleeping with one's head at the foot end of the bed could cause disruption.[89] There is a great individuality in the effect of potentially upsetting factors on different persons. One person may be unimpressed by a severe accident of fate and another is devastated by it. Personal peculiarities, innate sensibilities and acquired character and personality structure must be accounted for; evidence may include client upset over an examination, or anger and disappointment because of favoritism to a sibling; a child may experience anxiety due to believing that a parent or teacher is prejudiced against him; he may fear being discovered in a derilection or misdeed;[90] there may be evidence of severe trauma to infant or child due to hospitalization (constant crying, refusal of contact, loss of weight, slowing down of mobility, total or partial feeling that there is a threat to the child's existence); there may be evidence that the child has been battered by a parent (the child lies awake a long time before falling asleep, awakens unusually early, awakens suddenly with a cry, has been frightened by some awful image, is physically restless, or constantly turns in his sleep); a child may repeatedly call for his mother to make sure that she is nearby and tries to hold on to her and cries in order to keep her at bedside (this form of upset due to fear is quite different from that observed in the adult person, who usually suffers silently, alternating between lying awake, brooding and dozing). Some of this may be due to bad habits, efforts to adjust and obey, or to neurotic bedtime rituals[91]; it may be caused when sleep rituals are violated, after too heavy a dinner is consumed, with resulting intestinal disturbances, or when there is malfunctioning of body temperature control after too hot a bath or overexposure to sun; there may be an absence of accustomed warmth or quiet darkness, as well as fatigue; the client may experience lack of fatigue during days of sickness; he may be bored. A child may be so disturbed by the absence of accustomed circumstances as well as by experiencing strange impressions that he cannot fall asleep, or sleeps restlessly or interruptedly, or awakens before time; he may be a "spoiled child" growing out of improper direction and absence of loving limits—he may not want to go to bed and, above all, he may not want to sleep[92]. A client may drive late at night; he may worry about sleeplessness; there may be difficulty recognizing the difference between tension and relaxation; there may be an overestimation of sleep deficit as verified by EEG sleep length and pattern study; there may be a decrease in Stage 4 sleep with an increase in daytime stress while REM sleep may be unaffected; there may be evidence of change in work pattern from day to night shift; sleep onset may take longer than one-half hour; self- or physician-prescribed drugs or alcohol may have been used to reduce tension or anxiety, or induce sleep; there may be evidence of a life-disrupting situation such as death, illness, marital discord, or job problems, resulting in the heavy use of a caffeinated beverage, alcohol, drugs, and cigarette smoking. There may be sleep laboratory verification of sleep deficit related to length and diminished Stage 4 sleep. There may be evidence of a child being put to bed too early (he talks to animals, blanket, and recites nursery rhymes); teenagers may lie awake reviewing the day's events and fantasizing, as it may be the only time for them to be completely alone without disturbances (this may be a happy, pleasurable time); adults may think they have a sleep problem if they don't fall asleep instantly; the individual may overestimate the amount of time needed to fall asleep; he may perceive short awakenings as a continuation of wakefulness; if dream-starved, he may show subtle personality changes such as becoming increasingly abrasive and anxious and experiencing a diminished concentration level; and he may misinterpret acts and intentions of others. The person may have a racing mind, which is often associated with anticipation of future events or worry about past ones; he may be obese with occasional evidence of the Pickwickian syndrome (a disorder associated with respiratory insufficiency and sleep deprivation, thought to be caused by massive fatness in which symptoms are dramatically relieved with major reduction in body fat)[93]. Repetitive leg jerking during sleep (called nocturnal myoclonus) may be present, which disturbs the sleep of the sleeper as well as the sleep partner (perhaps more so). This is a rhythmic muscle twitching of the legs that can arouse the sleeper for 5 to 15 seconds anywhere from 100 to 400 times a night. The sleeper is rarely awakened by this disruption, but may awaken feeling that he didn't sleep a wink.[94] The nurse may observe commonly seen rhythmic tension outlets in children in the going-to-sleep period, including rocking on hands and knees and banging the head. These are often first noticed in children ages 1 to 2 years and may occur briefly; for others they may not occur until age 4 or older. At times this rocking is so vigorous that injury to the forehead may occur; the crib may bang against the wall or slide around the room. Some parents become angry and upset by this behavior, thereby disturbing their own sleep, although the behavior may have little or no effect on the child's sleep[95]; there may be difficulty in getting 13 to 16-year-olds up in the morning, whereas at an early growth and development stage children often arise discouragingly early. In some cultures, one does not go to bed unless absolutely clean—one takes a bath and has clean sheets and sleep clothing; in other cultures (many of them primitive), sleep problems do not exist because children are allowed to stay up with adults until they are sleepy and when asleep are put to bed. Changes in such cultural patterns result in sleep disruption. Regarding snoring, it has been found that both men and women snore due to allergies (as do some children), old age, swollen tonsils, nasal deformities, poorly fitting dentures, and excessive smoking, drinking, or eating, which aggrevates the condition. Many snorers are overweight. Snoring is caused by the vibration of the tongue and a flaccid soft palate and is brought on by relaxation of throat muscles. On rare occasions snoring may have an accompanying sleep apnea. In this situation there is a sudden explosive noise followed by an absence of breathing; this occurs intermittently and not with every breath.

Nursing Strategies

1. Advise the client that when an occasional late hour for sleep is needed, he should have a higher protein dinner to assure staying power; he should take a nap in advance of the late night; he should freshen up and change position frequently. Tell him to avoid caffeine products if they create sleeplessness so that no additional sleep will be lost when he finally goes to bed; use bouillon, orange juice, and nutritious snacks instead.
2. Remedy the cause. Offer support in grieving; provide diversional activities; support involvement in rituals related to death; and make referrals to clergy, lawyers, social workers, physicians, and sleep specialist as needed.
3. Promote reestablishment of sleep pattern rhythm by actually planning sleep time, and protecting the person from human and environmental disturbances.
4. Advise the client to refrain from overreacting to personal situations that prevent sleep. To prevent the establishment of a pattern of sleep deficit, maintain a stable sleep–wakefulness rhythm (as indicated by a superimposed 24-hour body temperature curve) so that alertness and efficiency are peaked during working and waking hours. This insures an easy onset of "good" sleep when it coincides with the drop in body temperature at certain hours of the evening and the low temperature during the night. The rhythm can be disrupted by irregularity, but can be fortified by one's schedule of work, meals, recreation, and sleep. Children, in particular, can be more easily induced to follow a repetitive routine of living. The ability to remain asleep much beyond one's customary awakening time indicates failure to establish and maintain a sleep–awake rhythm. "Whatever one's temperament and disposition may be, it should be remembered that the 24-hour rhythm is an individually acquired, learned process, depending upon the presence and functional participation of the cerebral cortex."[96]
5. Insure privacy for grieving, crying and the resolution of personal problems.
6. Encourage the client to keep a diary or log of activities related to sleep. This in itself may be therapeutic by allowing for more accurate (although subjective) determination of length and quality of sleep as well as situations and behaviors associated with sleep deficits.
7. Refer the client to a sleep center for diagnosis of prolonged or unabating sleep deprivation. To obtain information on the nearest sleep clinic, the nurse or the client may write to the American Association of Sleep Disorder Centers, University of Cincinnati Sleep Disorder Center, Christian R. Holmes Hospital, Eden and Bethesda Avenues, Cincinnati, Ohio 43215. A stamped, self-addressed envelope should be enclosed for the information.

8. Encourage the client to request work schedule adjustments if he is working on the night shift to allow for prolonged periods of night work to assure biologic rhythm readjustment and diminished disruption. Frequent shift changes or shift rotations within short time periods are hazardous to health and should be avoided.
9. Plan a dietary regime with the client (with the assistance of a nutritionist as needed) to assure that foods containing the protein tryptophan are included. After the ingestion and digestion of food containing this amino acid, it is changed to serotonin, a biochemical present in the brain that has been connected with the regulation of sleep patterns. Although the exact mechanism of action is not clear, tryptophan has been shown to facilitate normal sleep. Such foods as milk, cheese, peanut butter, and beans, to mention a few, contain tryptophan.
10. Advise the client to avoid taking a nap if it interferes with sleep at night. Naps are useful when used in addition to night sleep and if no further impairment of night sleep occurs with the nap.
11. Prevent the automatic and indiscriminate use of anxiety-reducing and sleep-inducing drugs, whether self or physician prescribed. Consultation with a clinical pharmacologist and a sleep specialist may be useful if short-term, very temporary medication is needed to cope with a crisis situation.
12. Oversee the gradual withdrawal from sleeping pills, considering full physical and emotional support for the client while he is awake and asleep. Be particularly attentive to meeting all other basic needs, the satisfaction of which may be in jeopardy during the withdrawal period.
13. When sleep deficits result for parents due to head banging and rocking of small children, suggest padding the crib, moving it away from the wall, and anchoring it on a heavy rug or thick foam rubber mat to prevent movement and reduce noise. Work out a plan with the child so that when a tap is made on the wall (or a similar signal) rocking or banging will stop. In addition, plan ahead with the child, expecting that he won't need to rock when he is moved to his own big bed (about age 3 or 4).[97]
14. In situations where there is a teenager who is very difficult to arouse in the morning, transfer the responsibility for getting himself up to the teenager. Avoid accepting that responsibility in order to offset the development of a serious dependency problem later. Provide an alarm clock and support the means the teenager develops to assume this responsibility.
15. If the sleep deficits result from a snoring partner, a sleep pattern diagnosis is needed to rule out pathology, such as sleep apnea, as well as a physical examination to rule out oral and respiratory problems. Otherwise, partial help to deaden the noise may be achieved by the use of ear plugs. Since some snoring can reach 69 decibels (compared with a 70 to 90 decibel level

for pneumatic drills used to break up concrete), only minimal results are achieved with earplugs. It has been found useful to have the snorer place a regular pillow well up under his chin, propping his mouth shut. Self hypnosis has been tried by some and found to be useful. Staggered bedtimes with the person who does not snore going to bed first so that he is fast asleep before the snorer commences sleep may be helpful. Most persons who are bothered by another's snoring complain about difficulty in getting to sleep rather than being awakened.[98] Increase the humidity in the room, control allergies, and avoid sniffing, since a cause of snoring is collapse of the nostril flares. Sleeping on one's side may be useful; arranging for the snorer to sleep alone in a separate room is another alternative.

16. Plan and practice a regimen of relaxation exercises as noted for the wellness sleep strategies. The conscious alternate tensing and relaxing of muscles while lying in bed, beginning with the toes and proceeding upward (muscle group by muscle group) to the head may be beneficial. Particular attention must be paid to the relaxation of the jaw, for clenched teeth are not likely to induce sleep due to the tension state that prevails. Advise the client to learn Yoga to promote tranquility and repose.
17. Plan an increase in exercise, although it is not to be done immediately before bedtime.
18. If the client is unable to sleep suggest that, rather than lying in bed concerned, he get up, read, watch television, or do some light work (clean some drawers) until he feels sleepy.
19. Encourage the client to think of pleasant, peaceful things. These will automatically push away worries so that only this one subject will occupy the mind at sleeptime.

Environmental Affronts

These include extremes of temperature and humidity; dripping faucets; loud noises (e.g., barking dogs, sirens, heavy traffic, noisy neighbors, too much light); strange noises; sensation of danger (e.g., creaking doors and floors); ringing telephone; crying infants; screams; and lightning and thunder.

Additional Data Base In addition to the general data base evident for sleep deprivation, the nurse will hear subjective complaints of the client's feeling of poor sleep. She may see direct evidence of a noisy room, an uncomfortable bed, or a lack of sleep area. There may be a poor, faulty, or nonexistent air conditioning system. There may be random awakenings by household members (spouse, children, neighbors); there may be loud stereo music systems, or the type of music played may be upsetting to the person; there may be a ringing telephone, sirens, fire crackers, or heavy traffic—ground and air; there may be evidence of decreased Stage 4 sleep and total sleep time; and the client may hear pneumatic drills, grass cutters, or general construction noises at inopportune times.

Nursing Strategies Advise the client to:

1. Eliminate the causative, noxious, and unpleasant noise problem. Repair faulty appliances; utilize a light signal to replace the ringing of the telephone; and confer with neighbors to plan for noise abatement. Police may be invited to assist with plans. Meet with businesses and city officials for broader plans for environmental noise abatement—air traffic, ground traffic, jackhammers; arrange for insulation of walls and padding to prevent banging noises. Move objects that vibrate (e.g., blenders, ice machines, refrigerators) away from walls a bit to prevent transfer and magnification of noise; provide a play area for children, preferably away from sleep areas (particularly important for those persons needing to sleep during the day because they work on the night shift); prepare infants and children for sleep appropriate to their needs to minimize prolongation and disruption at bedtime; keep radios, television sets, and stereo units at a volume to be heard only within the immediate vicinity of the appliance; use ear plugs to prevent annoyance to others, particularly at bedtime; promote use of lane dividers (particularly tree lined and grassy) to aid in traffic noise abatement; and encourage use of trees and shrubs to cut down street noises.
2. Eliminate noxious odors. Provide for effective cleanliness, encourage judicious use of odorless chemicals for cleaning and disinfection, quick and effective removal of causative items (food, pet odors), and judicious use of spray products; provide for effective ventilation (opening windows from top to bottom). In windowless environments restrict smoking, and install fans and air conditioning systems.
3. Minimize total noise and odor (fumes) input into immediate environment by turning off unused equipment, and by walking a reasonable distance rather than using car or bus.
4. Plan naptime or go to sleep earlier to offset previous deprivation. This is particularly needed if limiting environmental affronts is not fully successful or if selected affronts cannot be abated. The amount of naptime will be determined by the particular needs of the person, the age, and the broader arena of responsibilities during waking time.
5. Regulate the temperature and humidity. Little can be done to change barometric pressure. Utilize available temperature control measures available through use of a thermostat (have it repaired if it is non-functional); use fans (hand and electrical); minimize or add to the amount of clothing needed to protect

against temperature extremes—wool and flannel type fabrics to maintain heat, cottons and cotton blends and loose fitting clothing to promote coolness. Dress appropriately for the weather—this includes the appropriate dressing of infants; increase the humidity of the room by placement of pans of water at strategic points in the room, such as near windows and warming units; use of a humidifier is helpful, as well as a dehumidifier if needed and available; facilitate evaporation from skin for cooling. Maintain appropriate fluid levels—cool or warm liquids, warm or tepid baths as needed; minimize physical activity to reduce feelings of warmth. Redirect sun's rays for cooling; capitalize on use of sun's rays for room warming.

6. Take security precautions, such as installation of effective locks on doors and windows, keeping protective dogs, having a doorman; learn the art of self-protection; have emergency police number memorized; plan in advance a mode of escape if it should ever be needed.
7. Plan to have company if lightning and thunderstorms are predicted and these storms are feared. Plan involved activity to assure distraction during storms; comfort children during storms; explain mechanism for and purpose of thunder and lightning.
8. If a dripping faucet is creating an annoyance (even though the sound is monotonous, one's reaction is usually one of irritation, and this prevents sleep), get up and tie a string to the spigot so that the water will slide quickly into the basin. This action is temporary and should be followed by a call to a competent plumber in the morning.

Medical and Nursing Therapies (including hospitalization)

These include failure of physicians and nurses to recognize the need for sleep for the ill person; failure to provide periods of undisturbed sleep during hospitalization that are akin to the person's rhythmic sleep patterns; failure to control noise in the health care agency (particularly intensive care and coronary care units); lack of privacy; indiscriminate awakening for "routines"; inadequate or excessive lighting; placing no or low priority on the client's need for sleep; automatic or routine administration of sleep medication without attention to the needs of the client or the effect on his pattern of sleep; and failure to adjust timing of therapies to protect the biologic rhythm of the client, particularly the sleep cycle.

Additional Data Base Drug-induced illness is caused by treatment; in this situation the same pills used to regulate sleep profoundly disturb sleep, causing many awakenings and diminished total sleep; there is very little REM sleep or NREM Stages 3 and 4; there is a rebound of REM with drug withdrawal; there may be terrorizing nightmares and lessened total sleeptime. Drug dependency will develop rapidly from any drug in which tolerance to its sleep-inducing effects is shown.[99] Drugs, including barbiturates, nonbarbiturate hypnotics, nonprescription hypnotic drugs, antihistamines and histamine inhibitors, antidepressants, major tranquilizers (antipsychotic drugs), minor tranquilizers (antianxiety drugs), and stimulants (to stay awake), either alter or impair sleep quality, have no appropriate effect, or no untoward effect on sleep.[100] There is evidence to indicate that sleep deprivation may be caused by hospital environments with noises, movement, long waits, concerns and fears, limited information, questionable priority pattern, the automatic and routine approach of many health and nursing team members, and low priority placed on need to sleep to enhance physical and psychologic coping ability for an already stressed body system. Dlin et al. studied the problems of sleep and rest in the intensive care unit. They found that sleep deprivation factors included lights, noises, monitors, attitudes of the staff, and the individual client's personality. Clients responded either by emotional withdrawal or by hyperalertness (thought to be an attempt to participate in the environment in spite of illness). This latter behavior was shown to evoke staff hostility toward the client. Lack of sleep and rest during the crucial postoperative period for the clients who had undergone open heart surgery interfered with recovery. It was noted that while sleep is of major importance in the healing process, the longer the client was confined to the ICU, the more he suffered from lack of sleep. The diurnal cycle was grossly distorted; lights were on constantly. The client seemed to doze (lying quietly with eyes closed, but when the observer entered the sleeper's environment a speedup in the heart rate was noted on the monitor). The client who withdraws lies quietly with eyes closed, devoid of any facial expression. The hyperactive client is engrossed in his environment, fearful of just letting things happen to him. Uninterrupted sleep was not seen. Deterrents to sleep in order of importance were: activity and noise, pain and physical discomfort, nursing procedures, lights, vapor tents, and hypothermia. No attempt was made by the physician or the nurse to treat the need for sleep as a major aspect of therapy vital to the client's welfare. The client was not permitted to sleep more than 20 minutes at a time.[101] The effect of hospitalization on children (including sleep patterns) is well known. Often additional human need deficits are seen in conjunction with sleep deficits of hospitalized clients such as sensory deprivation, sensory overload, biologic dysrhythmia, as well as drug-induced sleep problems.

Nursing Strategies

1. Completely stop the use of sleep-inducing drugs such as barbiturates and alcohol to promote sleep. Refrain from abrupt withdrawal, especially if high doses have been used.

2. Refrain from administration of sleep medication unless an exact diagnosis of the sleep problem has been presented.
3. Provide an environment conducive to sleep—dim lights, quiet, and privacy.
4. Plan nursing and medical intervention in such a manner as to afford at least a four-hour period of undisturbed sleep for the ill client. Arrange the administration of treatments and medications to facilitate an undisturbed sleep time for as long a period of time as necessary to assure the experience of multiples of the 90-minute sleep cycles. Four or five sleep cycles comprise normal sleep. Orient health and nursing staff members to the client's sleeptime schedule and tolerate no violation. Even for the sickest of clients, time can be found to support the battered sleep system. In this day of electronic monitoring devices it is possible to obtain continuing physiologic data without undue disturbance of the client.
5. Refrain from automatically administering a drug to relieve every ill or discomfort experienced by the client.
6. Refrain from conversation about the client (particularly refrain from mentioning his name or the name of his loved ones) in the presence of the sleeping client. This will usually bring about an immediate arousal. Have a viable client identification system operational so that arousal for name identification will not be needed during the sleeptime.
7. Alleviate fear and discomfort by holding, cuddling, stroking (particularly the infant and child), and soothing the client. A warm bath, the physical presence of the nurse until the client sleeps, and the use of bedsides to prevent falls may be helpful. The appropriate adjustment of attached equipment will help to alleviate fear of falling or disconnection of needed equipment. Assure privacy by avoiding wholesale body exposure (failure to use curtains or screens). Do not negate territorial and personal space (a violation includes clients' beds being too close together).
8. Provide for visiting with a parent, family member, or significant person prior to sleeptime.
9. Provide for skin care, gentle back massage, position change, and clean dry linens to promote sleep.
10. Problem solve disruptions in client units (including removal or segregation of threatening sounds and other noxious noises and odors). Have a flashing light signal a telephone call during the night. Use an alternative to an active public address and paging system during the night.
11. Place high priority on the need for sleep and arrange all activities to assure that the sleep need is satisfied.
12. If allowed, give liquids and snacks that contain tryptophan to support sleep.
13. Plan orientation and staff development around the recognition of the need for

sleep and the methods available to meet the need. Alert staff to the infractions of need satisfaction and guard against continuing patterns of care that disregard sleep needs or that create problems for the already stressed client by imposing needless sleep deprivation.

14. Plan to touch or handle the client minimally if it is necessary to check diagnostic data when he is in Stage 4 sleep in order to minimize the danger of arousal.
15. Arrange that shift reports and conversations occur in an adjacent conference room.
16. Arrange for the repair of noisy or faulty equipment. Utilize insulation, partitions, soundproof walls and window covers to minimize noise that will disturb sleep.
17. Change existing attitudes that negated responsibility for and sensitivity to the need for sleep for the well and the ill client as well as for the nurse.
18. Provide continuous information to the client about his present state to reduce fear and minimize anxiety caused by lack of information on what to expect in self and from others.

Psychophysiopathologic States

These include cardiovascular problems resulting in pain, angina, dyspnea, and related symptoms that interfere with sleep; and high levels of stomach acids (HC1) for persons with a medical diagnosis of duodenal ulcers that may create pain during the night with resultant awakening.

Additional Data Base There may be pathology in the sleep state itself—difficulty falling asleep, frequent arousal during the night, awakening too early, rough and irregular transition from one sleep state to another (not induced by drugs); disturbance in the basic mechanism of circadian oscillation may be suspected. There may be juvenile depression caused by fear of being forgotten or abandoned by parents; in elderly clients there may be an unrealistic fear of destitution, or the client may be afraid that he not wake up (particularly evident in children and aged persons); thc presence of organic discomfort such as toothache, earache, or generalized or specific pain and discomfort will make sleep more difficult because of pathophysiologic and psychopathologic states. Sleep alterations are viewed as the cardinal early symptom in depression. Improvement in the quality and the length of sleep in the depressed person is often a reliable sign of recovery. Poor sleepers are known to have more emotional problems and to complain more often of physical ailments; one's view of and value of self may contribute to depression with subsequent sleep deprivation; less REM sleep and dreams and lessened Stage 4 sleep may be brought on by pathologic states as well as by the medical therapy applied to offset the pathology.

Sleep deprivation has been suggested as a mode of therapy for elderly depressed persons with some positive results.[102] In normal persons, Stage 4 deprivation resulted psychologically in depression and reduced functioning, whereas REM deprivation resulted psychologically in a state of higher irritability and lability. The sleep patterns of autistic children studied were not unusual. Disordered sleep (deprivation and disturbances) may be a precursor of many mental and physical ailments and is viewed as a promising clinical diagnostic entity. Most schizophrenics demonstrate normal sleep patterns. Some pathologic states may result in a change in the normal 90-minute sleep cycle (often decreased to as much as 30 minutes), and in an increase in the number of shifts from one sleep stage to another as well as an increase in the number of cycles during the night (an average of 9 in contrast to the normal 4 or 5). Disturbances in the sleep patterns of geriatric persons may be due to a degenerative process of the sleep system (or arousal system) involving cortical and subcortical areas of the brain.[103]

Sleep disruptions may be brought on by painful nerve and muscle diseases, arthritis, angina, asthma, migraine, and urinary disorders (disruption in the biorhythmic urine output associated with the sleep–awake cycle). Persons with duodenal ulcers whose stomach acid flow increases tremendously during REM dreams are likely to be awakened with pain. It is believed that the person with a stomach or duodenal ulcer secretes as much as 3 to 20 times more gastric acid during sleep than normal subjects.[104] Infections that invade the central nervous system are viral and bacterial in origin and may have an affinity for the hypothalamic region (encephalitis lethargica); effects of tumors and neoplasms on sleep are variable, depending on the area of involvement of the tumor and the amount of pressure exerted on the arousal or sleep centers of the brain. Some large growths may have actually no effect on sleep patterns whereas those in the midbrain area, particularly in the thalamic and hypothalamic regions, show hypersomnia. Head traumas may or may not have an impact on sleep patterns and the site of the damage will be influential, as noted above. It is important to distinguish deep coma from sleep—waking dysrhythmia. In many of these clients, the sleep–waking rhythm is maintained. An elevated temperature has an effect on sleep, causing fragmented sleep with increased awakening and some reduction in both Stages 3 and 4 sleep and REM sleep. Hypo- and hyperthyroidism affect the general activity levels during the waking hours. Hyperthyroid persons had light, fragmented sleep with lessened Stages 3 and 4, whereas hypothyroid persons had some lowering of Stages 3 and 4 sleep.[105]

Nursing Strategies

1. Plan nursing strategies to protect the integrity of the client's normal sleep system.
2. Collaborate with health and medical care specialists in the development of

medical therapies designed to eliminate the psychopathophysiologic state, with a focus toward protecting the sleep system and minimizing the disruptive impact on sleep that could accompany the therapy.

3. Refrain from automatically resolving manifestation of sleep problems with indiscriminate use of sleeping pills or the administration of inappropriately ordered sleep medications.
4. Plan care that allows time for a period of undisturbed sleep (at least 4 or 5 hours to assure the fullest experiences of the multiple 90-minute sleep cycles that comprise sleep).
5. Calculate the pain relief mechanism most appropriate for the client (whether positional, comforting, dietary, or pharmacologic) so that a minimum of discomfort is experienced by the client before relief can be achieved.
6. Plan to keep a diary or log of the ill client's sleep patterns, including incidents and situations that have an impact on sleep (encouraging or discouraging it).
7. Provide for a specified nap time for the client to offset nighttime sleep deficits.
8. Orient all health and nursing personnel to the client's nap- and sleeptime to assure that no disturbances occur.
9. Collaborate with the clinical pharmacist and sleep specialist to assure that prescribed sleep medication is appropriate to the sleep needs of the client and will enhance rather than hinder normal sleep patterns.
10. Arrange visits to the client by family and friends around the nap- and sleeptime.
11. Follow through with environmental and material factors as outlined previously to assure a wholesome environment for sleep.

Social and Economic Affronts

These include going to bed hungry; excessive eating; lack of a bed or territorial space for sleep; excessive partying, including drinking; life style that negates sleeptime; jet travel (east to west and back) for business, social, and recreational purposes; and working on the night shift or rotating work shifts too frequently.

Additional Data Base Workers employed at night (in the low point of their daily temperature cycle) expressed feeling physically miserable. Some had chills, felt dirty or sloppy, experienced more accidents, had impaired judgment, and slurred spoken words. This was typical for airline stewardesses, nurses, physicians, pilots, factory workers, city service employees, and military personnel. When the timing of this biological rhythm is modified, the original rhythm persists until a new rhythm occurs, which may take weeks or months. Even with an occasional dysrhythmia brought on by east–west jet travel, a biologic impact is experienced that may take as much as two weeks to resolve. The quality of day sleep may be inferior and it may be insufficient in quantity. Lack of appetite and digestion–elimination problems may present themselves. Diminished work output with an increase in errors has been noted.

Nursing Strategies

1. Demonstrate ways to enhance utilization of economic resources (particularly for a gambler or a compulsive buyer); provide information and establish supervised practice sessions if the client doesn't know how to manage money, or how to comparison shop, with the hope of offsetting sleepless nights brought on by money worries. Arrange for job counseling, vocational rehabilitation, and/or retraining to get the client back into the work force.
2. When planning work schedules for personnel, allow a prolonged period to facilitate biologic rhythm adaptation. Refrain from frequent and needless staff time changes to assure a high level of problem-solving ability on the part of personnel and safety for the client.
3. Advise the client that when he is traveling across time zones, he should arrange to arrive at the new destination at bedtime. This will facilitate adaptation and minimize sleep deprivation. Plan travel well in advance if possible to avoid undue stress and strain during the preparatory period. A minimum of this type of stress will enhance coping ability and adaptation in the new time zone and minimize REM sleep deprivation.
4. Advise the client to recognize the impositions on the body system (particularly the sleep system) resulting from time displacements and to plan accordingly.
5. Encourage the client to judiciously plan for social events with the goal of offsetting the anticipated deprivation by taking a nap, eating a nutritious dinner, and refraining from use of caffeine laden products.

Physiologic Miscalculation and/or Nonacceptance

These include failure of the client to appreciate his own biologic rhythms; underestimating or overestimating the amount of sleep needed; failure to appreciate changes in the amount and quality of sleep that normally occur during the aging process; comparing one's amount of sleep with a personal conception of a "normal" standard such as 8 hours per night; and preoccupation with sleep habits (amount, quality, time, and comparative differences).

Additional Data Base There is no prescribed set amount of sleep for all persons; each person has his own unique biologic rhythms, including sleep cycle. The client may be a naturally short sleeper needing only 5 or 6 hours of sleep; he may try to get what he thinks is "normal." "People do different things during their waking hours, yet when they show individuality as they sleep, others think they need medical help. This is not so."[106]

Sleep pattern diagnosis by EEG demonstrates normal pattern and consistency, with smooth transition from stage to stage, even though the quantity is less than 8 hours (5–6 hours); severity of sleepless complaint is often seen to have no relation to amount of sleep (as diagnosed in sleep laboratory).

Some persons are so-called "day" or "night" persons, depending on their body temperature cycle. Normally, when temperature is up, a person feels energetic and, when low, he feels tired and worn out.[107]

Nursing Strategies

1. Provide the client with information about the physiology of sleep, including the impact of age on the sleep system.
2. Arrange for sleep pattern study through EEG diagnosis in an approved local diagnostic sleep center.
3. Consult with sleep specialists and/or psychiatrists as needed based on diagnostic outcomes and client behavior.
4. Suggest that the client keep a diary or log of sleep habits as well as an overall biorhythm profile. This in itself may provide the client with evidence so that respect for his biologic rhythms will result.
5. Encourage the client to utilize nonsleep time for enjoyment, recreation, and work purposes.
6. Support the client's effort to accept the aging process with the accompanying sleep changes.
7. If excessive nap taking usurps night sleep, assist the client in arranging more active, fulfilling wake time.
8. Avoid the use of any sleep-inducing medication.

Causes of Sleep Disturbances

Immaturity

This applies particularly to children and has a familial tendency. It includes nightmares, enuresis, and horrifying dreams.

Data Base Sleepwalking is common; the person acts and moves as though he is in the real world, but consciousness is in the realm of sleep; he sleepwalks only during deep, slow wave sleep stage (Stage 4). More males than females walk in their sleep. Sleepwalking is associated with transition of sleep from Stage 4 to 3 to 2. When there are no REMs, the person is not acting out dreams; sleepwalking begins in childhood with a sudden burst of high voltage brain wave activity; sleepwalkers tend not to notice dangers—stairs, open windows, moving cars. Children outgrow the tendency within 2 to 3 years; if prolonged into adulthood, medical and psychotherapies may be needed. There is a tendency for children to walk in their sleep when parents argue a lot, after the death of a parent or loss of a pet, when they experience distress in school, move into a new house, or when there is a new baby. Adults tend to sleepwalk when in a new environment, or after the death of a loved one. If undisturbed they will complete a task and return to bed. Sleepwalking is episodic, and generally does not last longer than 10 minutes; it occurs one to two hours after falling asleep. The person gets out of bed, demonstrates coordination, and can avoid objects such as tables and chairs; he may go to the bathroom; and he moves in a confused manner.[108]

Night terrors (quite rare) and nightmares are classified as awake intrusion disturbances in which waking behavior disturbs sleep. The person awakes in a state of anxiety. The experience is abrupt and involuntary. These experiences are distinctly different from the common experiences of waking up and recalling an unpleasant dream. Some children go through a whole series of bedtime fears from age to age. At about 2½ years of age, fear of dark occurs, at 3½, fear of bugs and small animals occurs, at 5½, wild animals, at 6, fear of men under the bed (particularly for girls), fear of shadows, spies and ghosts, and of robbers in the closet. After this, fears diminish based on how they were handled and on the continuing growth and development of the child.[109]

Night terrors tend to run in families and differ from nightmares in that the child reports no frightening thoughts or dreams in association with these awakenings. A bloodcurdling screech brings distraught parents to the bedside to find a groggy and dazed offspring whose heart is racing and who cannot tell what is wrong because he cannot recall. The lack of frightening material is understandable because night terrors emerge from arousals from Stage 4 slow wave sleep and not from arousals from REM sleep. Night terrors do not result from bad dreams, but are awakenings from very deep sleep probably due to a rapid, radical shift in level of consciousness. These terrors usually disappear without treatment. Nightmares peak between the ages of 7 and 10. These awakenings are accompanied by frightening dream recalls and do evolve from frightening dreams associated with REM sleep.[110] Nightmares are a predictable and common consequence of drug withdrawal.

Bedwetting (enuresis) is the most prevalent sleep disorder for children past the age of 3. Five to 17 percent of the population from ages 3 to 15—more commonly males—are so afflicted. Bedwetting usually diminishes with maturation. The enuretic episode occurs approximately 1 to 2 hours after falling asleep, as the child is arousing from NREM Stages 3 to 4 sleep, but before he enters the REM

Stage. Sleep stage change is often associated with body movements and increased muscle tone followed by tachycardia, tachypnea, erection in males, and decreased skin resistance. Micturition occurs about 1 to 4 minutes after the start of the episode and in a moment of relative quiet. Immediately after urination, the child may be difficult to awaken and when awakened has total amnesia for the episode.[111] Parents often show an effect of sleep deficit resulting from these episodes. Hospitalization of the child with severe restriction of the presence and comforting of the parents may produce fears, nightmares, and bedwetting.

Nursing Strategies

1. Protect the sleepwalker from harming himself; he should sleep on the first floor; keep him away from dangerous objects and car keys; place him in a room close to the nurses' station; bedsides may not be a deterrent; check timing of Stage 4 sleep—expect sleepwalking and talking; do not awaken the client abruptly, but leave him alone to pass through the experience unless protection of the person is needed. If undisturbed he will complete his mission and return to bed. If the person must be wakened, do not seize him, but call his name, tell him where he is and reassure him that he is safe; do not scold; gently guide him back to bed. Refer the person to a sleep specialist if sleepwalking episodes last longer than 10 minutes.
2. Help children cope with fears at night. Comfort and cuddle the child. Handle the problem without undue concern. If the child needs help, a few supportive devices could be used temporarily (e.g., a flashlight under the pillow, allowing the child to see that the bed is free from bugs). Maximize the four-year-olds' readiness for novelty and expanded experiences to overcome bedtime fears.
3. Awaken the child with enuresis when bedwetting usually occurs, based on careful assessment. Assist the child to change wet nightclothing and bed linens. Minimize the embarrassment of the child who wets the bed. Provide protection for bed furnishings. The child may benefit by setting an alarm to be awakened to go to the bathroom. Review fluid intake patterns with the child, with adjustments made if most of the fluid intake occurs in the evening. Guard against overreacting to any inconvenience caused by bedwetting. Assist the parents to be supportive, minimizing the child's shame, guilt, and anxiety.
4. Explain the mechanism of nightmares and night terrors to parents who often show the sleep deficit symptoms. An overview of informational growth and development may be needed.
5. Alert members of the health care and nursing team to the client's sleepwalking, sleeptalking, nightmare and/or bedwetting problems. Develop a consistent, low-keyed mechanism to handle the situation and the feelings of the child.

Psychopathophysiologic Conditions

These include bacterial and viral infections affecting the brainstem, thalamus and other brain structures of the sleep center; tumors; circulatory disturbances (hemorrhage, aneurysms that impinge on or directly affect the sleep center); toxic states brought on by kidney disorders; skull fractures; penetrating wounds of the head (particularly the brain stem) which includes surgery; depression; manic depressive type behavioral alterations; drug and alcohol abuse; sleep apnea (respiratory cessation with event of sleep)—it could be minimal or excessive and may cause cardiovascular pathology if prolonged and untreated.

Data Base The problem may be due to a failure of the underlying sleep–waking system itself (small number of occurrences); there may be a diagnosis of accompanying illness with pathology identified—sleep disturbance as a result rather than a cause; the client's own behavior and belief system may contribute to fears and distress and thereby to sleep disturbances. Responses of children are frequently based on total or partial feeling of the existence of threat to the child's existence, as seen in the rejected child and the battered child.

Sleep apnea is a potentially fatal sleep disorder that may go undiagnosed except for a recognition of the accompanying sleep disturbance. Breathing stops, perhaps hundreds of times a night, for as long as 1½ minutes; the person awakes to start to breathe. In many situations, collapse of the upper air passages occurs. In some persons, the diaphragm stops moving. If prolonged and untreated, sleep apnea may result in high blood pressure, failure of the right side of the heart, highly abnormal heart rhythm, and even death. Sleep apnea victims who take sleeping pills may actually be killed by the drugs because they further impair breathing. There is speculation that sleep apnea may be a causative factor in crib deaths. Accompanying symptoms are those of sleep deprivation and excessive sleep—extreme sleepiness, exhaustion, irritability, and hazards related to driving and working.[112]

Sleep disturbance is one of the most common symptoms accompanying postpartum depression and sleep deprivation and disturbance may be the first clinical symptom to signal the onset of postpartum and other psychoses.

Nursing Strategies

1. Based on a full health assessment including physical examination performed in conjunction with the physician and/or physician and nurse specialists, and the formation of a nursing diagnosis and a medical diagnosis, plan to initiate nursing therapy and collaborate with medical therapies, assuring that there will be no further violation of the sleep system and maximizing the existing sleep cycle.
2. Plan for the protection of the rejected and/or abused child. Report the abuse

of the child to the proper authorities. Collaborate with colleagues such as social worker, police officer, and physician as needed.

3. Consult with the client, the sleep specialist, and the clinical pharmacist in relation to administration of therapeutic drugs—dosage and timing as well as quality of the drug to prevent violation of the sleep system.
4. Promote the sleep integrity of the client by planning interruptions and interventions in such a manner as to allow 4 to 5 hours of undisturbed sleep and a time for one or more naps. Keep in mind that a person normally experiences approximately five 90-minute sleep cycles during a night of sleep.
5. Plan the mechanism for relief of discomfort, breathing difficulty, urinary problems, pain, and other related nursing diagnoses so that waiting time is minimized and so that the nurse's use of herself in dietary strategies, positioning, and a multitude of other nursing and medical strategies brings about direct results. This is in contrast to an overdependence on and indiscriminate use of drugs as a panacea.
6. Orient health and nursing team members to the planned sleep periods (undisturbed) for the client.
7. Determine the most suitable environment for the client to enhance maximum recovery rate, facilitate coping, and capitalize on the physical and psychic strengths of the client. Nursing strategies explained previously may be applicable.
8. Support the client during experiences of upsetting dreams, restlessness, and frequent awakenings brought on by pathology directly or indirectly affecting the brain's sleep center.
9. Assist the client to care for his tracheostomy if this procedure was used to alleviate sleep apnea. Review the care of the skin, the care of the tube, and the daytime and the bedtime use of the tracheostomy.
10. Plan with family members and significant others the best visiting time and the best use of the time to assure undisturbed sleep and nap periods. Help explain client behavior resulting from sleep deprivation.

Drug Use and Abuse

This could be self- or physician-prescribed.

Data Base Evidence of sleep disturbance occurs with the abrupt withdrawal syndrome brought on by drug abstinence. This minimally involves jitters, apprehension about getting along without the drug, difficulty getting to sleep, and short REM rebound accompanied by highly fragmented and disrupted sleep with frequent vivid and horrid dreams. Such reactions may be followed by too much REM sleep per night; there is chronic REM suppression, and a history of taking sleeping pills, stimulants, antidepressants, and tranquilizers, both self and physician prescribed; there may have been excessive use of alcohol and the use of alcohol to induce sleep.

Sleeping pills produce delayed reaction time, confusion, and skin rashes; deformities can occur in unborn children when the pills are taken by pregnant women; a tolerance develops to increasing doses, or addiction may occur; cheap sleep of poor quality accounts for the hangover feeling. Delirium tremens (which follows acute alcohol withdrawal) is thought to be associated with severe sleep disturbance brought on by excessive use of alcohol. Most drugs significantly lower REM sleep—alcohol, amphetamines, barbiturates, MAO inhibitors, meprobamate, morphine, imipramine, and their derivatives. Those that generally increase REM sleep include reserpine and phenothiazines. A minimal or no significant effect on REM sleep was found with chloralhydrate, flurazepam, methaqualone, and chlordiazepoxide. All sleeping pills affect the person adversely for a minimum of 18 hours.[113] Contrary to popular belief, the use of alcohol to induce sleep may actually cause disturbed sleep by interfering with REM sleep. Barbiturates have been found to decrease Stage 1 as well as REM sleep and to reduce the frequency of movements and shifts of deep sleep.

Zung found that barbiturates inhibit the cerebral cortex, whose function is concerned with discriminative aspects of consciousness, the hypothalamus (regulation of negative and emotional functions), the limbic system (regulation of emotions), and the reticular formation (arousal system). Barbiturates stimulate the thalamus (the relay station to the cortex). Meprobamate inhibits the thalamus and the limbic system. Phenothiazines inhibit the hypothalamus, reticular formation, and neurohumoral depots (regulation of emotions) while stimulating the thalamus and limbic system.[114]

Drug use history usually includes the use of drugs to handle a crisis followed by quick tolerance and more and more drug. There may be a history of use of aspirin to relieve anxiety. Withdrawal brings about nightmares followed by resumption of the drug to reduce nightmares. It is not necessary to "take something" to assure a good night's sleep.[115] L-tryptophan is an essential amino acid and a natural physiologic precursor of serotonin. Researchers have noted that L-tryptophan has a prominent sedative effect. Research results have been variable on individuals taking L-tryptophan before sleep. An increase in REM sleep was noted with large doses. It is speculated that tryptophan may promote sleep by a direct effect on the brain, by conversion to protein or polypeptide, by a bulk effect on triggering a physiologic process, or by releasing a soporific hormone. Research continues.[116]

Alcohol was found to temporarily benumb one's sensations, causing a decrease in frequency of movement, which resulted in discomfort and increased motility during the latter portion of the night. When intoxication is too deep to allow for movement during the course of the night, the person awakens with muscle cramps, stiffness, and discomfort.[117]

Nursing Strategies

1. Support the client during *gradual* drug withdrawal; explain occurrences; use physical presence and touch to support the client, particularly during vivid and frightening dream experiences. Experts recommend a withdrawal pattern of one therapeutic dose every five days.[118] Total withdrawal may take weeks and months to accomplish.
2. Assist the client in determining and planning a more wholesome sleep–awake cycle in conjunction with his own biologic rhythms and free from any drug interference.
3. Suggest that the client keep a diary or log of sleep–awake patterns and activities.
4. Outline with the client and a nutritionist a balanced diet appropriate to the age, sex, living patterns, ethnicity, and socioeconomic background of the client to make certain that appropriate nutrients are available to offset past physical, emotional, and chemical affronts to the client's body and to assure that no nutritional deficit will provide an excuse for resorting to the use of drugs.
5. Determine the environmental factors that need adjustment and change. Nursing strategies prescribed earlier are applicable.
6. Make referrals, in conjunction with the client, with clergy, dentist, physician, psychiatrist, vocational counselor, community health nursing specialist, family therapist, etc., as needed to continue support therapy and psychotherapeutic therapies while drug withdrawal is in progress and after it has been completed.
7. Confer with family regarding overall basic human need maintenance. Arrange for follow-up home visit by the nurse or by the community health specialist, nursing colleague, or family nursing specialist.

Causes of Excessive Sleep

Previous Sleep Deprivation and Disturbances

Prolonged sleep may be needed to offset earlier deficits; naps may be needed during the day to offset nighttime deficits, particularly for persons with sleep apnea; and quality of sleep may be altered due to jet travel across time zones or working during the natural sleeptime.

Data Base Excessive sleep may occur following physical and psychologic disturbances in a child or an adult. Makeup sleep is longer in length and is characterized by REM rebound—longer REM periods to make up for previous lost REM sleep. Sleep deprivation (with the resultant need to sleep excessively) may be the result of sleep apnea (the inability to breathe with the onset of sleep), creating a broken sleep situation all night. Thus, the excessive need to sleep during the day results from a severe sleep deficit in order to accommodate the need for air. The central nervous system, which controls breathing, shuts down; the throat muscles collapse and the body undergoes a profound shock that awakens the person who gasps for air. The importance of the differential diagnosis of sleep apnea apart from other disorders is self-evident.

For persons who decide to sleep longer than usual on weekends or during vacations, etc., a groggy feeling may be evident. The person feels tired and has much more difficulty "getting started." This is probably due to an increase of REM sleep and dreams, particularly since they increase with the length of sleep span. Experiencing REM sleep is hard work and this accounts for the tired feeling.

Nursing Strategies

1. Provide an environment conducive to sleep as outlined previously.
2. Plan with the client the means to offset sleep deprivation and disturbances requiring prolonged sleep periods afterwards.
3. Determine with the client his own unique sleep pattern. This can be facilitated by keeping a diary or log or by designating a sleep–awake daily profile.
4. Plan with the client the methodology to implement a consistent pattern for sleeping and waking.
5. Refrain from suggesting the use of sleeping medication or alcohol to enhance sleep or psuedosleep and discourage the client's self-prescription of these drugs.
6. If the client has a tracheostomy that is plugged during the day and opened at night to relieve sleep apnea, a review of the methodology used by the client to care for the skin surrounding the tracheal opening, and the tube itself, as well as a means to maintain vigilance over sleep patterns, should be conducted.

Invasion of Sleep into Waking Time (Narcolepsy)

Sleep intrudes uncontrollably into awake time; it is brought on by laughter, crying, fear, shock, and boredom.

Data Base There is a dramatic intrusion of sleep into the waking state; this condition is commonly referred to as narcolepsy. While performing one's normal day-to-day activities, a person experiences a sudden, involuntary lapse into sleeping that can last from a few minutes to as much as 15 minutes. Narcolepsy is viewed by some authorities as a disorder of arousal and may be associated with neurologic immaturity, especially if it initially occurs in a young child. Other researchers see narcolepsy as a REM disorder. It has been found that the person with narcolepsy may begin a night of sleep with REM sleep and not with the normally expected NREM sleep. The wave of sleepiness cannot be prevented. A differential diagnosis in a sleep laboratory will rule out temporal lobe and other epileptic seizures which may mimic narcolepsy. Symptoms are paroxysmal in nature and are nonresponsive to the environment; they appear automatically in response to certain actions. Narcolepsy is accompanied by retrograde amnesia for the episode.[119] Other accompanying symptoms include catalepsy (muscle weakness ranging from subjective weakness to total inability to move), sleep paralysis (complete loss of muscle tone in transition between sleep and waking, but less often on awakening), unusual visual and auditory sensations at the onset of an attack, and attack is often precipitated by a heightened emotional response such as laughter, crying, anger. The likelihood of an occurrence increases with fatigue or after eating a heavy meal. Throughout most of the remainder of the waking period this person is normally alert. Approximately 2 to 5 persons in every thousand have this affliction, which seems to have an hereditary or genetic component and about three-fourths of the episodes of narcolepsy start between the ages of 15 to 25. Stimulants and drugs that suppress REM sleep have been found to be helpful in treatment.[120]

Nursing Strategies

1. Plan with the client periodic times during the day for sleep. Utilization of coffee break time and some of lunch time while on the job may be useful.
2. Assist the client to formulate the information base to provide a current or prospective employer regarding the condition.
3. Support the client's intention to have a media alert bracelet or information on his person in case of emergency.
4. Outline the use of specifically prescribed medication (based on EEG diagnosis) to minimize the intrusion of REM sleep into the awake state.
5. If excessive sleep is due to temporal lobe pathology, plan to maintain the integrity of the client's sleep system in conjunction with prescribed medical and nursing therapies.
6. Identify sleep inducing opportunities for the client with the objective of minimizing these conditions during the expected awake time, such as during heavy meals.
7. Plan how the client could anticipate a sleep attack, handle himself, and maintain safety during instantaneous bouts of sleep brought on by laughing or crying.

Psychopathophysiologic States

Sleep may be used as an escape from unpleasant and/or critical life situations; it may be due to damage to the arousal and/or sleep centers of the brain by bacteria, viruses, toxins, tumors, fractures, hemorrhages, and penetrating wounds (including surgery); it may result from excessive and/or indiscriminate use of anxiety reducing and sleep inducing drugs or from the excessive use of alcohol—all of which actually alter sleep both qualitatively and quantitatively.

Data Base Excessive sleep due to psychophysiopathologic states may occur in conditions like uremia, diabetes, brain concussion, and encephalitis; it may result from a brain tumor (distinguished from coma, which is not sleep); it may be used to escape overwhelming anxiety, with stumbling confusion lasting two hours after waking. Such conditions run in families; the person may seem lazy—can't awaken in the morning, and has an uncoordinated gait; he is late for work and falls asleep against his will; heart and respiratory rates are generally faster in these clients than in others.

The above kinds of behavior may be due to excessive and/or indiscriminate use of anxiety-reducing and sleep-producing drugs (including alcohol). These alter normal sleep patterns, creating a client condition requiring additional sleep time in an attempt to offset the drug impact, particularly if REM sleep deprivation results or if Stage 4 sleep is diminished.

Nursing Strategies

1. Assist the client to gradually withdraw from any and all sleep-inducing and/or anxiety-reducing drugs if they have been demonstrated to be the cause of the sleep problem. Suggest that the client consider using foods containing tryptophan, such as cottage cheese, yogurt, cheese, meats, nuts, and peanut butter, to bring about a sleep inducing effect.
2. Collaborate in the planning of medical and nursing therapies to remove the cause of excessive sleep due to uremia, diabetes, brain concussion, etc., mindful of the need to protect the integrity of the client's sleep cycle.
3. Plan judiciously the use of any drug that would increase or decrease the amount of sleep needed.
4. Calculate the pain relief mechanism most appropriate for the client, if needed, considering positional comforting, dietary, and pharmacologic strategies.
5. Assist the client in planning events during the waking period to enhance participation and wakefulness.
6. Assist the drug withdrawn client to work out a sleep–awake plan to enhance his individuality and life style while primarily recognizing and accounting for his individual sleep cycle and need for sleep.
7. Make referrals in conjunction with the client to other health care personnel

and agencies such as alcoholic and drug rehabilitation, the psychiatrist, clinical psychologist, clergy, and lawyer.

Following the designation of the nursing strategies that have been developed as a result of the data base (obtained through the health assessment and physical examination) with a particular focus on the need for sleep, the nurse implements the strategies appropriate for the client. She is ever mindful of the goal of problem resolution and the achievement of sleep integrity. In other words, the client's need for sleep is met as appropriate to his unique biologic sleep–awake rhythm cycle. Client data, the nursing strategies applied, and the response of the client are carefully and fully recorded on the client's record.

The nurse continues to collect data from and about the client, his family, and significant others to assure the correctness of the strategies. On full implementation, a thorough evaluation of all available data is made with the focus on determining whether sleep integrity has been achieved, if additional time is needed, or if new data dictate a reassessment, with replanning and implementation.

On meeting the need for sleep, the client should demonstrate behavior comparable to those data outlined for normal sleep, respecting the individuality of his biologic rhythms. If such a picture emerges, follow-up strategies to maintain sleep (as outlined for the well person) will be determined and implemented. If sleep alterations were the result of psychophysiopathologic states, the nurse continues to assure the highest level of sleep integrity while the client recovers from the pathologic state. The attention to meeting the client's sleep need can only enhance recovery from an accompanying illness.

When the client returns to optimal health, he continues the regimen to foster normal sleep, returning to the health care system at periodic intervals for verification of the health state or if problems are evident.

It is hoped that the reader will expand on the data offered as well as create additional and different sleep strategies to assure that a most fundamental and significant need is met—sleep.

References

1. Hernandez-Peon R: Attention, sleep, behavior: A mapping of an inhibitory system in the brain. In National Institute of Mental Health Research Project Summaries, No. 2, Washington, US Government Printing Office, 1965, pp 100–101
2. Ibid: p 101
3. Ibid: p 102
4. Ibid: p 103
5. Ibid: p 103

6. Ibid: p 97
7. Ibid: p 99
8. Bailey R: The Role of the Brain. New York, Time–Life Books, 1975, p 140
9. Ibid: p 141
10. Ibid: pp 143–144
11. Ibid: pp 144–145
12. Ibid: p 245
13. Sleep. Lancet 1 (7913):963, April 26, 1975
14. Webb W: Sleep: The Gentle Tyrant. Englewood Cliffs, New Jersey, Prentice-Hall, 1975, p 26
15. Dement W: Some Must Watch While Some Must Sleep. San Francisco, Freeman, 1974, p 114
16. Montagu A: The Direction of Human Development. New York, Hawthorn, 1970, p 131
17. Maslow A: Motivation and Personality. New York, Harper & Row, 1970, p 92
18. Kleitman N: Sleep and Wakefulness, Chicago, University of Chicago Press, 1963, p 71
19. Ibid: p 12
20. Ibid: pp 72–74
21. Linde SM, Savary LM: The Sleep Book. New York, Harper & Row, 1974, p 27
22. Dement W[15]: p 27
23. Linde SM, Savary LM[21]: p 29
24. Ibid: pp 29–30
25. Dement W[15]: p 29
26. Webb W[14]: p 69
27. Harms E: Problems of Sleep and Dreams in Children. New York, Pergamon, 1964, p 31
28. Dement W[15]: p 26
29. Ibid: p 26
30. Linde SM, Savary LM[21]: p 78
31. Harms, E[27]: p 67
32. Kleitman N[18]: p 8
33. Linde SM, Savary LM[21]: pp 78, 147
34. Kleitman N[18]: pp 85–91
35. Ibid: p 123
36. Ibid: p 16
37. Ibid: pp 49–50, 55
38. Ibid: pp 58, 67
39. Ibid: pp 67, 272
40. Linde SM, Savary LM[21]: p 40
41. Ibid: pp 27–28
42. Ibid: p 31
43. Webb W[14]: p 38
44. Dement W[15]: p 31
45. Linde SM, Savary LM[21]: pp 30–31
46. Ibid: p 76
47. Ibid: pp 20, 50
48. Webb W[14]: p 28

49. Harms E[27]: p 62
50. Ibid: p 64
51. Webb W[14]: p 25
52. Ibid: p 36
53. Ibid: p 37
54. Harms E[27]: p 67
55. Harms E[27]: pp 64, 66
56. Ibid: p 69
57. Webb W[14]: pp 54, 57
58. Linde SM, Savary LM[21]: pp 40, 50
59. Hartmann E (ed): Sleep and Dreaming. Boston, Little, Brown, 1970, p 67
60. Karacan I, Williams R: The relationship of sleep disturbances of psychopathology. In Hartmann E (ed)[59]: p 103
61. Foulkes D: Personality and dreams. In Hartmann E (ed)[59]: p 150
62. Linde SM, Savary LM[21]: p 48
63. Webb W[14]: p 26
64. Ibid: p 54
65. Ibid: p 43
66. Hartman E (ed)[59]: p 45
67. Webb W[14]: pp 44–45
68. Ibid: pp 46–50
69. Kleitman N[18]: p 8
70. Dement W[15]: pp 44–45
71. Ibid: pp 50, 71
72. Kleitman N[18]: p 72
73. Harms E[27]: p 41
74. Webb W[14]: pp 57–59
75. Ellis J: Noise: Stop it, before it stops you. Moneysworth, August 30, 1976, p 15
76. Aquino L: The Instant Sleep Method. Chicago, Playboy Press. 1976, pp 111–114
77. McKim R: Relaxed attention. In White J, Fadiman J (eds): Relax. New York, Confucian, 1976, p 92
78. Kleitman N[18]: p 207
79. Webb W[14]: pp 168–169
80. Kleitman N[18]: p 229
81. Ibid: p 223
82. Baekeland F, Hartmann E: Sleep requirements and the characteristics of some sleepers. In Harmann E (ed)[59]: p 34
83. Linde SM, Savary LM[21]: p 136
84. Ibid: p 133
85. Webb W[14]: pp 124–125
86. Ibid: p 133
87. Aquino L[76]: pp 94–95
88. Webb W[14]: p 134
89. Aquino L[76]: p 56
90. Adam R: Personality factors in children with sleep disturbance. In Harms E[27]: p 116
91. Ibid: pp 118–122
92. Vogl M: Sleep disturbances in neurotic children. In Harms E[27]: p 123
93. Crisp AH, Stonehill E: Sleep, Nutrition and Mood. New York, Wiley, 1976, p 17

94. Donofas CC: Insomnia: Fear of falling asleep. Moneysworth, June 20, 1977, p 14
95. Ames LB: Sleep and dreams in childhood. In Harms E[27]: p 23
96. Kleitman N[18]: p 317
97. Ames LB[95]: p 23
98. Cohen M: People who go zzzzzz in the night. Ladies Home Journal, October 1976
99. Dement W[15]: pp 80–81
100. Aquino L[76]: pp 105–107
101. Dlin B, Rosen H, Dickstein K, Lyons J, Fischer HK: The problems of sleep and rest in the intensive care unit. Psychosom 12(3):155–159, May–June, 1971
102. Cole MB, Muller HF: Sleep deprivation in the treatment of elderly depressed patients. J Am Geriatr Soc 24:308–313, July 1976
103. Zung W: The pharmacology of disordered sleep. In Hartmann E (ed)[59]: pp 129–135
104. Linde SM, Savary LM[21]: p 41
105. Webb W[14]: pp 81, 83
106. Aquino L[76]: p 41
107. Ibid: p 42
108. Linde SM, Savary LM[21]: p 136
109. Ames LB[95]: p 24
110. Webb W[14]: p 73
111. Anders TF: What we now know about sleep disorders in children. Med Times 104(4):77, April, 1976
112. Brody JE: Help for troubled sleepers. Family Circle, June 28, 1977, p 71
113. Linde SM, Savary LM[21]: pp 113–116, 119
114. Zung W: Insomnia and disordered sleep. In Hartman E (ed)[59]: p 136
115. Aquino L[76]: p 96
116. Wyatt RJ, Gillin JC: Biochemistry and human sleep. In Williams RL, Karacan I: Pharmacology of Sleep. New York, Wiley, 1976, p 252
117. Kleitman N[18]: p 91
118. Webb W[14]: p 113
119. Anders TF[111]: p 76
120. Webb W[14]: p 71

Supplementary References

1. Benson H: The Relaxation Response. New York, William Morrow, 1975
2. Binzley V: State: overlooked factor in newborn nursing. Am J Nurs 77:102–103, January, 1977
3. Cherry L: A new vision of dreams. The New York Times Magazine, July 3, 1977, pp 9–13, 34
4. Collins MB: Factors in evening care identified as contributing to patient comfort. Unpublished Masters Thesis. Washington, DC, School of Nursing, The Catholic University of America, 1968
5. Echols J: Development of an Observational Tool to Identify a Patient's Sleep Behavior. Unpublished Masters Thesis. Washington, DC, School of Nursing, The Catholic University of America, 1968
6. Fass G: Sleep, drugs and dreams. Am J Nurs 71:2316, December, 1971

7. Feinberg I: Changes in sleep cycle patterns with age. J Psychiatric Res 10(3–4):283–306, October, 1976
8. Foy AL: Dreams of patients and staff. Am J Nurs 70:80–82, January, 1970
9. Jouvet M: States of sleep. Sci Am 216:62, February, 1967
10. Kales A, Kales J: Sleep disorders. New Engl J Med 290(9): 487–499, February 28, 1974
11. Luce GG: Body Time. New York, Bantam, 1973
12. Ryzewski J: Factors associated with sleep. Unpublished Masters thesis. Washington, DC, School of Nursing. The Catholic University of America, 1967
13. Tackett LR: Identification of Sleep Behaviors of a Selected Group of Patients. Unpublished Masters thesis. Washington, DC, School of Nursing. The Catholic University of America, 1970
14. US Department of Health, Education and Welfare. Current Research on Sleep and Dreams. Washington, DC: US Government Printing Office, 1966.
15. White J, Fadiman J (eds): Relax. New York, Confucian, 1976
16. Williams RL, Karacan I: Pharmacology of Sleep. New York, Wiley, 1976
17. Woods NF, Falk SA: Noise stimuli in the acute care area. Nurs Res 23(2):144–150, March–April, 1974

Chapter Nine •

Epilogue

One of the purposes of the foregoing chapters was to demonstrate that the nursing process is the workable, cardinal mode of nursing practice. A second was to demonstrate that human needs—their maintenance, their fulfillment, their integrity—are the territory of nursing. A third was to provide a model for the operationalization of the nursing process into nursing practice. This model focused on wellness, as well as on illness, and it incorporated the range of data and strategies needed by the nurse, taking into consideration variables inherent in the client—gender (masculine or feminine), lifestyle, and cultural, ethnic, social, educational, and ethical dimensions. We feel that the purposes intended for this book have been realized through the dynamic group endeavor that produced it; contributors' support and enthusiasm for the purposes, despite some expected ambivalent feelings, have brought the framework proposed in the Preface to fruition.

The nursing process served as the arena for the contributors' creativity and intelligence, as it may also serve for nursing educators and nursing practitioners who use the process. Readers should note that while the basic structure of the nursing process was followed in all of the chapters, each contributor's own style and theoretical substance was drawn from the biological, physical, social, and behavioral sciences, and the humanities. The nurse's use of interdisciplinary material drawn from the arts as well as the sciences is designed to assure a more complete and integrated view of man and his world. Thus, the need for the nurse to have a broad general educational base in order to assure that she is an educated person as well as to provide the rationale for nursing intervention is fully supported in the presentation of each chapter. A focus limited to the biological and physical sciences would be inadequate to the full use of the nursing process.

The structure used in each of the chapters was an outgrowth of numerous experiences of nursing educators and nursing practitioners. Repeated nursing experiences over a period of time and a search of the current literature suggest that human needs and the nursing process have served consistently as the bases for nursing, whether or not labeled as such. Our early decision to develop the needs for nutrition, territory, activity, air, love, tenderness, and sleep proved to be a useful beginning and could serve as an example for the development of a host of additional human needs. Further, the recognition that one subject was common to all needs, namely biological rhythmicity, was supported throughout the book after its particular focus in Chapter 1.

Perhaps the most striking contribution of each of the chapters is the fact that the focus is on *nursing*. Though the relationship of pathophysiology and psychopathology is clearly seen, these fields, instead of predominating, are complementary and supportive to nursing. This constitutes a genuine nursing model.

These chapters provide direct evidence of the appropriateness of basic human needs as a useful and fruitful method to classify nursing diagnoses. Nurses have been actively searching for a suitable method or system to classify nursing diagnoses since 1974. Up to this time no one suitable system has been accepted. The contents of this book not only demonstrate support for the classification system, but provide examples of what constitute nursing diagnoses and how they can be developed.

The chapters also demonstrate the usefulness of the framework of human needs in developing data bases, nursing strategies for the wellness state, and the specified nursing diagnoses stemming from unmet needs. The use of the human needs framework for the operationalization of the nursing process requires a different mode of thinking, data gathering, and prescription of strategies than heretofore practiced by nurses. Each component of the nursing process is accounted for by extensive development of the knowledge the nurse needs before identifying wellness or sickness states and implementing strategies. The outcomes for the client were forecast, and effective, purposeful action suggested. Each of the chapters provides information needed by the nurse and should stimulate the reader to expand on each of the needs developed, bringing into play her own knowledge, as well as stimulating her to add to her practice and ensure a focus on strategic needs—the territory of nursing.

Several ideas and conclusions emerged as a result of this endeavor that may not be readily observed in the contents of the book, but which the editors believe have merit in being shared with the readers. These ideas are offered as the subject for future deliberations by nursing educators and practitioners who will duplicate and apply this model on a day-to-day basis. It is important that each of the eight contributors was convinced of the value to nursing of the framework adopted for this text, but each readily admitted that explaining the content with a strict nursing focus was not easy. The contributors suffered the same syndrome most nurses experience, namely, past reliance on other professional models. It was not easy to "shift gears" to assure a nursing focus. Nurses who are initiating the nursing process as their primary mode for practice can expect to experience some ambivalence and anxiety initially. But it is necessary, as one contributor stated, that "We really put our money where our mouth is!"

The identification of rhythmicity as the permeating element in human needs merits special attention. While it was overt in the discussion on sleep, probably due to the obvious cyclic activity of sleep in every human person, it was covert in a number of other presentations and inferred in all of them. Nurses need to be alert to the outcomes of research related to rhythmicity and to apply the outcomes of this research in practice as they strive to maintain the integrity of the fulfillment of human needs for the client and for themselves.

Each chapter portrays the individuality of the contributor's application of the nursing process. The independence afforded each of the contributors in developing a particular need within the need–nursing process framework in her own style and in keeping with her education and experiences demonstrates the flexibility inherent in the framework. Further, no nurse needs to feel that her full use of self is thwarted as she engages in the utilization of the framework. On the contrary, the fullness of her personality and experience is required. The successful production of each chapter confirmed the belief that the concept of human needs operating within the nursing process framework is a legitimate basis for nursing education and nursing practice.

It was suggested in several chapters that a log be kept of one's own parameters of human need fulfillment so that a baseline of normality could be known about one's self. Since this suggestion arose independently from several contributors, there may be some validity for implementing it; certainly the potential for such a recording system should be examined. Such an approach supports the belief that as a person becomes more knowledgeable about himself and is more consciously aware of his own ranges of activity, he becomes more responsible for his own care and the voice of the client in turn becomes a more integral part of the client's care.

A conclusion that was voiced by every contributor and which could have been inferred from chapter content is that a great deal was learned through participation in this endeavor. A sense of pleasure and satisfaction was experienced and it is expected that nurses willing to duplicate and apply this model will experience similar feelings. Involved in this enterprise is the satisfaction of rendering a more knowledgeable, goal-directed nursing service to the client, and there are the rewards to the nurse and the client that result from quality service.

To conclude, the contributors have shared in their support of and gratification in the nursing process format. They have stated that the experience was professionally and personally beneficial—increasing the depth of understanding of self and others and opening an entirely new vista for nursing knowledge and intervention. The editors believe more firmly than ever that the classification of nursing diagnoses within the framework of human needs is most useful and fruitful. It is hoped that the readers will be stimulated to revamp their thinking as a result of these chapters and to participate fully in the nursing process with its heavy demand on the intellectual, interpersonal, and technical skills needed for independent and interdependent nursing practice. It is hoped that additional human needs and the nursing process will be developed in subsequent volumes.

Index